EMERGENC ...

EDITORS

WILLIAM A. WOODS, M.D., FAAP
Assistant Professor of Emergency Medicine and Pediatrics
University of Virginia Health System
Charlottesville, Virginia

JEFFREY S. YOUNG, M.D., FACS
Associate Professor of Surgery and Emergency Medicine
Director, University of Virginia Trauma Center
University of Virginia Health System
Charlottesville, Virginia

J. SCOTT JUST, M.D.
Chief Resident
Department of Emergency Medicine
University of Virginia
Charlottesville, Virginia

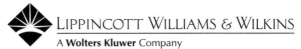

LIPPINCOTT WILLIAMS & WILKINS
A **Wolters Kluwer** Company
Philadelphia • Baltimore • New York • London
Buenos Aires • Hong Kong • Sydney • Tokyo

Editor: Elizabeth Nieginski
Managing Editor: Marette D. Magargle-Smith
Development Editor: Melanie Cann
Marketing Manager: Aimee Sirmon

351 West Camden Street
Baltimore, Maryland 21201-2436 USA

530 Walnut Street
Philadelphia, Pennsylvania 19106 USA

Printed in the United States of America

Libary of Congress Cataloging-in-Publication Data

Emergency medicine recall / editors, William A. Woods, Jeffrey S. Young, J. Scott Just.
    p. ; cm.—(Recall series)
    Includes index.
    ISBN 0-683-30610-3
    1. Emergency medicine. 2. Emergency medicine—Examinations, questions, etc.
I. Woods, William A. (William Anthony), 1963-II. Young, Jeffrey S. (Jeffrey Seth)
III. Just, J. Scott (Joseph Scott) IV. Series.
    [DNLM: 1. Emergency Medicine—Examination Questions. 2. Emergencies—Examination Questions. WB 18.2 E529 2000]
RC86.7 .E57848 2000
616.02'5'076—dc21

                                    99-057934

                                  04 05
                        3 4 5 6 7 8 9 10

Contributors

Lisa Andolina, M.D.
Devin Bateman, M.D.
Michael Baylor, M.D.
Danny Benjamin, M.D.
William J. Brady, M.D.
Christopher Chase, M.D.
Erica Chen, M.D.
Melissa Clark, M.D.
Todd Kenkinger, M.D.
Brian Doyle, M.D.
Russell Ford, M.D.
Mary Frazier, M.D.
Andy Kagel, NREMTP
Curtis Lehman, M.D.
James Lowry, M.D.
Christopher Moore, M.D.
Antonette Morris-Chatman, M.D.
Mark Mullins, M.D.
Sarah Ogrosky, M.D.
Thomas Pollehn, M.D.
Edward Ullman, M.D.
Gia Viscardi, M.D.

Dedication

To my daughters, Sarah and Maggie

William A. Woods

To my beautiful wife, Denise Young, M.D., FACOG, and my three children, Andrew, Steven, and Brian. You make all the work worthwhile.

Jeffrey S. Young

To my first teachers, Joe and Charlene, for their love and guidance; to my grandmother, Lillie, for her unconditional love and support; to my grandfather, Robert, for his camaraderie; and to Elizabeth, for her friendship and encouragement.

J. Scott Just

Contents

Preface xi
Figure Credits xiii

SECTION 1
MEDICAL EMERGENCIES 1

1	Signs and Symptoms	3
2	Resuscitation	34
3	Cardiovascular Emergencies	48
4	Pulmonary Emergencies	74
5	Gastroenterologic Emergencies	88
6	Urologic and Nephrologic Emergencies	116
7	Obstetric and Gynecologic Emergencies	135
8	Infectious Disease and Immunologic Emergencies	162
9	Hematologic, Oncologic, and Post-Transplant Emergencies	207
10	Endocrinologic and Metabolic Emergencies	246
11	Neurologic Emergencies	258
12	Psychiatric Emergencies	289
13	Toxicologic Emergencies	309
14	Environmental Emergencies	344
15	Pediatric Emergencies	365
16	Dermatologic Emergencies	392

SECTION 2
SURGICAL EMERGENCIES 403

17	Initial Evaluation of the Surgical Patient	405
18	Trauma	408
19	Emergency Medical Services	439
20	Emergency Procedures and Wound Care	445
21	General Surgical Emergencies	462
22	Vascular Emergencies	474
23	Unique Injuries	481
24	Burns	484
25	Otolaryngologic and Dental Emergencies	492
26	Ophthalmologic Emergencies	499

Preface

Emergency Medicine Recall, a member of the popular *Recall* series, is written for third- and fourth-year medical students who are completing their emergency medicine clerkships, and for junior housestaff. The goal of this book is to provide you with the information necessary to answer four basic questions:

- What illnesses are typically seen in patients who come to the emergency department?
- What is a broad differential diagnosis for this patient's particular complaint?
- What signs, symptoms, and laboratory findings can help to narrow the differential?
- What initial therapy must be provided in the emergency department?

The ability to answer these questions is critical in order to provide problem-focused care to the patient in the emergency department. *Emergency Medicine Recall* presents you with the information necessary to answer these questions and, through repetition and its unique "rapid-fire" question-and-answer format, reinforces the information that has been presented. Although *Emergency Medicine Recall* is not intended to be a replacement for textbook study, it will enable you to provide better patient care in the emergency department by reinforcing important concepts and providing a framework for focusing your thoughts before and after seeing a patient.

Our hope is that you will find Emergency Medicine Recall useful; we consider this a "work in progress" and would welcome your comments.

Figure Credits

Chapter 7: Figure reprinted from Beckmann CRB, Ling FW, Herbert WNP, et al: *Obstetrics and Gynecology,* 3rd ed. Baltimore, Williams & Wilkins, 1998, p 112. Granted with permission of Lippincott Williams & Wilkins.

Chapter 18: Figures reprinted from Blackbourne LH: *Surgical Recall,* 2nd ed. Baltimore, Williams & Wilkins, 1998, pp 567–568, 641, 644–647. Granted with permission of Lippincott Williams & Wilkins.

Chapter 20: Figures reprinted from Blackbourne LH: *Surgical Recall,* 2nd ed. Baltimore, Williams & Wilkins, 1998, pp 56–58, 64–66, 87–90, 531. Granted with permission of Lippincott Williams & Wilkins.

Chapter 24: Figure reprinted from Plantz SH, Adler JN: *NMS Emergency Medicine.* Baltimore, Williams & Wilkins, 1998, p 557. Granted with permission of Lippincott Williams & Wilkins.

Section 1

Medical Emergencies

1   Signs and Symptoms

CHEST PAIN

TYPES OF CHEST PAIN

Name the two types of chest pain.
Somatic pain and visceral pain

Describe somatic chest pain.
Somatic pain is generally sharp and easy to localize.

Why is somatic pain easily localized?
Because somatic pain is caused by focal stimulation of one nerve root

Can somatic pain that is reproducible by palpation be serious?
Yes. Studies report that 5%–15% of patients with reproducible somatic pain have ischemic heart disease.

Describe visceral chest pain.
Visceral chest pain is indistinct and difficult to localize. It generally radiates to other regions of the body.

Why does visceral pain radiate?
Because multiple nerve roots innervate the stimulated tissue

Describe the innervation of visceral pain.
Visceral afferent nerves enter both sides of the spinal cord at several levels, causing midline pain.

Where are visceral nerves found?
In the visceral pleura, pericardium, aorta, diaphragm, and esophagus

Is the location of pain helpful in arriving at a diagnosis?
If the pain is sharp and easy to localize, then it is more likely to be musculoskeletal pain. Visceral pain, which is not as easily localized, may only suggest a diagnosis.

EVALUATION OF THE PATIENT WITH CHEST PAIN

**What are five life-threaten-
ing causes of chest pain?**

1. Myocardial infarction
2. Pulmonary embolism
3. Aortic dissection
4. Pneumothorax
5. Unstable angina

**Name nine other conditions
that may cause chest pain.**

1. Muscular pain
2. Costochondritis
3. Esophageal spasm or reflux
4. Pericarditis
5. Pleuritis
6. Herpes zoster
7. Anxiety
8. Peptic ulcer disease
9. Pneumonia

**What is the best approach
to the patient with chest
pain?**

Assume the patient has a life-threatening
illness until proven otherwise. Start an IV
and oxygen, and put the patient on a
cardiac monitor (IV, O_2, monitor).

**What is the most important
component in evaluating
the patient with chest pain?**

Taking a thorough history

**What are five characteris-
tics to include in the history
of the patient with chest
pain?**

PQRST
Precipitation and **P**alliation
Quality
Radiation
Severity
Timing

Physical examination findings

**What type of pain does
tenderness on palpation
suggest?**

Musculoskeletal pain

**Blood pressure asymmetry
between the upper and
lower extremities suggests
what life-threatening
condition?**

Aortic dissection

**What conditions does fever
suggest?**

Pericarditis, pleuritis, or pneumonia

Absence of breath sounds suggests what?	Pneumothorax
Describe Hamman's sign.	A crunching sound, heard on auscultation of the heart, caused by pneumomediastinum
What does Hamman's sign suggest?	Esophageal rupture
Pericardial friction rub suggests what condition?	Pericarditis
What studies are helpful in identifying the cause of chest pain?	Electrocardiogram (EKG), chest x-ray, arterial blood gases (ABGs), and cardiac enzyme measurements

DYSPNEA

What is dyspnea?	Dyspnea, which may be acute or chronic, is the patient's subjective and unpleasant awareness of his own breathing (often described as "shortness of breath").
What causes dyspnea?	Primarily pulmonary, cardiac, and neurologic conditions
What are the pulmonary causes of dyspnea?	**Traumatic:** Pneumothorax, hemothorax, pulmonary contusion, rib fractures, diaphragm rupture **Atraumatic:** Pulmonary embolism, asthma, pneumonia, pleural effusion, aspiration, airway foreign bodies, acute lung injury **Chronic pulmonary problems:** Chronic obstructive pulmonary disease (COPD), interstitial fibrosis, lung cancer
What are the cardiac causes of dyspnea?	**Acute:** Congestive heart failure (CHF) exacerbation; acute myocardial infarction or ischemia; arrhythmia **Chronic:** Valvular heart disease; congenital heart disease; severe, compensated CHF; arrhythmia
What are the neurologic causes of dyspnea?	**Acute:** Guillain-Barré syndrome, ascending tick paralysis, myasthenia gravis,

spinal cord injury, organophosphate poisoning, snake envenomation, botulism, black widow spider bites, Lyme disease

Chronic: Polio, polymyositis, amyotrophic lateral sclerosis (ALS), stroke, multiple sclerosis, phrenic nerve dysfunction

Are any other causes important to consider when evaluating the patient with dyspnea?

Psychogenic dyspnea and "pulmonary embarrassment" from obesity, ascites, or pregnancy

How is the patient with dyspnea managed?

Evaluate and support the patient's airway, breathing, and circulation (ABCs). Then, identify and treat the underlying cause of the dyspnea.

ABDOMINAL PAIN

TYPES OF ABDOMINAL PAIN

What are the three types of abdominal pain?

Referred, somatic, and visceral

Referred pain

What is referred pain?

Pain felt at a site distant from the disease process

What is the mechanism of referred pain?

Convergence of multiple pain afferents in the posterior horn of the spinal cord

Name the classic locations of referred pain from:

    Nephrolithiasis?   Groin or testicles

    Splenic injury?   Left shoulder (Kehr's sign)

    Liver injury or abscess?   Right shoulder

    Pancreatitis?   Mid-back

    Cholecystitis?   Right infrascapular region or epigastrium

    Early appendicitis?   Periumbilical region

Myocardial infarction?	Mid-epigastrium
Leaking abdominal aortic aneurysm (AAA)?	Back

Somatic pain

Describe somatic abdominal pain.	Sharp, localizable pain caused by irritation of the parietal peritoneum

Visceral pain

Describe visceral abdominal pain.	It is an indistinct, crampy, colicky pain that is difficult to localize but is generally perceived in the midline

EVALUATION OF THE PATIENT WITH ABDOMINAL PAIN

Physical examination

What five life-threatening conditions must be considered during evaluation of abdominal pain?	1. Perforation 2. Mesenteric ischemia 3. Leaking aortic aneurysm 4. Ectopic pregnancy 5. Myocardial infarction
What aspects of the physical examination are frequently forgotten?	A rectal examination and a thorough genitourinary examination for pelvic pathology and hernias
Is the duration of pain helpful in arriving at a diagnosis?	Pain lasting longer than 48 hours is less likely to be surgically correctable.
What are five signs of peritoneal pain?	Extreme tenderness, rebound tenderness, guarding, rigidity, and absent bowel sounds
Why are peritoneal signs important?	Peritoneal signs suggest that the patient has a condition requiring evaluation by a general surgeon.
What is Murphy's sign?	Pain and cessation of inspiration elicited by palpation of the right upper quadrant (RUQ) during inspiration; a sign of appendicitis
What is Rovsing's sign?	Pain in the right lower quadrant (RLQ) felt during palpation of the left lower quadrant (LLQ); also a sign of appendicitis

Give the differential diagnosis of abdominal pain by quadrants:

LUQ?

Gastrointestinal: Splenic injury or abscess, hypersplenism, peptic ulcer disease, gastritis, pyelonephritis, pancreatitis, nephrolithiasis
Cardiopulmonary: Myocardial infarction or ischemia, left lower lobe pneumonia
Neurologic: Herpes zoster

RUQ?

Gastrointestinal: Cholecystitis, hepatic injury or abscess, hepatitis, pyelonephritis, nephrolithiasis, peptic ulcer disease, gastritis, choledocholithiasis, appendicitis (in pregnant patients, when the appendix is behind the cecum), cholangitis, pancreatitis
Cardiopulmonary: Pericarditis, right lower lobe pneumonia
Neurologic: Herpes zoster

RLQ?

Gastrointestinal: Appendicitis, nephrolithiasis, hernia, diverticulitis, intussusception, Meckel's diverticulum
Cardiopulmonary: Leaking aneurysm
Genitourinary: Gonadal torsion, ectopic pregnancy, endometriosis, ovarian cyst, pelvic inflammatory disease (PID)

LLQ?

Gastrointestinal: Diverticulitis, volvulus, hernia, leaking aneurysm, nephrolithiasis, inflammatory bowel disease, carcinoma of colon, colonic perforation
Genitourinary: Ectopic pregnancy, endometriosis, ovarian cyst, PID, gonadal torsion

Name causes of diffuse abdominal pain.

Intestinal obstruction, porphyria, uremia, diabetic ketoacidosis (DKA), pancreatitis, ischemic bowel disease, sickle cell pain crisis, leaking aortic aneurysm, aortic dissection, black widow spider bite, gastroenteritis, and lead poisoning

Laboratory tests

What test should be performed on every woman of childbearing age with abdominal pain?

A pregnancy test [beta human chorionic gonadotropin (β-hCG)]

What laboratory tests are helpful in making a diagnosis in the patient with abdominal pain?

Tests should be guided by patient history and physical examination. A complete blood count (CBC); serum biochemistry panel; urinalysis; and serum β-hCG, amylase, lipase, bilirubin, lactic acid, and cardiac enzyme levels can be helpful.

Imaging studies

What imaging studies are helpful in the diagnosis of abdominal pain?

A chest x-ray (flat and upright plain films), ultrasound, and CT scan can be helpful.

What findings can be seen on plain abdominal x-rays?

Flat plate?

Renal stones, aortic aneurysm (if calcified), pancreatic calcifications (in chronic pancreatitis), biliary stones (occasionally)

Upright abdominal films?

Abnormal air–fluid levels, air in the biliary tree, hollow viscus perforation with free air, volvulus, appendicitis (if an appendicolith is noted)

Upright chest films?

Perforation (if free air is seen), pneumonia, or abnormal air–fluid levels

What diagnoses may be identified by performing an abdominal ultrasound?

Cholecystitis, choledocholithiasis, pancreatitis, hydronephrosis, ovarian torsion, ovarian cyst, and ectopic pregnancy; also appendicitis, aortic aneurysm

When is an abdominal CT scan indicated?

When abscesses or masses are suspected; if the patient has sustained a traumatic injury; or to make a diagnosis that can also be made by ultrasound

Surgical evaluation

If a patient with abdominal pain may require surgery, should she receive pain medication before surgical evaluation?

Yes. Use a short-acting narcotic (e.g., fentanyl).

What is the management of the patient requiring abdominal surgery?	Obtain timely surgical consultation; maintain ABCs; IV, O_2, monitor; control pain and emesis; and administer antibiotics as indicated.
What are the two most common reasons for abdominal surgery?	Obstruction and appendicitis

SHOCK

What is the definition of shock?	Shock is the inadequate delivery of oxygen and metabolites to the tissues.
What metabolic error results in shock?	The inability of the cardiovascular system to meet the metabolic demands of body tissues
What is the difference between compensated and uncompensated shock?	Blood pressure remains normal in compensated shock. In uncompensated shock, the early cardiovascular compensatory mechanisms are unable to prevent compromise of the cardiovascular system, kidneys, or brain.
What four components are necessary for adequate tissue perfusion?	Intact vascular system, adequate oxygenation, adequate cardiac function, and adequate blood volume
What are the best indicators of tissue perfusion?	Urine output and mental status
Name seven signs of shock.	Altered mental status, tachycardia, tachypnea, pallor, diaphoresis, decreased urine output, and hypotension
What is the initial management of any patient in shock?	Establish ABCs; IV, O_2, monitor; control hemorrhage.

TYPES OF SHOCK

What are the five major categories of shock?	1. Hypovolemic shock (caused by hemorrhage or dehydration) 2. Neurogenic shock (caused by spinal cord injury) 3. Cardiogenic shock (caused by left ventricular failure) 4. Septic shock (caused by infection)

5. Distributive shock (caused by anaphylaxis or "third spacing")

Which type of shock is also known as "warm shock"?

Septic shock

Hypovolemic shock

Why does hypovolemic shock occur?

Hypovolemic shock results from inadequate intravascular volume.

What types of hemorrhage may cause hypovolemic shock?

Trauma, gastrointestinal bleeding, aneurysms, vaginal bleeding, and ectopic pregnancy

Other than hemorrhage, name five causes of hypovolemic shock.

Burns, vomiting or diarrhea, DKA, pancreatitis, and ascites

What is the earliest sign of hypovolemic shock?

Tachycardia

Name four other early signs of hypovolemic shock.

Tachypnea, narrowed pulse pressure, anxiety, and diaphoresis

What is a late sign of hypovolemic shock?

Hypotension

How is hypovolemic shock treated after ABCs are established?

Correct the underlying hypovolemia and replace fluids.

What fluid should be used initially for resuscitation of the patient with hypovolemic shock?

Isotonic crystalloid (normal saline or lactated Ringer's)

What should be monitored to evaluate the treatment plan for the patient with hypovolemic shock?

Heart rate, mentation, and urine output

What other factors are useful to monitor treatment of the patient with hypovolemic shock?

Central venous pressure, hematocrit levels, and blood pressure

Neurogenic shock

How can spinal cord injury result in shock?

The loss of sympathetic tone leads to vasodilation, which leads to hypoperfusion.

At what level would the spine have to be injured for bradycardia to occur?

An injury to the cervical spinal cord would result in loss of cardiac sympathetic tone.

Can neurogenic shock be caused by anything other than spinal cord injury?

Yes, it can be caused by spinal anesthesia.

What are the signs and symptoms of neurogenic shock?

Lightheadedness, weakness, neurologic deficits, hypotension, and often bradycardia

What is the initial treatment for neurogenic shock?

Maintain ABCs; IV, O_2, monitor; and consider other causes of shock.

What drugs are used to treat neurogenic shock?

α-Agonists (e.g., phenylephrine) and high doses of dopamine

Cardiogenic shock

Name five causes of cardiogenic shock.

Myocardial infarction, arrhythmias, trauma, pulmonary embolism, and valvular abnormalities

What are three traumatic causes of cardiogenic shock?

Myocardial contusion, tension pneumothorax, and cardiac tamponade

What is the most common cause of cardiogenic shock?

Myocardial infarction

What are the possible causes of shock in myocardial infarction?

Papillary muscle rupture, left ventricular failure, and right ventricular failure

What are the clinical findings in cardiogenic shock?

Tachypnea, tachycardia, rales, altered mental status, possibly a new murmur, and a third heart sound (S_3) gallop

How are cardiogenic shock and hypovolemic shock differentiated?

By patient history and presentation. The patient with cardiogenic shock presents with jugular venous distention, rales, and murmur or gallop; the patient with hypovolemic shock has flat neck veins and clear breath sounds.

What tests are useful in the diagnosis of cardiogenic shock?	Chest radiography, electrocardiography, and echocardiography (if available)
How is right ventricular failure identified?	Check right-sided EKG leads for a right ventricular infarction.
What is the management of cardiogenic shock caused by myocardial infarction?	Maintain ABCs; IV, O_2, monitor; and identify the cause of the shock (i.e., papillary muscle rupture, left ventricular failure, or right ventricular failure).
What is the treatment for right ventricular failure?	Cardiac output is dependent upon preload; intravenous fluids and dobutamine should be given.
How is left ventricular failure treated?	Administer intravenous fluids and dopamine for pressure support.
How does dopamine affect myocardial oxygen demand?	Dopamine increases myocardial oxygen demand.
What other options are available for treating cardiogenic shock?	Dobutamine (for mild hypotension) or balloon pump.

Septic shock

What is the most common cause of septic shock?	Infection with Gram-negative organisms
Why does the patient develop shock?	Vasodilation and intravascular volume depletion occur as a result of abnormal capillary permeability.
Who is at risk for septic shock?	People who are immunocompromised, the elderly and the very young, and people with diabetes
What are the signs of septic shock?	The patient may or may not be febrile. Tachycardia, hypotension, tachypnea, and other symptoms may be seen, depending on whether presentation is early or late.
What are the characteristics of early septic shock?	Warm skin, increased cardiac output, and normal urine output

What are the characteristics of late septic shock?	Cold skin, vasoconstriction, decreased cardiac output, and decreased or absent urine output
The patient with septic shock is at risk for what other condition?	Disseminated intravascular coagulation (DIC)
What laboratory tests and imaging studies are helpful in making the diagnosis of septic shock?	CBC; serum biochemistry panel; chest x-ray; blood cultures and Gram stain; urinalysis and culture; prothrombin time (PT) and partial thromboplastin time (PTT)
What is the treatment for septic shock?	Maintain ABCs; IV, O_2, monitor; administer empiric antibiotics and dopamine for pressure support (if needed).

SHOCK IN CHILDREN

What is the blood volume of an infant?	80 ml/kg; by comparison, adult blood volumes are approximately 60 ml/kg in men, and 70 ml/kg in women.
What is adequate urine output for an infant?	0.5–1 ml/kg/hour
What is the procedure for volume resuscitation in a child?	Administer intravenous fluid boluses (10–20 ml/kg) until urine output is established or signs of volume overload are noted.
What three types of shock occur most commonly in children?	Hypovolemic shock, distributive shock, and cardiogenic shock
In children, what are the typical causes of:	
Hypovolemic shock?	Vomiting and diarrhea (most common); also blood loss, fluid loss from burns, or diuresis from DKA
Distributive shock?	Sepsis (most common); also spinal shock or anaphylaxis
Cardiogenic shock?	Drug ingestions, myocarditis, congenital heart disease, or metabolic abnormalities

What is the most common type of shock seen in children?

Hypovolemic shock from vomiting and diarrhea

What are the most common causes of bacteremia in children younger than 2 months?

Group B streptococci, gram-negative *Escherichia coli,* and *Listeria* species (least likely)

Which organism is most likely to cause bacteremia in the child 3 months to 3 years of age?

Streptococcus pneumoniae

Children with sickle cell disease are susceptible to what kind of organisms?

They are susceptible to encapsulated organisms such as *Streptococcus pneumoniae, Neisseria meningitidis,* and *Salmonella* species.

What is the usual choice of empiric antibiotics for the neonate younger than 4 weeks with a fever or shock?

Ampicillin and gentamycin have shown *in vitro* evidence of synergy when used to treat group B streptococci.

What three common types of congenital heart disease can present as shock in the newborn?

Tetralogy of Fallot, hypoplastic left heart syndrome, and transposition of the great vessels

What endocrinologic disorder may present as shock in a newborn boy?

Congenital adrenal hyperplasia

What two metabolic derangements are seen in children with congenital adrenal hyperplasia?

Hyperkalemia and hyponatremia

What laboratory data are needed to diagnose an inborn error of metabolism in a newborn presenting in shock?

Anion gap; serum levels of lactate, ammonia, and glucose; urine for reducing substances

How is an anion gap calculated?

$Na - (HCO_3 + Cl)$; normal range is 10–14 mEq/L.

Can shaken babies exhibit signs of shock?

Yes. They may also have apnea, hypothermia, bradycardia, and seizures.

CYANOSIS

What is cyanosis?	A bluish color of the skin and mucous membranes resulting from the concentration of deoxyhemoglobin (reduced hemoglobin) or hemoglobin derivatives in the capillary blood
On what areas of the body is cyanosis usually seen?	The lips, nail beds, malar eminences, ears, conjunctivae, and tongue
What increases deoxyhemoglobin in the capillary blood?	Decreased oxygen delivery, increased uptake of oxygen in the periphery, or abnormal hemoglobin
How much reduced hemoglobin is required to produce cyanosis?	5 g of reduced hemoglobin per 100 ml of capillary blood
Is the tendency toward cyanosis higher or lower in the patient with low hemoglobin levels?	The tendency toward cyanosis is lower in patients with anemia.
Why?	Cyanosis is caused by the absolute quantity of reduced hemoglobin. If the initial hemoglobin level is 15 mg/dl, cyanosis (5 mg/dl deoxygenated blood) is evident at an oxygen saturation of 67% $[(15 \text{ mg/dl} - 5 \text{ mg/dl}) \div 15 \text{ mg/dl}]$. If the initial hemoglobin level is 10 mg/dl, cyanosis is evident at a saturation of 50%.
What are the two types of cyanosis?	Peripheral and central
What causes peripheral cyanosis?	1. Decreased cardiac output 2. Arterial occlusion 3. Venous obstruction 4. Exposure to cold 5. Central redistribution of blood flow
What causes central cyanosis?	1. Decreased oxygen saturation 2. Hemoglobin abnormalities
What factors may decrease the oxygen saturation?	1. Decreased atmospheric pressure 2. Alveolar hypoventilation 3. Impaired oxygen diffusion 4. $\dot{V}/\dot{Q}$ mismatch

5. Congenital heart defect
6. Intrapulmonary shunt
7. Hemoglobin with a low affinity for oxygen

What is the most common congenital heart defect associated with cyanosis?

Tetralogy of Fallot [characterized by ventricular septal defect (VSD) and pulmonary outflow obstruction]

Other than deoxyhemoglobinemia, what hemoglobin abnormalities produce cyanosis?

1. Sulfhemoglobinemia, defined as 0.5 g of sulfhemoglobin per 100 ml of capillary blood
2. Methemoglobinemia, defined as 1.5 g of methemoglobin per 100 ml of capillary blood

What causes sulfhemoglobinemia?

Exposure to acetanilid or phenacetin

What causes methemoglobinemia?

Exposure to benzocaine, nitrates, nitrites, or sulfonamides

When should methemoglobinemia be treated?

When signs of hypoxia are present

How are levels of sulfhemoglobin and methemoglobin determined?

Cooximetry (to detect type of hemoglobin) in addition to standard ABGs

Are methemoglobinemia and sulfhemoglobinemia reversible?

Methemoglobinemia is reversible, but sulfhemoglobinemia is not.

What is the treatment for methemoglobinemia?

Administer methylene blue in a 1% solution, 1–2 mg/kg intravenously over 5 minutes

What physical examination finding may be seen along with cyanosis in a patient with a hemoglobinopathy or congenital heart disease?

Clubbing

SYNCOPE IN ADULTS

Define syncope.

The transient loss of consciousness with associated loss of postural tone

Name the five types of syncope.

1. Vasomotor
2. Cardiac
3. Central nervous system (CNS)
4. Metabolic
5. Psychogenic

What is vasomotor syncope?

Transient hypotension from abnormal vascular tone or hypovolemia

Name four kinds of vaso-motor syncope.

Vasovagal syncope, postural hypotension, hypovolemia, and autonomic insufficiency

What are historical clues to hypovolemia?

Thirst, decreased intake by mouth, melena, and dysfunctional uterine bleeding

What are common causes of postural syncope?

Diabetic neuropathy, deconditioning, and alcoholic neuropathy

What aspects of the patient's history suggest vasovagal syncope?

Reports of dizziness, nausea, stress, and diaphoresis before the syncopal episode

What causes cardiac syncope?

Arrhythmias (fast or slow)

What historical clues point to a cardiac etiology?

The abrupt loss of consciousness without other symptoms before the syncopal episode

What are CNS etiologies of syncope?

Transient ischemic attack (TIA), sub-arachnoid hemorrhage, and vertebral-basilar insufficiency

What is the most common cause of metabolic syncope?

Hypoglycemia

The possible causes of syncope are numerous; name a few.

Subclavian steal syndrome
Drugs
Pulmonary embolism
Carbon monoxide inhalation
Coughing
Micturition

When is subclavian steal suspected?

When syncope occurs after upper extremity exertion

What categories of drugs contribute to syncope?

Beta blockers, calcium channel blockers, diuretics, nitrates, and alcohol

How often is the cause of syncope identified in the emergency department (ED)?

A cause is identified in about 50% of patients with syncope presenting to the ED.

How is seizure distinguished from syncope?

Syncopal patients generally wake up quickly without a postictal period.

How is the diagnosis of syncope usually made?

The diagnosis is made by history more than 50% of the time.

What other studies are helpful in making a diagnosis?

EKG, glucose testing, and hematocrit determination; possibly CT scan of the head or Holter monitoring

How is syncope managed?

Ensure ABCs; IV, O_2, monitor; assess vital signs; and examine the patient for trauma caused by the syncopal episode.

What patients with syncope should be admitted?

Patients at high risk for complications:
Those older than 60–70 years
Those having significant cardiac risk factors
Those experiencing recurrent syncope
Those with a serious underlying illness

What patients are at low risk for serious complications of syncope?

Young patients without cardiac disease

How is presyncope different from syncope?

In presyncope, there is never a complete loss of consciousness.

In the ED, is presyncope approached differently from syncope?

No.

SYNCOPE IN CHILDREN

What are the structural causes of cardiac syncope?

Severe aortic or pulmonic stenosis
Idiopathic hypertrophic subaortic stenosis (IHSS)
Mobile atrial myxoma
Mitral valve prolapse

What feature of the patient history suggests a cardiac cause of syncope?

Syncope occurring during or shortly after physical exertion

What EKG abnormalities at rest predispose the patient to cardiac syncope?

Prolonged QT interval; short PR interval and wide QRS complex [typical of Wolff-Parkinson-White (WPW) syndrome]

What EKG abnormality is seen in patients with WPW?

A delta wave (gradual upsloping of the QRS complex)

What is the most common acquired heart disease in children?

Kawasaki disease

What cardiac abnormality is seen in Kawasaki disease?

Coronary artery aneurysms leading to myocardial infarction

What four murmurs should raise suspicion of a cardiac cause of syncope?

Diastolic
Holosystolic
Continuous
Systolic murmur grade above 3/6

What two other sounds should raise suspicion of a cardiac cause of syncope?

A click or heave
A fixed or single second heart sound (S_2)

Does IIHS always present with a murmur on examination?

No

How is IIHS diagnosed?

By performing cardiac ultrasonography

What conduction abnormality is associated with a family history of deafness?

Long QT syndrome

How is a corrected QT interval calculated?

Divide the QT interval by the square root of the R-R interval.

What conduction abnormality occurs in an infant whose mother has lupus?

Atrioventricular (AV) dissociation

What are some metabolic causes of syncope?

Hypoglycemia, anemia, carbon monoxide poisoning

Describe the characteristics of hysterical syncope.

Histrionic-type patient falls gracefully to the floor, typically in front of an audience.

Name three respiratory causes of syncope.

Hyperventilation
Coughing (tussive syncope; often occurs in children with asthma or pertussis)
Breath-holding spells

Describe the two classic types of breath-holding spells.

1. A crying child holds his breath at end-exhalation until he becomes cyanotic, unconscious, and limp. Several clonic contractions also may occur.
2. A child cries once or twice after a sudden painful stimulus, turns pale, and becomes limp.

Which type of breath-holding spell is more common?

The cyanotic variety

How common are breath-holding spells in children?

Approximately 5% of children experience them.

In what age group do they typically occur?

In children 6–18 months old

How can breath-holding spells be differentiated from seizures?

1. Breath-holding spells never occur during sleep, only after appropriate stimuli.
2. Cyanosis occurs late in a seizure, but at the onset of breath-holding syncope.
3. More than one cry is uncommon before a seizure.
4. There may be a family history of breath-holding spells.

Which children with syncope should have an EKG performed?

Children whose syncope does not have an obvious cause
Children with a family history of sudden death or hearing problems

When should the child receive neurologic evaluation?

When breath-holding spells occur repeatedly
When the diagnosis is unclear

GASTROINTESTINAL BLEEDING IN ADULTS

Name the two types of gastrointestinal bleeding.

Upper and lower gastrointestinal bleeding

UPPER GASTROINTESTINAL BLEEDING

What are the signs of upper gastrointestinal bleeding?

Shock, positive guaiac test for occult blood, signs of underlying liver disease (e.g., spider angiomata, gynecomastia, or jaundice)

What are the symptoms of upper gastrointestinal bleeding?

Abdominal pain, melena, syncope, altered mental status, hematemesis, shock, hematochezia, coffee-ground emesis

Name some of the risk factors for upper gastrointestinal bleeding.

Alcohol abuse, tobacco use, liver disease, use of aspirin or nonsteroidal anti-inflammatory drugs (NSAIDs), sepsis, trauma, burns, admission to the intensive care unit (ICU), steroid use, vomiting

What are the most common causes of upper gastrointestinal bleeding?

Peptic ulcer disease: 45%–50% (of these, 20% are gastric ulcers and 25%–30% are duodenal ulcers)
Gastritis: 20%
Esophageal varices: 10%–20%
Mallory-Weiss syndrome: 10%

What are some of the less likely causes of upper gastrointestinal bleeding?

Arteriovenous malformations; malignancies; aortoenteric fistulas; pancreatitis; and epistaxis masquerading as gastrointestinal bleeding

What laboratory studies should be used in evaluating the patient with upper gastrointestinal bleeding?

Serum biochemistry panel, serum bilirubin level, liver function test, amylase test, blood type and crossmatch, PT/PTT, CBC

What other studies may be useful?

Chest x-ray to look for free air; EKG

What diagnostic study is useful in identifying and treating the source of bleeding?

Esophagogastroduodenoscopy (EGD)

EGD will not identify what bleeding site?

Bleeding distal to the duodenum

What diagnostic study should be used in the presence of ongoing upper gastrointestinal bleeding not seen with EGD?

Angiography or radiolabeled erythrocyte scanning

Angiographic demonstration of upper gastrointestinal bleeding requires what bleeding rate?

0.5 ml/min. At this bleeding rate, patients are transfusion dependent.

Radiolabeled erythrocyte scanning requires what blood loss rate for detection?	0.1 ml/min
What is the initial management of the patient with upper gastrointestinal bleeding?	Maintain ABCs; IV, O_2, monitor; perform nasogastric suction; insert a Foley catheter; and perform an endoscopy.
What drug therapy is available for upper gastrointestinal bleeding?	Vasopressin has been used intravenously at a dosage of 0.1–0.9 units/min.
What are the side effects of vasopressin?	Hypertension, arrhythmias, myocardial and splanchnic ischemia, local skin necrosis due to infiltration
What measure should be taken to prevent myocardial infarction while using vasopressin?	Nitroglycerin should be infused.
Is there a role for intravenous administration of histamine-2(H_2) antagonists?	They have not been proven to improve rebleeding, surgery, or mortality rates.
Which consultants should be involved in the evaluation of the patient with upper gastrointestinal bleeding?	A gastroenterologist and a surgeon
What percentage of patients have upper gastrointestinal bleeding that stops spontaneously?	80%–85%
What is the mortality rate for patients with a first episode of bleeding?	4%–5%
What percentage of patients with upper gastrointestinal bleeding experience bleeding again after admission?	25%

What is the mortality rate for patients with subsequent episodes of bleeding?	30%–35%
What causes melena?	The reaction of blood with hydrochloric acid produces hematin and yields black, tarry, and sticky stool.
How much bleeding is necessary to produce melena?	60 ml of blood in the gastrointestinal tract
What can simulate melena?	The ingestion of iron or bismuth
What can simulate hematochezia?	The ingestion of certain foods (e.g., beets)
Do iron, bismuth, or beets cause a positive result on fecal occult blood testing?	No.
Are there confounding variables that may yield a positive result on fecal occult blood testing?	Dietary peroxidases and vitamin C
Differentiate upper gastrointestinal bleeding from lower gastrointestinal bleeding.	Coffee-ground emesis or hematemesis suggests bleeding proximal to the ligament of Treitz. Melena suggests a bleeding site proximal to the right colon. Hematochezia suggests either a more distal colorectal bleed or brisk bleeding proximal to the ligament of Treitz.
Does performing nasogastric suction help differentiate upper from lower gastrointestinal bleeding?	Only if the aspirate appears bloody, red-tinged, or like coffee grounds. A negative result on nasogastric suction does not rule out upper gastrointestinal bleeding.

LOWER GASTROINTESTINAL BLEEDING

What is the definition of lower gastrointestinal bleeding?	Bleeding distal to the ligament of Treitz
What are the signs of lower gastrointestinal bleeding?	Abdominal distention or masses; bright red blood per rectum; peritoneal signs;

shock; orthostasis; positive results on fecal occult blood test

List five symptoms of lower gastrointestinal bleeding.

Abdominal pain, melena, hematochezia, syncope, fatigue, shortness of breath

What is the most common cause of lower gastrointestinal bleeding?

Upper gastrointestinal bleeding; a proximal source should be sought.

Name some of the other causes of lower gastrointestinal bleeding.

Diverticulosis (most common), angiodysplasia, carcinoma, hemorrhoids, inflammatory bowel disease, polyps, anal fissures, Meckel's diverticulum, infectious gastroenteritis, intussusception, volvulus, ischemic colitis, infarcted bowel, strangulated hernia, and radiation injury

Why does diverticulosis cause bleeding?

Erosion into a penetrating artery of the diverticulum results in painless bleeding.

How frequently does diverticular bleeding stop spontaneously?

Bleeding stops spontaneously in 75%–90% of cases; however, most patients require a transfusion.

What is angiodysplasia?

Angiodysplasia is an arteriovenous malformation usually found in the right colon of elderly patients. It is associated with hypertension and aortic stenosis.

Why is a rectal exam important in the diagnosis of lower gastrointestinal bleeding?

To rule out local pathology such as hemorrhoids, fissures, or proctitis

What laboratory tests are used to evaluate the patient with lower gastrointestinal bleeding?

Blood type and crossmatch; CBC; serum biochemistry panel; and PT/PTT.

What is the management of the patient with lower gastrointestinal bleeding?

The treatment is the same as for upper gastrointestinal bleeding: maintain ABCs; IV, O_2, monitor; insert a nasogastric tube to look for upper gastrointestinal source of bleeding; perform colonoscopy and anoscopy; consider arteriography or infusion of vasopressin.

If the site of lower gastro-intestinal bleeding is known and infusion therapy fails, what is the standard treatment?

If infusion therapy fails, the standard treatment is surgical: a hemicolectomy.

What percentage of patients with lower gastrointestinal bleeding stop bleeding spontaneously?

75%

What is the mortality rate for patients having a first occurrence of lower gastro-intestinal bleeding?

10%

GASTROINTESTINAL BLEEDING IN CHILDREN

UPPER GASTROINTESTINAL BLEEDING

What are the most common causes of upper gastro-intestinal bleeding in:

  Newborns?

Swallowed maternal blood, esophagitis, stress ulcers, bleeding diathesis

  Infants and children younger than 5 years?

Mucosal abnormalities: esophagitis, Mallory-Weiss syndrome, gastritis, stress ulcer

  Children older than 5 years?

Mucosal abnormalities and peptic ulcer disease

What test distinguishes swallowed maternal blood from fetal blood?

The Apt test

Why should vitamin K be given to newborns in the nursery?

To prevent hemorrhagic disease of the newborn (rare)

What congenital abnormalities can present as upper gastrointestinal bleeding?

Vascular malformation, intestinal duplications, and bleeding abnormalities

Ingestion of what drugs can cause gastrointestinal bleeding?

Aspirin, steroids, NSAIDs, iron, alcohol

What causes esophageal varices in children?	Extrahepatic obstruction, such as portal vein thrombosis, is very common. Hepatic disease from cystic fibrosis, biliary cirrhosis (from biliary atresia), and hepatitis can cause portal hypertension.

LOWER GASTROINTESTINAL BLEEDING

What are five common causes of lower gastrointestinal bleeding in newborns?	Swallowed maternal blood, milk allergy, colitis, midgut volvulus, nodular lymphoid hyperplasia
Name four uncommon but serious causes of lower gastrointestinal bleeding in newborns.	1. Necrotizing enterocolitis 2. Hirschsprung's disease 3. Intussusception 4. Meckel's diverticulum
Name some conditions that cause lower gastrointestinal bleeding in infants and toddlers.	Anal fissures; colitis [inflammatory bowel disease (IBD), infectious colitis, pseudomembranous colitis]; milk allergy; Meckel's diverticulum; intussusception; hemolytic-uremic syndrome (HUS); juvenile polyps.
What are some common causes of lower gastrointestinal bleeding in preschool children?	Anal fissures; colitis; juvenile polyps; Henoch-Schönlein purpura; HUS; IBD; angiodysplasia; intussusception
What signs and symptoms are seen in children with malrotation and midgut volvulus?	These children experience bilious vomiting, pain, and abdominal distention. Blood in the stool implies ischemia.
When should intussusception be suspected?	When a child between the ages of 3 months to 1 year presents with intermittent colicky pain, often followed by periods of lethargy, "currant jelly" stools, and systolic hypertension. A negative result on a guaiac test for occult blood in the stool does not rule out the diagnosis.
What signs would be seen in a child with polyps?	The child with polyps usually presents with painless rectal bleeding. Fragments of polyp tissue can often be found in the stool.

How is malrotation diagnosed in children?	By means of a barium enema or upper gastrointestinal study
How is Meckel's diverticulum diagnosed in children?	These children present with painless rectal bleeding. Diagnosis is done by means of a Meckel's scan (a technetium scan to identify ectopic gastric mucosa). (Remember, a Meckel's scan cannot be performed immediately after a barium enema.)
What are the typical signs and symptoms of Crohn's disease in children?	Children with Crohn's disease often present with chronic abdominal pain, intermittent bloody diarrhea (which may be massive or minimal), failure to thrive, and an elevated erythrocyte sedimentation rate (ESR). Toxic megacolon is a life-threatening presentation.

HEMOPTYSIS

What is hemoptysis?	Expectoration of blood
What is considered massive hemoptysis?	The expectoration of at least 600 ml of blood during a 24-hour period
Name six causes of hemoptysis.	1. Trauma 2. Tuberculosis 3. Bronchitis 4. Carcinoma 5. Bleeding from the oropharynx or nasopharynx 6. Cardiac disorders (e.g., CHF, mitral stenosis) 7. Pulmonary embolus
What is the most common cause of hemoptysis?	Chronic bronchitis
How often is hemoptysis seen in patients with pulmonary emboli?	Hemoptysis occurs in about 30% of patients with pulmonary infarction.
What symptoms are associated with hemoptysis?	Cough and dyspnea

What additional symptoms are associated with hemoptysis in patients with:

Tuberculosis?   Fever and night sweats

Carcinoma?   Persistent cough and weight loss

What tests are useful in the work-up of a patient with hemoptysis?   Chest radiography, sputum analysis, CBC, PT, PTT, platelet count, blood type and cross match

What other studies are potentially useful?   Computed tomography (CT) scan and bronchoscopy

How is massive hemoptysis treated in the ED?   Maintain the ABCs: IV, O_2, monitor, and intubate (or perform selective intubation of the unaffected bronchus) to protect the airway.

What patient position may decrease the severity of lung injury?   Position the patient on her side, with the affected lung down

ALTERED MENTAL STATUS

Name three types of altered mental status.   Dementia, delirium, and coma

What is required for normal consciousness?   The reticular activating system (RAS), both cerebral hemispheres, and their connections all must be functioning normally.

What center mainly controls wakefulness?   The RAS

Describe coma.   Unresponsiveness due to abnormal arousal and content functions

What is the differential diagnosis for altered mental status?   **TIPS AEIOU:**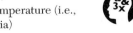
Trauma or **T**emperature (i.e., hypothermia)
Infection
Psychiatric (diagnosis of exclusion)
Stroke, **S**ubarachnoid hemorrhage, **S**pace-occupying lesion, **S**eizure, or **S**erotonin syndrome

Alcohol (Wernicke-Korsakoff syndrome)
or Ammonia (hepatic encephalopathy)
Electrolyte imbalances or an Endocrine
disorder
Insulin excess (hypoglycemia)
Oxygen, Overdose, or Opiates
Uremia

What is dementia?

The failure of content portions of
consciousness while alerting functions are
preserved

**Distinguish delirium from
dementia.**

Delirium has a more abrupt onset with
more variability in cognitive function.

**What is the classic history
of dementia?**

Chronic, progressive loss of short-term
memory. Dementia is generally seen in
elderly patients.

**What are the most common
causes of dementia?**

Alzheimer's disease and multiple cerebral
infarcts

**What are the potentially
treatable causes of dementia
or delirium?**

DEMENTIA:
Drugs (anticholinergics, narcotics,
sedatives, or phenothiazines)
Electrolyte imbalances, Eye or Ear
difficulties (deafness or blindness)
Metabolic disorders (thyroid, hepatic)
Emotional disorders(depression)
Nutritional deficiencies (e.g., folate, B_{12},
B_1; Wernicke-Korsakoff syndrome)
Trauma or Tumor
Infections or Inflammation
Alcohol

What is pseudodementia?

Depression that imitates dementia

**What is the key component
when evaluating the patient
with altered mental status
in the ED?**

A thorough patient history is vital.

**If the patient is comatose,
how can the history be
obtained?**

The history may be obtained by
questioning paramedics, family, and
bystanders, and by checking the patient's
wallet or pill bottles.

What are the key components of the physical examination of the patient with altered mental status?

Assess vital signs (including temperature), evaluate mental status, perform a neurologic exam for focal deficits or asymmetry, and examine the eyes.

What are the pupillary findings in a patient with altered mental status caused by toxins or metabolic disorders?

Small, reactive pupils

Are there exceptions to this finding?

Yes, a patient taking anticholinergic drugs will have dilated pupils.

What bedside tests can help to establish the causes of altered mental status?

Pulse oximetry, glucose levels, and vital signs

What is the ED management of the patient with altered mental status?

Maintain ABCs; IV, O_2, monitor

What is the initial treatment for altered mental status of unknown cause?

After ensuring ABCs, correct any abnormalities detected by bedside testing. Some measures that may be taken include applying oxygen, administering glucose as needed, and intravenous administration of 100 mg of thiamine and 2 mg of naloxone hydrochloride.

What areas of the patient evaluation would raise suspicion of a structural brain lesion?

A history of trauma, focal deficits found on the neurologic examination, or abnormal pupillary findings

Which patients should receive a CT scan?

Patients believed to have increased intracranial pressure (ICP) or a structural lesion

What is the treatment for increased ICP?

Maintain ABCs; sedate the patient and induce paralysis; administer mannitol at a rate of 1 g/kg; and obtain a neurosurgical consult.

What other tests are helpful to narrow the differential diagnosis?

CBC, chemistries, urinalysis, chest x-ray, lumbar puncture, and serum levels of ammonia and ethyl alcohol

When is a lumbar puncture indicated?

When CNS infection is suspected and there is no evidence of elevated ICP, or if subarachnoid hemorrhage is suspected and head CT findings are negative.

What other x-rays are helpful?

If trauma is suspected, cervical spine x-rays should be obtained.

If a patient has had a seizure and has not awakened appropriately in 25–30 minutes, what should you consider?

Nonconvulsive status epilepticus

How is nonconvulsive status epilepticus diagnosed?

Obtain a neurology consultation and perform an electroencephalogram (EEG).

FEVER

Oral temperature is how much lower than rectal temperature?

0.5°C

Axillary temperature is how much lower than oral temperature?

0.5°C

What is a hectic fever?

A hectic fever has a large variation between the peak and nadir.

What is an intermittent fever?

An intermittent fever returns to normal each day.

What are examples of conditions in which relapsing fever occurs?

Hodgkin's disease, malaria, rat-bite fever

What associated characteristics are suggestive of infection?

High fever with sudden onset, constitutional symptoms, abnormal white blood cell (WBC) count, meningeal symptoms, urinary symptoms

What temperature suggests an invasive bacterial illness in:

Neonates younger than 8 weeks?

38.0°C or greater

Children 3 months to 3 years?	39.5°C or greater
Name some of the infectious causes of prolonged fever.	Abscesses, prostatitis, osteomyelitis, mycobacterial illness, sinusitis, endocarditis, fungal infections, tuberculosis, malaria (parasitic diseases), spirochetal infections, hepatitis, mononucleosis, rickettsial disease
What other diseases may cause prolonged fever?	Neoplasms, connective tissue disease (e.g., rheumatic fever, rheumatoid arthritis, lupus), granulomatous disease (e.g., Crohn's disease, sarcoidosis)

2 ___

Resuscitation

RESUSCITATION IN ADULTS

AIRWAY

What four factors are evaluated during an examination of the airway anatomy?

1. Mandible size and mobility
2. Cervical spine mobility
3. Size of the oropharynx
4. Midface stability

What landmarks should you seek when you look inside a patient's open mouth?

The uvula, soft palate, and tonsilar pillars

What does visualization of these landmarks predict?

Easier intubation

Why is midface stability important?

Midface stability is important in case it becomes necessary to bag-valve-mask ventilate a patient who becomes apneic.

Name two airway adjunct devices.

Oropharyngeal airway and nasopharyngeal airway

When is an oropharyngeal airway used?

In a spontaneously breathing, unconscious patient

When is a nasopharyngeal airway used?

In a spontaneously breathing, semiconscious or conscious patient

List eight options for airway control.

1. Nasopharyngeal airway
2. Oropharyngeal airway
3. Orotracheal intubation
4. Nasotracheal intubation
5. Cricothyrotomy
6. Tracheostomy
7. Retrograde intubation
8. Percutaneous transtracheal ventilation

Intubation

What drugs commonly used in resuscitation situations can be administered via an endotracheal tube?

NAVEL
Naloxone
Atropine
Valium
Epinephrine
Lidocaine

Rapid sequence induction (RSI)

What is RSI?

RSI is a series of steps that are taken to facilitate intubation. RSI involves sedation and paralysis of the patient to minimize the risk of complications as a result of intubation.

Why is chemical paralysis useful?

Chemical paralysis enhances mechanical ventilation, thereby improving oxygenation, which controls the intracranial pressure (ICP). In addition, chemical paralysis can decrease peak airway pressures and provide pharmacologic restraint.

Why is succinylcholine used for paralysis?

It has a rapid onset of action (30–60 seconds) and a short duration of action (5–6 minutes).

What complications are associated with the use of succinylcholine?

Hyperkalemia; sudden, brief increases in the ICP; increased intragastric pressure; increased intraocular pressure; myalgias; arrhythmias

What characterizes conscious sedation?

Depressed consciousness with intact respiration

What are its components?

Sedation and anesthesia

How many people does it take to perform a procedure (e.g., fracture reduction, chest tube placement) and monitor the patient's sedation?

Two

What questions should be asked prior to inducing sedation?

AMPLE
Allergies?
Medications?
Past history?
Last meal?
Events of injury? (Not essential)

Describe the presedation physical examination.

The patient's baseline cardiac, respiratory, and mental status is assessed, and the airway anatomy is evaluated.

What vital signs must be monitored before, during, and after sedation?

Heart rate, respiratory effectiveness (evaluated by assessing the pulse rate and using pulse oximetry), and blood pressure

What equipment and medications must be available before sedation is attempted?

Oxygen with an appropriate mask, suction equipment, and an intravenous fluid bolus

Why is intravenous administration of sedatives preferred to intramuscular injection?

Intravenous administration is associated with more reliable effects.

What class of medications is used for analgesia?

Narcotics (e.g., meperidine, fentanyl)

What side effects are associated with narcotics?

Respiratory depression, hypotension, histamine release, urinary retention

What is one side effect of meperidine?

Seizures (especially in patients with sickle cell disease or renal failure)

What are the advantages of fentanyl?

It has a quick onset and short duration of action.

What is ketamine?

A dissociative anesthetic agent

What side effects are associated with ketamine?

Bronchodilation, increased ICP, vomiting, increased salivation, unpleasant sensations or dreams following the procedure

Name four types of sedatives.

Benzodiazepines, barbiturates, propofol, chloral hydrate

What advantage does ketamine have over benzodiazepines?

The respiratory drive is maintained.

What are the side effects of:

    Benzodiazepines?   Respiratory depression, hypotension

    Barbiturates?   Respiratory depression, decreased ICP

    Propofol?   Respiratory depression, hypotension, burning at the site of injection

    Chloral hydrate?   Prolonged sedation

When can continuous cardiopulmonary monitoring be stopped?   When the patient is awake, able to respond to questions, and able to protect his airway, and when the peak effects of the drugs have passed

Orotracheal intubation

List three potential complications of orotracheal intubation.

1. Endobronchial or esophageal intubation with subsequent hypoxia
2. Obstruction of the tube secondary to a bulging cuff, secretions, kinking, or biting
3. Arytenoid cartilage displacement

What size endotracheal tube should be used in:

    Women?   7.0–8.0 mm

    Men?   8.0–8.5 mm

Following intubation, what areas should be auscultated?   The axillary region and over the stomach

What does detection of breath sounds on only the right side suggest?   Right main stem bronchus intubation

List five ways of ensuring that the endotracheal tube is in the right place.

1. Observation (fogging and clearing of the tube, bilateral breath sounds, bilateral chest expansion)
2. Laryngoscopy (visualization of the tube passing through the cords)
3. Capnography
4. Fiberoptic visualization
5. Chest radiograph (reveals bronchial, but not esophageal, placement)

How does a Miller laryngo-scope blade differ from a Macintosh laryngoscope blade?

The Miller blade directly and physically lifts the epiglottis, while the Macintosh blade rests in the vallecula above the epiglottis and lifts it indirectly.

Nasotracheal intubation

What are the advantages of blind nasotracheal intuba-tion (BNTI)?

Paralysis of the patient is not necessary, and the procedure can be performed with the patient in a semi-upright position.

List six situations when BNTI might be appropriate.

1. Clinical situation makes it difficult to perform laryngoscopy
2. Neuromuscular blockade would be risky
3. Cricothyrotomy unnecessary
4. Patient unable to lie supine [e.g., as a result of chronic obstructive pulmonary disease (COPD), asthma, agitation]
5. Patient has sustained oral trauma
6. Patient has trismus

Where is the endotracheal tube most likely to be when it is placed incorrectly during BNTI?

The pyriform fossa

How can improper place-ment of the tube during BNTI be detected?

Look at and palpate the lateral aspect of the neck.

Cricothyrotomy

What is a cricothyrotomy?

Creation of a temporary airway by inserting a breathing tube (either a #7 or #8 endotracheal tube, or a #8 tracheos-tomy tube) through the cricothyroid membrane

List five indications for cricothyrotomy.

1. Ongoing tracheobronchial or oral hemorrhage
2. Massive midface trauma
3. Inability to control the airway using less invasive procedures
4. Oral or pharyngeal edema (e.g., as a result of infection, anaphylaxis, or inhalation injuries)
5. Inability to remove blood or vomitus secondary to trismus

Why should a cricothyroid-otomy be converted to a formal tracheostomy at the earliest opportunity?

Because of the proximity of a cricothyroidotomy to the subglottic region, significant airway stenosis may occur with long-term use of a cricothyroid airway; thus, a cricothyroidotomy should be converted to a formal tracheostomy at the earliest opportunity in the operating room by a surgical team.

How does a cricothyroid-otomy differ from a tracheostomy?

The cricothyroidotomy was designed to allow access to the trachea with a minimal amount of dissection and exposure. A tracheostomy involves the placement of a tube below the second tracheal ring. This almost always involves dissection around the thyroid gland and operating in a deeper portion of the neck, which requires proper lighting and exposure. Tracheostomy should not be performed in an emergency situation by non-surgeons, and even trained neck surgeons would most likely place the emergency airway through the cricothyroid membrane initially and convert it to a tracheostomy at a later time.

BREATHING

How is respiration assessed?

1. Examination (note the respiratory rate and effort; look for cyanosis, which indicates profound hypoxia)
2. Pulse oximetry
3. Arterial blood gases (ABGs)

What are the signs of respiratory failure?

Tachypnea, deep respirations, retractions, nasal flaring, patient anxiety, decreasing level of consciousness

List three limitations of pulse oximetry.

1. Requires perfusion of the probe site
2. Does not measure ventilation (i.e., the $PaCO_2$)
3. Does not detect methemoglobin or carboxyhemoglobin

What is the normal $PaCO_2$ in a tachypneic patient?

Less than 40 mm Hg. Normocarbia suggests respiratory failure.

What does upper airway obstruction sound like?	Inspiratory stridor
List four causes of upper airway obstruction.	1. Infection (e.g., croup, epiglottitis) 2. Upper airway edema (e.g., anaphylaxis, trauma) 3. Foreign body aspiration 4. Congenital or anatomic disorders (e.g., laryngomalacia, large tongue, tumor or cyst, vocal cord paralysis)
List seven supplemental oxygen delivery systems that are available.	1. Nasal cannula 2. "Blow by" oxygen 3. Oxygen mask (simple, partial rebreather, or nonrebreather) 4. Face tent 5. Oxygen hood 6. Bag-valve-mask ventilation 7. Tracheal intubation
When is it important to apply cricoid pressure?	When using bag-valve-mask ventilation or when intubating a patient, in order to minimize the risk of aspiration and gastric inflation

CIRCULATION

Volume resuscitation

What is the defining feature of "decompensated shock?"	Decreased blood pressure
What is the normal blood volume of a:	
Woman?	70 ml/kg
Man?	60 ml/kg
Name three sites for obtaining central venous access.	1. Femoral vein 2. Internal jugular vein 3. Subclavian vein
Why is the femoral vein preferred for obtaining central venous access?	1. The femoral vein is "out of the way" (i.e., farther away from where resuscitation activity is taking place). 2. Catheterization of the femoral vein is associated with a lower complication

rate than catheterization of the
internal jugular or subclavian veins.

**Name two complications
that can result from
femoral venous access
attempts.**

1. Retroperitoneal bleeding (as a result
   of achieving access above the inguinal
   ligament)
2. Femoral artery puncture

**Name four large peripheral
veins.**

1. Basilic vein
2. Cephalic vein
3. External jugular vein
4. Saphenous vein

Rhythm restoration

**What is the primary treat-
able rhythm encountered
in cardiac arrest?**

Ventricular fibrillation

**What is the treatment for
ventricular fibrillation?**

Electrical defibrillation at 200 J, 200–300 J,
and 360 J

**What is the first-line treat-
ment for persistent ventricular fibrillation?**

Epinephrine, 1 mg intravenously,
followed by defibrillation

**List five second-line agents
that can be considered (in
conjunction with defibrillation) if epinephrine plus
defibrillation does not work.**

1. Lidocaine
2. Bretylium
3. Magnesium sulfate
4. Procainamide
5. Amiodarone

**What is the therapy for
asystole?**

Epinephrine and atropine; treatment of
the underlying cause (if one can be
identified)

**Name some reversible
causes of asystole.**

Hypoxia, hypo- or hyperkalemia, drug
overdose, hypothermia

**Name ten reversible causes
of pulseless electrical
activity (PEA).**

1. Pulmonary embolism
2. Severe metabolic acidosis
3. Tension pneumothorax
4. Cardiac tamponade
5. Drug overdose (e.g., β blockers,
   digoxin, calcium channel blockers,
   tricyclic antidepressants)
6. Massive myocardial infarction
7. Hypovolemia

8. Hypothermia
9. Hypokalemia
10. Hypoxia

What feature on an electrocardiogram (EKG) distinguishes a wide QRS complex tachycardia from a narrow QRS complex tachycardia?

A narrow QRS complex spans less than three small boxes (i.e., is less than 0.12 msec in duration), while a wide QRS complex spans more than three small boxes (i.e., is more than 0.12 msec in duration). One small box on an EKG represents 0.04 msec.

What is the most likely site of origin of a:

Wide QRS complex tachyarrhythmia?

Below the atrioventricular (AV) node

Narrow QRS complex tachyarrhythmia?

Above the AV node

What is the differential diagnosis in a patient with a wide QRS complex tachycardia?

1. Ventricular tachycardia
2. Sinus tachycardia with left bundle branch block
3. Supraventricular tachycardia with aberrant conduction

What features in the patient's history would suggest ventricular tachycardia?

Age greater than 50 years and features suggestive of underlying ischemic heart disease

What EKG findings would suggest ventricular tachycardia?

Fusion beats, extreme left axis deviation, AV dissociation, and a QRS complex with a duration of more than 0.14 second

What feature in the patient's history would suggest a supraventricular tachycardia with aberrant conduction?

Age younger than 35 years

What EKG findings would suggest supraventricular tachycardia with aberrant conduction?

Normal axis and QRS complexes preceded by P waves

What are the signs and symptoms of an "unstable" tachyarrhythmia?	Ischemic chest pain, dyspnea as a result of pulmonary edema, an altered level of consciousness, systemic hypotension
What is the treatment for an unstable tachyar-rhythmia?	Electrocardioversion (in most instances)
What is the treatment for a stable wide QRS complex tachyarrhythmia?	Assume ventricular tachycardia and treat with lidocaine (1–1.5 mg/kg).
What drug is contra-indicated in patients with a wide QRS complex tachyar-rhythmia, and why?	Verapamil, because it may cause hypo-tension, ventricular fibrillation, or asystole
What is the treatment for a narrow QRS complex tachyarrhythmia?	Vagal maneuvers (e.g., carotid massage, the Valsalva maneuver), adenosine, a calcium antagonist (e.g., verapamil or diltiazem), and a β-adrenergic antagonist (e.g. esmolol or metoprolol)
What are possible causes of atrial fibrillation?	Ethanol intoxication ("holiday heart"), cardiomyopathy, chronic hypertension, hyperthyroidism, myocardial infarction, pulmonary embolus, and valvular heart disease
Patients with atrial fibril-lation or atrial flutter may present with which symptoms?	Chest pain, hypotension, palpitations, and syncope
What is the initial treatment goal in patients with symp-tomatic atrial fibrillation or atrial flutter?	Rate control
What drugs can be used to treat atrial fibrillation and atrial flutter?	Calcium antagonists (e.g., verapamil, diltiazem), β-adrenergic antagonists (e.g., esmolol, metoprolol), digoxin, procaina-mide, quinidine, ibutilide, propafenone
How do patients with sick sinus syndrome typically present?	With palpitations, syncope, or both

Is it usually possible to diagnose sick sinus syndrome in the ED?	No.
What is the electrocardiographic sign of first-degree atrioventricular (AV) block?	Prolongation of the PR interval
What is second-degree AV block?	Intermittent nonconduction of an atrial impulse
What are the two types of second-degree AV block?	Mobitz type I (Wenckebach) AV block and Mobitz type II AV block
What is the electrocardiographic appearance of a:	
Mobitz type I AV block?	Progressive prolongation of the PR interval until a QRS complex is dropped
Mobitz type II AV block?	Intermittently dropped QRS complexes with no change in the RR interval
Which type of second-degree AV block is a marker for impending AV dissociation?	Mobitz type II AV block
What is third-degree AV block?	Complete AV dissociation
What is the treatment for bradyarrhythmia?	Atropine, glucagon, transcutaneous pacing
Describe how dopamine/ dobutamine drips and epinephrine drips are mixed.	The procedure is the same for both dopamine/dobutamine drips and epinephrine drips. Multiply the patient's weight (in kilograms) by 6 to get the dosage (in milligrams). Add the drug to a crystalloid solution to achieve a total volume of 100 milliliters. Administer at a rate of 1 ml/hr (1 μg/kg/min).
What is the exception to the hierarchy of management described by the ABCs (i.e., airway, breathing, circulation)?	A patient with witnessed arrest in ventricular fibrillation or ventricular tachycardia should be defibrillated immediately.

RESUSCITATION IN CHILDREN

How does the pediatric airway differ from the adult airway?	Overall, the diameter of the airway is smaller, and the subglottic region is the narrowest part of the airway. The larynx is relatively cephalad. The occiput and tongue are larger than in adults.
How should one select an endotracheal tube for children?	If the child is younger than 8 years, use an uncuffed endotracheal tube. Estimate the correct diameter by matching the diameter of the patient's little finger or by using the following formula: (child's age + 16)/4.
Why pretreat with atropine before pediatric intubation?	Pretreatment with atropine can prevent vagal stimulation (which can lead to bradycardia).
How is cardiopulmonary arrest different in children (as opposed to in adults)?	In children, arrests are usually respiratory, whereas in adults, they are primarily cardiac in nature.
Where is the easiest place to detect a pulse in a child younger than 1 year?	The brachial artery
What formula is used to calculate the lower limit of normal for the systolic blood pressure in a child older than 2 years?	$70 + (2 \times$ the child's age)
Why does it take longer for children to become hypotensive (as compared with adults)?	In children, cardiac output is more rate-dependent than volume-dependent.
What is the normal blood volume of a pediatric patient?	80 ml/kg
How many attempts should be made to achieve peripheral intravenous access in a pediatric patient?	Two

If peripheral intravenous access cannot be achieved, what type of access should be attempted next?	Intraosseous access
Where is an intraosseous line placed?	At the anterior medial tibial plateau, 1–3 cm below the tibial tuberosity
Why is it best to use short tubing with a large diameter?	Decreasing resistance allows faster infusion of fluid.
What solution is used for pediatric boluses?	An isotonic solution, such as normal saline or lactated Ringer's solution (20 ml/kg)
What defines adequate urine output in a child?	At least 1–2 ml/kg/hr

RESUSCITATION IN NEONATES

What is the slowest adequate heart rate for a newborn?	100 beats/min
What indicates good respiratory effort for a newborn?	Crying without grunting or nasal flaring
How do you stimulate spontaneous ventilation in a newborn?	By rubbing the infant's back and the soles of her feet
What is the minimum resuscitation effort that must be made for every newborn?	Warm and dry the infant, and consider suctioning of the oral and nasal secretions.
Where do you palpate the pulse of a newborn?	At the inferior portion of the umbilical stump or at the brachial artery
What causes newborn bradycardia?	Respiratory insufficiency
How can intravenous access be achieved in a newborn?	Through the umbilical vein
How many vessels does the umbilical cord contain?	Three—two arteries and one vein

What is most crucial to administer during newborn resuscitation?	Oxygen
What else may be needed?	Epinephrine, naloxone, fluid bolus
What is the treatment for meconium aspiration syndrome in newborns (evidenced by meconium staining of the amniotic fluid)?	Suctioning of the meconium from the infant's mouth and nasopharynx following delivery of the infant's head, but before delivery of the body (i.e., at the perineum)

3 ____ Cardiovascular Emergencies

ACUTE CORONARY SYNDROMES

What are the acute coronary syndromes?

1. Myocardial infarction
2. Unstable angina pectoris
3. Variant (Prinzmetal's) angina

What is the fundamental pathophysiologic problem in acute coronary syndromes?

An oxygen supply/demand mismatch—Infarction occurs when the mismatch is severe enough to cause the death of cardiac myocytes.

What factors determine myocardial oxygen demand?

The preload, the afterload, the heart rate, and the heart contractility

What factors can increase myocardial oxygen demand?

The myocardial demand for oxygen is increased by exertion, inotropic substances (e.g., cocaine, catecholamines), tachycardia, and cardiac hypertrophy.

What factors determine cardiac oxygen supply?

The perfusion and oxygen-carrying capacity of the blood

At which point in the cardiac cycle does cardiac perfusion occur?

During diastole

What factors influence cardiac blood flow?

The aortic diastolic blood pressure, the duration of diastole, and the coronary artery vascular resistance

What are the risk factors for coronary artery disease?

1. Age
2. Male gender
3. Family history of coronary artery disease
4. Smoking
5. Diabetes mellitus
6. Hypertension
7. Hyperlipidemia

Describe the Canadian Cardiovascular Society (CCS) classification scheme for angina pectoris.

Class I: No angina with normal physical activity; strenuous or prolonged exertion may produce angina
Class II: Angina slightly limits normal physical activity
Class III: Angina markedly limits normal physical activity
Class IV: Any physical activity results in angina; angina may be present at rest

What is stable angina?

Stable angina is chest pain that occurs after a predictable amount of exertion, lasts 5–15 minutes, and is relieved by rest.

What causes stable angina?

A fixed obstruction of the coronary arteries by a stable atheromatous plaque

What is unstable angina?

Cardiac pain of new onset; cardiac pain that occurs at rest; or cardiac pain that is more severe, of longer duration, or unrelieved by the usual dose of nitroglycerin

What is the cause of unstable angina?

The cause is the same as that of acute myocardial infarction—thrombus formation and acute narrowing of an epicardial coronary artery's lumen, inflammatory intimal swelling, or hemorrhage into an atheromatous plaque

What is variant (Prinzmetal's) angina?

Chest pain resulting from spasm of an epicardial coronary artery

What are the clinical features of Prinzmetal's angina?

The pain usually occurs at rest, and often in the morning. Electrocardiographically, ST segment elevation is seen during the spasm episode.

What percentage of patients with Prinzmetal's angina have occluded coronary arteries?

Approximately 66%; the remaining third have clean coronary arteries

What is the incidence of myocardial infarction?

In the United States, two million people per year experience myocardial infarction. One third of these infarctions are fatal, and 50% of the fatalities occur outside the hospital.

How many acute myocardial infarctions went clinically unrecognized in the Framingham Study?	25%
Can patients with occluded coronary arteries survive?	Yes. Slow occlusion induces sufficient collateral circulation.
Can patients with minimal coronary artery disease have fatal heart attacks?	Yes. Even hemodynamically insignificant plaques may rupture. In some patients, the first sign of heart disease may be a massive infarction.
What coronary artery is affected in most cases of myocardial infarction?	The right coronary artery (80% of cases); in the remaining cases, the left circumflex artery is usually involved
What are the two general types of complications in myocardial infarction?	Electrical disturbances (i.e., arrhythmias) and heart failure
What is the Killip-Kimball classification system?	A means of correlating the degree of heart failure as a result of myocardial infarction with mortality
Describe the Killip-Kimball classification scheme.	**Class I:** No heart failure **Class II:** Mild heart failure **Class III:** Frank pulmonary edema **Class IV:** Cardiogenic shock
What is the approximate mortality rate associated with each class?	**Class I:** 5% **Class II:** 20% **Class III:** 35% **Class IV:** 80%

DIAGNOSIS

What are the symptoms of acute coronary syndromes?	Typically, patients complain of a sensation of substernal or left-sided chest pressure or pain that radiates to the left or right arm, the throat, the neck, the jaw, the teeth, or the abdomen (but not below the umbilicus). The pain may be non-radiating.
What are typical associated symptoms?	Nausea, vomiting, malaise, profuse sweating, shortness of breath, dizziness, syncope, and indigestion

What are the signs of heart failure?

Rales, neck vein distention, a third heart sound (S_3), peripheral edema, a new or changing murmur

What tests are indicated in the work-up of a patient with a suspected acute coronary syndrome?

1. Electrocardiogram (EKG)
2. Serum troponin levels, creatinine phosphokinase MB isoenzyme levels, or both
3. Serum chemistry panel
4. Complete blood count (CBC)
5. Stool guaiac (prior to heparinization or thrombolysis)
6. Urinalysis
7. Blood type and screen (in case thrombolytic therapy may be indicated)

For how long should serial creatinine phosphokinase MB isoenzyme levels be monitored to rule out infarction?

For at least 8–12 hours after the onset of pain

What condition may also cause elevated serum creatinine phosphokinase levels?

Renal failure

Which marker stays elevated for a longer period after myocardial infarction occurs?

Troponin

What percentage of patients with an acute myocardial infarction have a normal EKG on initial presentation?

3%–7%

How many patients with acute myocardial infarction have diagnostic changes on their first EKG in the emergency department (ED)?

Only 50%; therefore, serial EKGs are essential

What part of the heart is not well represented by the EKG?

The posterior wall of the left ventricle (usually fed by the circumflex artery) and the right ventricle

How can these areas be
better studied using electrocardiography?

Add posterior precordial leads (V_8 and
V_9) and right precordial leads (V_2R
through V_4R) to a standard 12-lead EKG
to increase the study's sensitivity for
ischemia in these areas.

**Describe how the EKG
leads correlate with the
myocardial anatomy:**

Left ventricular antero-
lateral wall?

Leads V_1 through V_6, I, and aVL

Left ventricular lateral
wall?

Leads V_5, V_6, I, and aVL

Left ventricular antero-
septal wall?

Leads V_1 through V_4

Left ventricular inferior
wall?

Leads II, III, and aVF

Left ventricular posterior
wall?

Leads V_8, V_9, and reciprocal changes in
V_1 through V_3 (all R-wave with ST
depression)

Right ventricle?

Leads V_2R through V_6R

**Describe how the EKG
leads correlate with the
vascular anatomy:**

Left anterior descending
artery?

Leads V_1 through V_6 (proximal); leads V_1
through V_4 (distal)

right coronary artery?

Leads II, III, and aVF

Left circumflex artery?

Leads II, III, and aVF, especially when a
large R wave is seen in lead V_1 Note, the
correlation between EKG leads and
vascular anatomy is less predictable than
that between EKG leads and myocardial
anatomy.

What aspects of an EKG
always require attention?

1. The patient's name
2. The date and the time that the EKG
   was obtained

3. The machine settings (i.e., the speed and amplitude)
4. The heart rhythm
5. The heart rate
6. The axis
7. The intervals (i.e., PR, QRS, and QT)
8. The waves (i.e., P, Q, U, R)
9. The ST segment
10. The QRS amplitude
11. Ectopy

What do Q waves suggest?

An old infarct or a late-stage acute transmural infarct

What is a non–Q wave myocardial infarction?

A myocardial infarction that is diagnosed by finding serum concentrations of myocardial enzymes (released when the myocytes undergo necrosis), as opposed to finding diagnostic changes on an EKG

In a patient with acute chest pain, what is the significance of:

ST segment elevation?

Myocardial infarction

ST segment depression?

If the EKG abnormality resolves with therapy (e.g., oxygen, nitroglycerin), then the patient has ischemia (i.e., angina). If the defect is not reversible, it may be a sign of infarction. ST segment depression may represent ischemia distant from the leads (reciprocal change), or it may suggest ischemia in an electrically silent area of the heart.

Give an example of ST segment depression as a result of ischemia that is not represented by standard EKG leads.

Anterior ST segment depression as a result of posterior ischemia

What is reciprocal change?

ST segment depression in leads opposite those with ST segment elevation

What is pseudonormalization?

Chronically inverted T waves flatten or became upright, implying cardiac ischemia

When can the computer interpretation of an EKG be trusted?	Never.

THERAPY

List the indications for admission to a cardiac care unit.	1. Acute myocardial infarction after thrombolytic therapy 2. Unstable angina pectoris accompanied by worrisome EKG changes 3. Hemodynamic instability (including unstable hypertension) 4. Unstable arrhythmias or ongoing chest pain
What are the physiologic goals of therapy when treating a patient with an acute coronary syndrome?	Increase oxygen delivery, decrease myocardial oxygen demand, and prevent or reverse thrombus formation
What treatments have been shown to reduce mortality in patients with acute myocardial infarction?	1. Thrombolytic agents [e.g., tissue plasminogen activator (t-PA), streptokinase] 2. Aspirin 3. Supplemental oxygen 4. Nitroglycerin 5. β blockers (e.g., esmolol, metoprolol) 6. Heparin (intravenous heparin with t-PA, subcutaneous heparin with streptokinase) 7. Angiotensin-converting enzyme (ACE) inhibitors (subacutely) 8. Magnesium (in patients with hypomagnesemia)
What is the goal of endotracheal intubation in the setting of myocardial infarction?	Endotracheal intubation decreases the work of breathing, which decreases myocardial oxygen demand. It decreases pulmonary edema and increases oxygenation.

Increasing oxygen delivery

Name three methods of increasing oxygen delivery.	1. Supplemental oxygen 2. Nitroglycerin 3. Red blood cells (RBCs)
What is the minimum hematocrit in patients with an acute coronary syndrome?	30% or more, to optimize the blood's oxygen-carrying capacity

Decreasing myocardial oxygen demand

Name three methods of decreasing myocardial oxygen demand.	1. β blockers 2. ACE inhibitors 3. Morphine
Does the use of β blockers have a proven positive effect on the mortality rate?	Yes; they reduce the mortality rate when administered acutely after infarction.
When should β blockers be withheld?	Absolute contraindications include hypotension, bradycardia, pulmonary vascular congestion, severe chronic obstructive pulmonary disease (COPD), and heart block. Asthma and diabetes are relative contraindications.

Preventing or reversing thrombus formation

Name four methods of preventing or reversing thrombus formation.	1. Aspirin 2. Heparin 3. Thrombolytic agents 4. Platelet glycoprotein IIb/IIIa receptor inhibitors
Why is aspirin an essential therapy for any patient with an acute coronary syndrome?	It reduces the mortality rate in patients with acute myocardial infarction by 24%. The effect is additive when aspirin is combined with a thrombolytic agent.
What agent should be administered to patients with an acute coronary syndrome who are allergic to aspirin?	Ticlopidine

Thrombolytic therapy

What is a "red" clot?	A thrombus composed mainly of RBCs trapped in a mesh of insoluble fibrin
How do thrombolytic agents work?	They convert endogenous plasminogen to plasmin, a protease that hydrolyzes fibrin into small pieces that are subsequently eaten by macrophages.
What are the indications for thrombolytic therapy?	1. Acute myocardial infarction within the past 12 hours 2. EKG findings that suggest candidacy for thrombolytic therapy

In the presence of chest pain and a diagnosis of myocardial infarction, what EKG findings suggest candidacy for thrombolytic therapy?

1. New left bundle branch block
2. ST segment elevation of 1 millimeter in two or more contiguous pericardial leads
3. ST segment elevation of 2 millimeters in two or more contiguous limb leads

What are the absolute contraindications to thrombolytic therapy?

1. Internal bleeding
2. Aortic dissection
3. Central nervous system (CNS) arteriovenous malformation (AVM) or tumor
4. History of intracranial hemorrhage
5. Status less than 2 months post CNS surgery or less than 2 weeks post major surgery
6. Blood pressure greater than 200/120 mm Hg
7. Allergy to the agent
8. Pregnancy
9. Hemophilia
10. Recent head trauma
11. Cardiogenic shock [when percutaneous transluminal coronary angioplasty (PTCA) is available within 60 minutes]

What are the relative contraindications to thrombolytic therapy?

1. History of nonhemorrhagic cerebrovascular accident
2. Warfarin, ticlopidine, or enoxaparin therapy
3. Status greater than 2 weeks but less than 2 months post non-CNS surgery
4. History of chronic uncontrolled hypertension
5. Subclavicular or internal jugular intravenous lines

How are bleeding complications as a result of thrombolytic therapy treated?

1. Immediately discontinue administration of the thrombolytic agent, aspirin, and heparin (administer protamine if the heparin was started within the past 4 hours)
2. Obtain a blood type and cross-match, and evaluate the platelet count, the prothrombin time (PT) and partial thromboplastin time (PTT), and the fibrinogen levels.

3. Initiate volume replacement with a crystalloid solution.
4. Apply prolonged direct pressure if the bleeding is superficial.

What measures should be taken if the patient is hemodynamically unstable?

Administer 10 units of cryoprecipitate and then recheck the fibrinogen level. If the fibrinogen level is less than 1 g/L, administer another 10 units of cryoprecipitate. If it is greater than 1 g/L but the patient is bleeding, administer 2 units of fresh frozen plasma along with aminocaproic acid. If the bleeding time is longer than 9 minutes, administer 10 units of platelets.

What measures should be taken in the event that the patient develops an intracranial hemorrhage as a result of thrombolytic therapy?

Stop therapy with all anticoagulant agents and administer 10 units of cryoprecipitate, 2 units of fresh frozen plasma, 10 units of platelets, and aminocaproic acid. Obtain an urgent neurosurgical consultation.

When is PTCA superior to thrombolytic therapy?

When it can be performed within 1 hour of presentation

What are the indications for PTCA?

1. Acute myocardial infarction in a patient with contraindications to thrombolysis
2. Equivocal EKG changes in a patient when the clinical suspicion of infarction is high
3. Cardiogenic shock
4. Persistent chest pain, ST segment elevation, or both following thrombolytic therapy in a patient with acute myocardial infarction (this is called "rescue PTCA").

Patients with which type of infarct may benefit the most from rescue PTCA?

A large anterior infarct

Platelet glycoprotein IIb/IIIa receptor inhibitor therapy

What is a "white" clot?

A thrombus composed mainly of platelets linked by fibrinogen

How do platelet glycoprotein IIb/IIIa receptor inhibitors work?

They block the attachment of fibrinogen to platelets, decreasing platelet aggregation

Under what circumstances should the use of a platelet glycoprotein IIb/IIIa receptor inhibitor be considered?

1. In a patient with unstable angina and continuing pain despite maximal antianginal therapy
2. In a patient with a myocardial infarction who is not a candidate for thrombolytic therapy
3. When urgent or emergent inter-ventional angiography is anticipated

What are the contraindica-tions to the use of a platelet glycoprotein IIb/IIIa receptor inhibitor?

1. Bleeding diathesis
2. Major surgery within the previous 6 weeks
3. Gastrointestinal bleeding within the previous 30 days
4. A history of intracranial hemorrhage
5. Nonhemorrhagic stroke within the previous 30 days
6. Uncontrolled hypertension
7. A PT greater than 1.2 times control
8. A hematocrit less than 30%
9. A platelet count less than 100,000 cells/μl^3
10. Pregnancy
11. Hemodialysis
12. Allergy to the platelet glycoprotein IIb/IIIa receptor inhibitor

Treating complications

When should lidocaine use be considered in the setting of an acute myocardial infarction?

In the presence of frequent premature ventricular contractions (PVCs), ventricular fibrillation, or ventricular tachycardia (three or more beats of wide complex tachycardia)

What are the indications for temporary pacing in the setting of an infarction?

Indications for temporary pacing in the setting of a myocardial infarction include symptomatic sinus bradycardia, second-degree heart block (Mobitz type II), third-degree heart block, right bundle branch block with left ventricular block, left bundle branch block with first-degree heart block, alternating bundle branch block, and asystole.

Name two possible indica-tions for overdrive pacing in the setting of a myocar-dial infarction.

Torsades de pointes and atrial flutter

What is cardiogenic shock? Left ventricular failure causing pulmonary edema and systemic hypotension

Does thrombolytic therapy improve the mortality rate in patients who develop cardiogenic shock as a result of myocardial infarction? No. These patients require emergent revascularization procedures, such as PTCA or intra-aortic balloon counterpulsation.

How is cardiogenic shock treated? With emergent intubation, the administration of fluids and dopamine, and emergent PTCA or intra-aortic balloon counterpulsation

If emergent revascularization cannot be performed, what treatment should be offered to patients with cardiogenic shock? Thrombolytic therapy

What is the initial treatment for hypotension without pulmonary edema? The administration of fluids, followed by dopamine

What is the treatment for pulmonary edema without hypotension? Nitrates, diuretics, oxygen, morphine, and dobutamine

CONGESTIVE HEART FAILURE (CHF)

What are the causes of CHF?
1. Cardiac ischemia
2. Valvular disease
3. Cardiotoxicity (e.g., that caused by alcohol or cocaine)
4. Thyroid disorders
5. Cardiac tamponade
6. Constrictive pericarditis
7. Severe hypertension
8. Severe anemia
9. Myocarditis

What is the most common cause of CHF? Hypertensive cardiomyopathy combined with myocardial ischemia or infarction

Describe three ways of categorizing CHF.
1. Systolic versus diastolic
2. Left ventricular versus right ventricular
3. High-output

What is systolic heart failure?	Systolic heart failure results when the heart's ability to contract is compromised. It is characterized by a decreased ejection fraction.
What is diastolic heart failure?	Diastolic heart failure results when the heart's ability to relax is compromised, which means that adequate filling during diastole cannot take place. It is character-ized by a normal or increased ejection fraction.
What is high-output cardiac failure?	In high-output cardiac failure, the cardiac output may be several times higher than normal but is still not adequate to ade-quately perfuse the tissues.
Name four causes of high-output cardiac failure.	1. Anemia 2. Thyrotoxicosis 3. Pregnancy 4. Atrioventricular shunting

DIAGNOSIS

What are the symptoms of:

Left ventricular CHF?	Dyspnea on exertion, paroxysmal nocturnal dyspnea (PND), orthopnea, decreased urine output during the day and increased urine output at night (i.e., nocturia)
Right ventricular CHF?	Lower extremity edema

What are the signs of:

Left ventricular heart failure?	Diaphoresis and cool, clammy skin Tachycardia, an S_3, and rales and wheezes Tachypnea and Cheyne-Strokes respirations Pulsus alternans
Right ventricular heart failure?	Jugular venous distention, lower extremity edema, hepatosplenomegaly, and hepatojugular reflex
What findings may be noted on a chest radiograph in patients with CHF?	Cardiomegaly, pulmonary venous congestion, plural effusions, Kerley B lines, and cephalization

What are the EKG findings in:

    Chronic CHF?   Atrial enlargement and left ventricular hypertrophy

    Acute CHF?   Ischemia or infarction

TREATMENT

How is CHF treated in the ambulatory setting?

In the ambulatory setting, treatment regimens for CHF focus on reducing the preload and afterload and improving contractility; patients usually take furosemide, digoxin, and an ACE inhibitor.

In the ED, what are the mainstays of therapy for CHF?

Oxygen, nitroglycerin, furosemide, morphine, and continuous positive airway pressure (CPAP)

In the setting of CHF, what is an indication for:

    Dobutamine?

CHF without hypotension (dobutamine produces a mild increase in myocardial oxygen demand with increased contractility)

    Dopamine?

CHF with hypotension

When should patients who present to the emergency department (ED) with CHF be admitted to the hospital?

Whenever the CHF is newly diagnosed

HYPERTENSIVE EMERGENCY

What is the definition of hypertension?

Hypertension is arbitrarily defined as a sustained blood pressure of greater than 140/90 mm Hg.

What are the causes of hypertension?

In 90% of cases, the hypertension is idiopathic (essential hypertension). The remainder of cases are secondary to some other process.

What processes can lead to secondary hypertension?

1. Renovascular or renoparenchymal disease

2. Aldosteronism
3. Glucocorticoid excess (e.g., Cushing's disease)
4. Catecholamine excess (e.g., pheochromocytoma)
5. Hyperparathyroidism
6. Pregnancy
7. Coarctation of the aorta
8. Drugs [e.g., nonsteroidal anti-inflammatory drugs (NSAIDs), steroids, sympathomimetics, cocaine]

What can cause increased sensitivity to catecholamines, precipitating a hypertensive emergency in a hypertensive patient?

Withdrawal from antihypertensive agents (especially calcium channel blockers and β blockers) and clonidine

What drugs cause increased adrenergic stimulation?

Monoamine oxidase inhibitors (MAOIs), tricyclic antidepressants (TCAs), amphetamines, cocaine

How is essential hypertension treated on an outpatient basis?

With diuretics, β blockers, ACE inhibitors, calcium channel blockers, α-adrenergic antagonists, and nitrates (either alone or in combination)

What is a hypertensive emergency?

New or acutely progressive end-organ injury (i.e., injury to the brain, heart, or kidneys) in the presence of severe hypertension

What signs and symptoms suggest a CNS hypertensive emergency?

Nausea or vomiting, seizures, headache, coma, altered mental status, Cushing's response [i.e., bradycardia and hypertension as a result of increased intracranial pressure (ICP)]

What is the pathophysiology of hypertensive encephalopathy?

Hypertensive encephalopathy occurs when the increased mean arterial blood pressure overwhelms the brain's autoregulatory mechanism, leading to dilatation of the arterioles, an increased capillary pressure, the leakage of fluid into the perivascular space, and cerebral edema.

How do patients with hypertensive encephalopathy present?

With headache, altered mental status, nausea or vomiting, coma, seizures, papilledema, fundal exudates, and renal hemorrhage

What signs and symptoms suggest a cardiovascular hypertensive emergency?

Chest pain or dyspnea in the face of acute hypertension with or without neurologic changes

What constitutes evidence of a renal hypertensive emergency?

Increased blood pressure with laboratory findings suggestive of acute renal failure [i.e., elevated blood urea nitrogen (BUN) and creatinine levels, proteinuria, microscopic hematuria]

What laboratory and imaging studies are indicated for patients with suspected hypertensive emergency?

1. Urinalysis
2. BUN and creatinine levels
3. Serum electrolyte panel
4. CBC
5. An EKG and possibly a head computed tomography (CT) scan

What is the goal in the treatment of hypertensive emergencies?

To effect a gradual decline in the blood pressure to "normal" levels within 1 hour of presentation, with improvement of signs and symptoms related to hypertension

What is the treatment for hypertensive encephalopathy?

Sodium nitroprusside drip or labetalol boluses

What is the pharmacology of labetalol?

Labetalol is a β_1, β_2, and α_1 receptor antagonist that decreases the blood pressure, heart rate, and myocardial oxygen demand concomitantly.

How is hypertension in patients with aortic dissection treated?

With labetalol

PULMONARY EMBOLISM

What are the risk factors for pulmonary embolism?

1. Advanced age
2. Smoking
3. Oral contraceptive use
4. Immobilization
5. Deep venous thrombosis (DVT)

6. Lower extremity injury
7. Surgery
8. Pregnancy

When is the diagnosis of pulmonary embolus made in most patients?

After they have already died

DIAGNOSIS

What are the typical symptoms of pulmonary embolus?

Chest pain of sudden onset (often pleuritic), dyspnea, cough, syncope, hemoptysis, anxiety, and diaphoresis

What are the signs?

Tachypnea, tachycardia, hypotension, low-grade fever, distended neck veins, focal lung findings on auscultation, thrombophlebitis, and lower extremity edema

What are the most common EKG findings in patients with pulmonary embolus?

The EKG may be normal, or the following may be seen:
Tachycardia
A large S wave in lead I, a large Q wave in lead III, and an inverted T wave in lead III ($S_1Q_3T_3$)
ST changes
Inverted T waves
Right-axis deviation or strain

Can a patient with pulmonary embolus have a normal chest radiograph?

Yes.

Does a normal chest radiograph in a patient with acute dyspnea increase suspicion for a pulmonary embolus?

Yes.

List five abnormal chest radiograph findings that may be seen in a patient with pulmonary embolus.

1. Elevated hemidiaphragm
2. Atelectasis
3. Wedge-shaped infiltrates
4. Westermark's sign
5. Hampton's hump

What is Westermark's sign?

Sudden cut-off of dilated pulmonary vessels

What is Hampton's hump?   A pleural-based, wedge-shaped or rounded density pointing to the hilum, demonstrating an area of infarction

What is the gold-standard study for diagnosing pulmonary embolism?   Pulmonary angiography

What other studies are helpful in diagnosing pulmonary embolism?   Pulmonary function testing, arterial blood gases (ABGs), ventilation–perfusion ($\dot{V}/\dot{Q}$) scanning, computed tomography, and studies used to diagnose DVT (i.e., lower extremity ultrasound, venography)

What is a common finding on ABG testing?   A widened alveolar-arterial (A–a) gradient

How is an A–a gradient calculated?

$$\text{A–a gradient} = \text{FIO}_2 \times (\text{barometric pressure} - 47) - \frac{5\,(\text{PaCO}_2)}{4} - \text{PaO}_2$$

How is this equation simplified when it can be assumed that the patient is breathing room air at sea level?

$$\text{A–a gradient} = 150 - \frac{5\,(\text{PaCO}_2)}{4} - \text{PaO}_2$$

In a patient with a suspected pulmonary embolus and no evidence of DVT, what should be done?   A $\dot{V}/\dot{Q}$ lung scan

Is $\dot{V}/\dot{Q}$ lung scanning contraindicated in pregnant women?   No.

How is a $\dot{V}/\dot{Q}$ lung scan useful in diagnosing pulmonary embolus?   It allows identification of areas of $\dot{V}/\dot{Q}$ mismatch

What disorders can cause abnormal results on perfusion scanning?   Pneumonia, COPD, lung tumor, CHF

What information is obtained from the ventilation portion of the study?   Pulmonary embolus is suggested if no other obvious causes for the mismatch between ventilation and perfusion can be identified.

What study should be performed if the V̇/Q̇ lung scan is indeterminate?	Pulmonary angiography

TREATMENT

How is pulmonary embolus managed in the ED?	Anticoagulation therapy is initiated, typically with intravenous heparin. Supportive care entails maintenance of the ABCs, including the administration of fluids and dopamine to counteract hypotension.
What other therapy can be considered in patients who do not respond to anti-coagulation therapy and supportive care?	Thrombolytic therapy

VALVULAR HEART DISEASE

MITRAL VALVE DISORDERS

What is the most common cause of mitral stenosis?	Rheumatic heart disease
What are the symptoms of mitral stenosis?	Left-sided heart failure and pulmonary hypertension lead to dyspnea, orthopnea, and hemoptysis.
What are the cardiac findings in patients with mitral stenosis?	1. A loud first heart sound (S_1) 2. An opening snap in early diastole followed by a low-pitched, rumbling diastolic murmur at the apex that is increased by exertion 3. Atrial fibrillation
What are the most common causes of mitral insufficiency (regurgitation)?	Rheumatic heart disease, infective endocarditis, and myocardial ischemia
What are the signs and symptoms of:	
Acute mitral insufficiency?	Dyspnea, pulmonary edema, tachycardia, and an apical harsh systolic murmur
Chronic mitral insufficiency?	Atrial fibrillation and exertional dyspnea

AORTIC VALVE DISORDERS

What is the most common form of congenital heart disease?	Bicuspid aortic valve
What are the two most common causes of aortic stenosis?	Bicuspid aortic valve and rheumatic heart disease
What are the symptoms of aortic stenosis?	Dyspnea, syncope, and angina
Describe the murmur of aortic stenosis.	A harsh systolic ejection murmur
What blood pressure abnormality is found in patients with aortic stenosis?	A narrowed pulse pressure
Why does exertional syncope occur in patients with aortic stenosis?	Peripheral vasodilation decreases the mean arterial pressure.
What complication may occur with afterload reduction?	Hypotension
What are the causes of aortic insufficiency (regurgitation)?	**Acute:** Endocarditis and aortic dissection **Chronic:** Rheumatic heart disease, syphilis, and ankylosing spondylitis
What conditions are associated with:	
Acute aortic insufficiency?	Dyspnea and acute pulmonary edema
Chronic aortic insufficiency?	Uncomfortable feeling accompanied by tachycardia or palpitations, especially noticeable when the patient is supine Chest pain Dyspnea on exertion and PND (late findings suggestive of left ventricular failure)
Describe the murmur of aortic insufficiency.	A high-pitched blowing, decrescendo, diastolic murmur

What other physical examination findings are seen in patients with aortic insufficiency?

Water-hammer pulses, Quincke's sign, Duroziez's murmur, diminished S_1

What is Quincke's sign?

Alternate blanching and perfusion of the nail bed, elicited by pressing on the end of the nail

What is Duroziez's murmur?

A to-and-fro murmur heard over the femoral artery

Does afterload reduction improve the symptoms of acute aortic insufficiency?

Yes.

TRICUSPID VALVE DISORDERS

What is the cause of tricuspid stenosis?

Rheumatic heart disease

What physical examination findings are noted in patients with tricuspid stenosis?

Hepatosplenomegaly, jugular venous distention, and a diastolic murmur along the left sternal border that increases with inspiration

What are the causes of vcuspid insufficiency (regurgitation)?

Rheumatic heart disease, endocarditis, and pulmonary hypertension

What physical examination findings are noted in patients with tricuspid insufficiency?

Hepatomegaly, hepatojugular reflux, peripheral edema, jugular venous distention, and a holosystolic murmur along the left sternal border

ENDOCARDITIS

What are risk factors for endocarditis?

1. Rheumatic heart disease
2. Intravenous drug use
3. Congenital heart disease
4. Prosthetic heart valve
5. History of endocarditis

What are the most common causes of:

    Left-sided infective endocarditis?

Staphylococcus aureus, Streptococcus viridians, Enterococcus species, and fungi

Right-sided infective endocarditis?	*S. aureus, Streptococcus pneumoniae,* Gram-negative organisms, and fungi
What physical examination finding is present in most patients with infective endocarditis?	Most, but not all, patients with infective endocarditis have a murmur.
What are the symptoms of subacute infective endo-carditis?	The patient may complain of night sweats, fever, anorexia, arthralgia, weakness, and embolic symptoms (e.g., hematuria, neurologic changes, hemoptysis, melena).
What physical examination findings are typical of sub-acute infective endocarditis?	The patient appears chronically ill. Fever, tachycardia, petechiae, splinter hemor-rhages (in the nail bed), and Osler's nodes may be found on examination.
Describe the clinical pre-sentation of acute infective endocarditis.	The classic presentation is fever, chills, petechiae, Roth's spots (retinal hemor-rhages), and Janeway lesions (erythe-matous lesions on the palms or soles) in a patient who has recently had a suppura-tive infection.
Describe the symptoms of right-sided infective endo-carditis.	Patients complain of a high fever of several weeks' duration, pleuritic chest pain, hemoptysis, dyspnea on exertion, and malaise.
What chest x-ray finding is typical in patients with right-sided infective endo-carditis?	A peripheral wedge-shaped pulmonary infiltrate with cavitation
How many sets of blood cultures should be obtained if infective endocarditis is suspected?	Three or more
Do patients with suspected infective endocarditis require hospital admission?	Yes.

MYOCARDIAL DISEASES

MYOCARDITIS

What is myocarditis?	Inflammation of the heart muscle
What are common viral causes of myocarditis?	Coxsackie B virus, HIV, influenza virus, Epstein-Barr virus, and adenovirus
What are common bacterial causes of myocarditis?	*Borrelia burgdorferi* (i.e., the organism responsible for Lyme disease), *Streptococcus* species, and *Mycoplasma* species
What are the clinical findings in patients with myocarditis?	Cardiac failure, fever, myalgia, substernal chest pain, and a pericardial friction rub
What EKG changes may be seen in a patient with myocarditis?	Tachycardia, prolongation of the QT interval, nonspecific ST and T wave changes, ST segment elevation, or atrioventricular (AV) block
What conduction abnormality is seen in patients with myocarditis as a result of Lyme disease?	AV block
What is the main differential diagnosis for myocarditis?	Myocardial infarction or ischemia; the pain of myocarditis is easily confused with ischemic chest pain.
Are cardiac enzyme levels elevated in patients with myocarditis?	They may be.
What complications can lead to death in patients with myocarditis?	Heart failure, tachyarrhythmias, and heart block

CARDIOMYOPATHY

What are the three types of cardiomyopathies?	Dilated, hypertrophic, and restrictive

Dilated cardiomyopathy

List six causes of dilated cardiomyopathy.	1. Viral infections, including HIV 2. Myocarditis

3. Postpartum status
4. Amyloidosis and sarcoidosis
5. Myocardial ischemia

What are the symptoms of dilated cardiomyopathy?

Patients usually have CHF and dyspnea on exertion. Mural thrombi can cause embolic symptoms.

What murmurs may be detected in a patient with dilated cardiomyopathy?

The holosystolic murmur of mitral or tricuspid regurgitation, or a diastolic rumble

Hypertrophic cardiomyopathy

What are the presenting symptoms of hypertrophic cardiomyopathy?

Chest pain, dyspnea, angina, exertion-related sudden death or syncope

What are the cardiac findings in patients with hypertrophic cardiomyopathy?

A fourth heart sound (S_4) and a harsh crescendo–decrescendo mid-systolic murmur that increases when a Valsalva maneuver is performed or when the patient stands up, and lessens when the patient squats or performs an isometric handgrip maneuver

What EKG findings may be found in a patient with hypertrophic cardiomyopathy?

The EKG is usually normal, but left ventricular hypertrophy, left atrial hypertrophy, and inferior and lateral Q waves may be seen in some patients.

Do patients with hypertrophic cardiomyopathy tolerate atrial fibrillation?

No. Effective diastolic filling is necessary to maintain cardiac output.

Restrictive cardiomyopathy

List three causes of restrictive cardiomyopathy.

Amyloidosis, hemachromatosis, and sarcoidosis

What are the signs of restrictive cardiomyopathy?

Tender hepatomegaly, an elevated jugular venous pressure that increases with inspiration, dependent edema, and ascites

PERICARDIAL DISEASE

PERICARDITIS

List seven causes of pericarditis.

1. Uremia
2. Tuberculosis

3. Myocardial infarction
4. Malignancy (primary or metastatic)
5. Collagen vascular disease
6. Radiation (most often, exposure is a result of therapy for Hodgkin's lymphoma)
7. Coxsackie virus infection

What malignancies are most often associated with pericarditis?

Breast and lung tumors

What is the classic description of the chest pain caused by pericarditis?

The pain originates in the center of the chest, and radiates to the back and trapezius ridge. It is pleuritic and is alleviated by sitting upright and leaning forward. It may be constrictive and radiate to both arms.

Is the pain of pericarditis similar to that of ischemia?

Yes.

What other signs and symptoms may be present in a patient with pericarditis?

A pericardial friction rub, tachycardia, fever, an elevated WBC count, and dyspnea

What EKG changes may be seen in a patient with pericarditis?

Diffuse ST segment elevation, followed days later by T wave inversion

What is the creatinine phosphokinase MB isoenzyme level in a patient with pericarditis?

Elevated or normal

What causes an elevated creatinine phosphokinase MB isoenzyme level in patients with pericarditis?

Ischemia or myopericarditis

What complication can occur if the pericarditis is misdiagnosed and anticoagulant therapy is initiated?

Hemorrhagic pericarditis

PERICARDIAL EFFUSION

List four causes of peri-cardial effusion.	1. Viral infection 2. Malignancy 3. Uremia 4. Radiation
What EKG finding may occur with a pericardial effusion?	Electrical alternans (i.e., fluctuating QRS amplitude)

CARDIAC TAMPONADE

What is cardiac tamponade?	Cardiac tamponade can occur following pericardial effusion when the fluid volume in the pericardium compresses the heart, decreasing ventricular filling and leading to decreased cardiac output.
What blood pressure abnormality is associated with tamponade?	Pulsus paradoxus
How is pulsus paradoxus detected?	Measure the patient's arterial systolic pressure during inspiration. A decrease of 10 mm Hg or more (pulsus paradoxus) suggests cardiac tamponade but is not pathognomonic.
What is Beck's triad?	Beck's triad represents the classic physical examination findings in patients with cardiac tamponade: hypotension, muffled heart sounds, and jugular venous distention.
How is cardiac tamponade treated?	With pericardiocentesis
What complications can be associated with pericardiocentesis?	1. Myocardial injury 2. Laceration of a coronary or internal mammary artery 3. Dysrhythmias 4. Pneumothorax or hemothorax 5. Liver laceration 6. Hemopericardium

4

Pulmonary Emergencies

ASTHMA

What is asthma?

A chronic disease of heightened airway responsiveness that leads to obstructive symptoms

Describe the pathophysiology of asthma.

Hypertrophy of the bronchial smooth muscle, mucus plugging of the respiratory epithelium, and inflammation of the airways leads to obstructive symptoms.

Asthma occurs in what percentage of the population?

Asthma occurs in 5% of the population in the United States.

Are hospitalization and deaths owing to asthma decreasing?

No, they are increasing.

Why are age and socio-economic status significant when evaluating the patient with asthma?

Of patients with asthma, 50% develop the disorder before 20 years of age, and 70% before 40 years of age. Asthma occurs more frequently in black men living in cities, and less frequently in white women living in rural areas.

What are the risk factors for early-onset asthma?

1. Atopy
2. Positive skin tests
3. History of neonatal lung disease
4. Genetic predisposition (people with asthma often have a family history of the disease)
5. Respiratory infection, particularly with respiratory syncytial virus (RSV)

Is asthma exacerbated only by allergic disorders?

No. Asthma exacerbations may be caused by either allergic or nonallergic conditions.

What are nonallergic causes of an exacerbation?

Exercise, upper respiratory tract infection, dust, smoke, smog

What are five essential elements of the history for every patient with an asthma exacerbation?

1. The cause of the exacerbation
2. Previous admissions to the intensive care unit (ICU) for treatment of asthma
3. Previous intubations
4. Timing of recent steroid use
5. Frequency of asthma medication use

What aspects of the patient history help to delineate the child at high risk for an asthma exacerbation?

1. Prior intubation or admission to a pediatric intensive care unit (PICU)
2. Multiple hospital admissions
3. Multiple visits to the emergency department (ED) within the previous year

What are the signs and symptoms of an asthma exacerbation?

Tachypnea, nasal flaring, cyanosis, shortness of breath, coughing, altered consciousness, use of accessory muscles, expiratory wheezing, speaking in fragments, and pulsus paradoxus

What is the differential diagnosis of wheezing:

In an adult?

1. Asthma
2. Pneumonia
3. Congestive heart failure (CHF)
4. Chronic obstructive pulmonary disease (COPD)
5. Pulmonary embolus
6. Upper airway obstruction (e.g., foreign body, epiglottitis, tumor)
7. Anaphylaxis

In an infant?

1. Asthma
2. Recurrent colds
3. Foreign body
4. Tracheoesophageal fistula
5. Congenital heart disease
6. Cystic fibrosis
7. Immunodeficiency
8. Vascular ring

How is the severity of an acute asthma exacerbation assessed?

1. Physical examination, including assessment of the patient's vital signs (pulsus paradoxus is ominous)
2. Pulse oximetry
3. Pulmonary function testing [peak expiratory flow rate (PEFR), forced expiratory volume in 1 second (FEV_1)]
4. Arterial blood gases (ABGs)
5. Assessment of the patient's response to treatment

In which patients would ordering a chest radiograph be an appropriate course of action?

1. Patients with fever, a first episode of wheezing, or asthma that is refractory to treatment

2. Asthmatic patients in whom pneumothorax or pneumomediastinum is suspected

What findings may be present on the chest x-ray?

Bronchial wall thickening, hyperexpansion, and shifting atelectasis

What is the medical treatment for an acute exacerbation of asthma?

1. Maintain ABCs.
2. Administer oxygen to maintain an oxygen saturation of more than 91% [more than 95% in pregnant patients and patients with coronary artery disease].
3. Administer inhaled β_2 agonists (e.g., albuterol), systemic steroids, and ipratropium bromide.

Which patients should receive corticosteroids?

Patients with moderate or severe acute exacerbations of asthma should be given corticosteroids to decrease the late-phase inflammatory response.

What measures should be considered if these treatments do not work?

1. Administration of continuous nebulized albuterol or inhaled general anesthetics
2. Administration of anticholinergics, magnesium, or ketamine
3. Intubation for respiratory failure
4. Cardiopulmonary bypass and extracorporeal oxygenation for extreme cases

CHRONIC OBSTRUCTIVE PULMONARY DISEASE (COPD)

What is COPD?	Airflow obstruction owing to chronic bronchitis or emphysema
How prevalent is COPD?	The disease affects 15% of adults in the United States.
What are "pink puffers" and "blue bloaters?"	Patients with emphysema are referred to as "pink puffers," whereas patients with chronic bronchitis are characterized as "blue bloaters."
What symptoms are typically seen in a "pink puffer?"	The "pink puffer" has prominent emphysema and must hyperventilate to adequately oxygenate. Cardiac output is decreased, and lung volumes are increased.
What symptoms are typical of a "blue bloater?"	The "blue bloater" has chronic bronchitis. In this patient, increased mucus production and inflammation cause decreased ventilation and a compensatory increase in cardiac output, followed by pulmonary hypertension.
What studies are included in the emergency department (ED) work-up of a COPD exacerbation?	Pulse oximetry, ABGs, pulmonary function testing (to evaluate the PEFR), chest radiography, electrocardiography, and serum chemistries
What is seen on the chest radiograph of the patient:	
With emphysematic COPD?	Barrel chest, small heart, decreased pulmonary vasculature
With bronchitic COPD?	Enlarged heart, normal lung volumes with prominent pulmonary vasculature, generous soft tissue
What are the typical ABG results in both forms of COPD (i.e., emphysematic and bronchitic COPD)?	Hypoxemia is a typical ABG result. It is eventually followed by hypercapnia and respiratory acidosis.
What life-threatening conditions must be considered in a patient with a presumed COPD exacerbation?	1. Foreign body aspiration 2. Pneumothorax 3. CHF exacerbation 4. Pure asthma

5. Acute myocardial infarction
6. Pulmonary embolus
7. Pneumonia
8. Toxic inhalation

What measures should be taken when treating a patient with a COPD exacerbation?

Maintain ABCs; administer broncho-dilators, anticholinergics, and possibly antibiotics.

Is it dangerous to administer oxygen to someone with hypoxic drive?

No, oxygen should be administered to correct the oxygen saturation to 90%.

What is the best test for determining the severity of COPD?

ABGs. A pH less than 7.3 or an increasing arterial carbon dioxide tension ($PaCO_2$) suggests acute respiratory compromise.

How is the PEFR useful in monitoring the management of COPD?

Sequential PEFR measurements demonstrate improving or worsening airway obstruction.

What complications are possible in patients with COPD?

1. Pneumothorax
2. Adrenal crisis (in patients receiving steroids for chronic disease)
3. Pulmonary embolus

INTERSTITIAL LUNG DISEASE

What is interstitial lung disease?

Inflammation and eventual scarring of the alveolar walls

What causes interstitial lung disease?

1. Inhalation of asbestos and inorganic and organic dusts
2. Sarcoidosis or collagen vascular disorders
3. Adult respiratory distress syndrome
4. Radiation
5. Chemotherapy

What is the most common interstitial lung disease?

Idiopathic pulmonary fibrosis

What are the initial clinical manifestations of interstitial lung disease?

Dyspnea on exertion and a dry cough

What are two common later symptoms of interstitial lung disease?

Weight loss and anorexia

What physical findings are suggestive of interstitial lung disease?	Tachypnea, clubbing, coarse rales, and (in severe disease) cor pulmonale
Should chest radiographs be included in the evaluation of the patient with interstitial lung disease?	Yes. Chest radiographs can be helpful in making the diagnosis.

What is seen on the chest radiograph in a patient with:

Early-stage interstitial lung disease?	A reticular or "ground-glass" appearance
Late-stage interstitial lung disease?	A reticular–nodular pattern or "honeycomb" appearance
How is the diagnosis of interstitial lung disease obtained?	For a definitive diagnosis, the patient should be referred to a pulmonologist for pulmonary function tests and possibly biopsy.
What is the ED treatment for patients with interstitial lung disease?	Administer oxygen as needed; administer bronchodilators and possibly steroids; and obtain a pulmonology consult.

PNEUMONIA

What types of organisms can cause pneumonia?	Bacteria, fungi, and viruses
What are the two major types of bacterial pneumonia?	Community-acquired and hospital-acquired (nosocomial)
What are the two types of community-acquired pneumonia?	Typical and atypical
Which patients are most susceptible to pneumonia?	Children, elderly patients, and immunocompromised patients
How often is pneumonia fatal?	Pneumonia is the sixth leading cause of death in the United States.

Which bacteria are the most common causes of community-acquired pneumonia in:

Otherwise healthy adults?

Streptococcus pneumoniae, Haemophilus influenzae, Mycoplasma pneumoniae, Legionella pneumophila

Debilitated adults (e.g., those with alcoholism)

Klebsiella pneumoniae, Staphylococcus aureus, Moraxella catarrhalis, and anaerobes

Patients with HIV infection?

S. pneumoniae, M. pneumoniae

Infants younger than 2 months?

Group B streptococci

Which organisms cause atypical pneumonias?

M. pneumoniae, Chlamydia pneumoniae, and *M. catarrhalis*

What pathogens are the most common causes of nosocomial pneumonia?

Pseudomonas species, *K. pneumoniae, Escherichia coli, Serratia* species, and *S. pneumoniae*

What fungal infections can cause pneumonia in susceptible patients?

Histoplasmosis, blastomycosis, and coccidioidomycosis

What is the classic presentation of typical (pneumococcal) community-acquired pneumonia?

Pneumococcal pneumonia classically presents with the sudden onset of a single shaking chill (versus multiple rigors), fever, and a productive cough with rust-colored sputum.

What are the presenting symptoms of atypical community-acquired pneumonias?

Patients may present with a flu-like illness characterized by a sore throat and a nonproductive cough or a cough productive of clear or purulent sputum.

Is it easy to distinguish typical community-acquired pneumonia from atypical community-acquired pneumonia using the clinical presentation as a basis for making the distinction?

No, because symptoms frequently overlap.

What physical findings are commonly found in patients with bacterial pneumonias?

Fever, tachypnea, tachycardia, and signs of consolidation (e.g., increased tactile fremitus, whispered pectoriloquy, focal rales)

What is consolidation?

A condition occurring in the patient with pneumonia in which the lung becomes firm as exudate fills the air spaces

Describe tactile fremitus.

An intense vibration can be felt by placing the hand on the chest wall while the patient is speaking.

Describe whispered pectoriloquy.

Whispered words can be heard through the patient's chest wall.

Why are increased tactile fremitus, whispered pectoriloquy, and focal rales noticeable in the patient with consolidation?

Because sound is transmitted more clearly through consolidated areas than through air-filled spaces

Who gets *Pneumocystis carinii* pneumonia (PCP)?

Patients with HIV infection and other immunocompromised patients.

What is the duration of symptoms prior to diagnosis of PCP?

Typically longer than 2 weeks

What tests are helpful in the work-up of a patient with suspected pneumonia?

1. Oxygen saturation
2. CBC
3. Chest x-ray (posteroanterior and lateral views)
4. Sputum Gram stain and culture
5. Blood cultures
6. ABGs (in patients with respiratory failure)

What complications can be associated with pneumonia?

Respiratory failure, sepsis, empyema, and pulmonary abscess

How frequently is bacteremia associated with pneumococcal pneumonia?

Of patients with pneumococcal pneumonia, 30% develop bacteremia.

What are the criteria for hospital admission?

1. Age younger than 6 months or older than 65 years
2. Underlying immunocompromising illness

3. Debilitated condition
4. Hypoxia
5. Multilobar pneumonia
6. Empyema

How is pneumonia treated in the ED?

Administer oxygen and empiric antibiotics.

What is the basis for choosing an antibiotic?

The antibiotic is chosen based on the suspected bacterial cause of pneumonia.

What causes pneumonia and hypoxia immediately after aspiration of gastric contents?

Chemical pneumonitis

What is the potential role for antibiotics in patients with aspiration pneumonia?

As prophylaxis against secondary bacterial infection

What organisms cause lung abscesses?

Anaerobes, Gram-positive and Gram-negative organisms, and parasites

TUBERCULOSIS

What are the two main classifications of tuberculosis?

Primary infection and reactivation

How is tuberculosis spread?

By transmission of aerosolized particles, especially among people who live or work in crowded conditions

Who is at highest risk for tuberculosis?

1. Prison inmates
2. Residents of nursing homes
3. Residents of homeless shelters
4. HIV-infected patients
5. Immigrants from high-prevalence areas
6. Intravenous drug abusers

Are many patients with tuberculosis also infected with HIV?

Yes. HIV testing should be encouraged for all patients with newly diagnosed tuberculosis.

What are the symptoms of primary tuberculosis?

Nonspecific respiratory symptoms, including a cough

What tests are useful in the work-up of a patient with suspected tuberculosis?

1. Chest x-ray
2. Purified protein derivative (PPD) skin test
3. Sputum analysis

What are the two classic chest x-ray findings in a patient with primary tuberculosis?

1. A Ghon complex (i.e., a calcified lung granuloma accompanied by hilar adenopathy)
2. Infiltrates with unilateral adenopathy

What age group is more likely to have adenopathy?

Children

How are the results of PPD skin testing interpreted?

The PPD skin test is considered positive based on the diameter of the induration (swelling) around the injection site. The specific diameter necessary to qualify as a "positive" result depends on the patient's risk factors for tuberculosis and whether or not the patient has an underlying disease (e.g., HIV infection).

In what patients is the PPD test considered positive if the diameter of the indurated area is:

≥ 5 mm?

HIV-positive patients; patients in close contact with a patient with tuberculosis; patients with signs of tuberculosis on chest x-ray

≥ 10 mm?

Patients in high-risk living situations; intravenous drug users

≥ 15 mm?

Anyone

Response to PPD is mediated by what type of immunity?

Cell-mediated immunity

What disease states may cause a false-negative PPD test?

1. Overwhelming tuberculosis
2. Other active infection
3. Lymphoma
4. Sarcoidosis
5. Renal failure

What other factors may cause a false-negative result on a PPD test?	1. Extremes of age (i.e., very young or elderly) 2. Recent surgery 3. Use of corticosteroids
What other test should always be performed with a PPD test?	An anergy panel
What is reactivation tuberculosis?	Reactivation tuberculosis occurs when the immune system can no longer contain the disease.
What are the symptoms of reactivation tuberculosis?	Malaise, weight loss, night sweats, fever, cough

In patients with reactivation tuberculosis:

What percentage have disease at extrapulmonary sites?	15%
What percentage have a positive PPD skin test?	80%
Disseminated tuberculosis is most common in what anatomic locations?	1. The posterior portion of the upper lobe 2. The superior segment of the lower lobe 3. The adrenal glands 4. The epiphyses of the long bones 5. The vertebrae (Pott's disease) 6. The meninges
What characteristic is common to all of the anatomic locations of disseminated tuberculosis?	They all have a relatively high oxygen tension.
What are typical findings on cerebrospinal fluid (CSF) analysis in patients with tuberculous meningitis?	Monocytes, low glucose levels, very high protein levels
What electrolyte abnormalities are seen in patients with tuberculous meningitis?	Because the syndrome of inappropriate secretion of antidiuretic hormone (SIADH) is common, hyponatremia may be present.

What are three classic findings on urinalysis in patients with renal tuberculosis?	Sterile pyuria, hematuria, and albuminuria
What is miliary tuberculosis?	Diffuse disease following the hematogenous spread of *Mycobacterium tuberculosis*
What are the symptoms of miliary tuberculosis?	Fever, cough, anorexia, weight loss, hepatosplenomegaly, lymphadenopathy
What laboratory abnormalities are seen with miliary tuberculosis?	Anemia, thrombocytopenia, neutropenia, thrombocytosis, leukocytosis, hyponatremia
What is scrofula?	Tuberculous lymphadenitis, usually affecting the cervical nodes
Should the masses resulting from tuberculous lymphadenitis be incised and drained?	No, they should not, because sinus formation and prolonged drainage may occur.
What antibiotics typically may be used to treat tuberculosis?	Rifampin, isoniazid, pyrazinamide, and ethambutol, in various combination
What are the possible complications of:	
Rifampin therapy?	Hepatitis, thrombocytopenia
Isoniazid therapy?	Hepatitis, neuritis, central nervous symptoms (CNS) symptoms, metabolic acidosis
Pyrazinamide therapy?	Hepatitis, arthralgias
Ethambutol therapy?	Optic neuritis
What is the disposition of patients with newly diagnosed active disease?	These patients should be admitted, unless outpatient follow-up can be guaranteed.

PNEUMOTHORAX

What is a pneumothorax?	Collapse of a lung with accumulation of air in the pleural space

Name the three types of pneumothoraces.	1. Simple 2. Open 3. Tension
When does a pneumothorax become life threatening?	1. When pulmonary reserve is inadequate 2. When tension pneumothorax develops
Name four causes of pneumothorax.	1. Blunt or penetrating chest trauma 2. Iatrogenic 3. Spontaneous 4. Pulmonary disease (e.g., pneumonia)
What are four iatrogenic causes of pneumothorax?	1. Central venous pressure line placement 2. Mechanical ventilation 3. Thoracentesis 4. Intercostal nerve block
Who is most likely to develop a spontaneous pneumothorax?	Tall men between the ages of 20 and 40 years who smoke
What other patient population is at risk for spontaneous pneumothorax?	Patients with COPD
What are the most common pneumonias associated with pneumothorax?	Pneumonias caused by *S. aureus, M. tuberculosis, P. carinii,* and *K. pneumoniae*
What are the most common symptoms of pneumothorax?	Dyspnea and chest pain
What physical findings suggest pneumothorax?	Tachypnea, decreased breath sounds, obvious trauma, and subcutaneous emphysema
What is the best study to identify a pneumothorax?	Expiratory chest x-ray
What findings on chest x-ray would raise your suspicion for pneumothorax?	Pneumomediastinum and subcutaneous emphysema
What physical findings suggest tension pneumothorax?	Severe respiratory distress, hypotension, tracheal deviation, and jugular venous distention

What is the treatment for tension pneumothorax?

Needle decompression (i.e., needle thoracostomy) followed by chest tube placement

Where is the needle placed for needle thoracostomy of a:

Tension pneumothorax?

In the second intercostal space along the midclavicular line

Traumatic pneumothorax?

In the fifth intercostal space along the anterior axillary line

What is the treatment for a simple pneumothorax in a symptomatic patient?

Chest tube placement

Can a pneumothorax be observed?

Yes. If the patient is asymptomatic, he may be observed.

What can speed the resolution of a pneumothorax that is being observed?

Administration of high-concentration oxygen

5

Gastroenterologic Emergencies

ESOPHAGEAL DISORDERS

What are the esophageal emergencies?

Esophageal hemorrhage and esophageal perforation

What are the categories of blood loss?

Mild blood loss: < 10% of the total blood volume
Moderate blood loss: 10%–20% of the total blood volume
Major blood loss: 20%–40% of the total blood volume
Massive blood loss: > 40% of the total blood volume

What are the usual causes of:

Mild blood loss?

Capillary bleeding or an intermittent arterial bleed

Moderate blood loss?

Laceration of an artery or a nondistended vein in the esophagus

Major and massive blood loss?

A ruptured esophageal varix or an eroded artery (as a result of peptic ulcer disease)

What are the signs and symptoms of esophageal hemorrhage?

Possible signs and symptoms include hematemesis, hematochezia, "coffee ground" emesis, heme-positive stools, melena, and anemia of chronic disease. The signs and symptoms depend on the rate and duration of the bleeding.

What is the differential diagnosis for esophageal hemorrhage?

All other possible sources of upper gastrointestinal tract bleeding must be ruled out—duodenal ulcer, gastric ulcer, acute gastritis, esophagitis, gastric cancer, gastric volvulus, hemobilia, duodenal diverticula, aortoenteric fistula, paraesophageal hiatal hernia, epistaxis, angiodysplasia, and irritation as a result of nasogastric tube placement.

What is the initial management strategy for a patient with acute blood loss?

Placement of two large-bore intravenous lines, coagulation studies [i.e., prothrombin time (PT) and partial thromboplastin time (PTT)], blood type and cross match

What is the treatment for:

Mild blood loss?

Intravenous administration of crystalloid, close follow-up, and possibly elective endoscopy

Moderate blood loss?

Intravenous administration of crystalloid; patient may require packed red blood cells (packed RBCs) and admission for diagnostic evaluation

Major blood loss?

Resuscitation and prompt fiberoptic endoscopy; consider fresh frozen plasma, vitamin K, and a surgery consult

What is the mortality rate associated with an acute, major esophageal bleed?

Approximately 50%

What causes esophageal perforation?

Esophageal trauma

List five causes of esophageal trauma.

1. Ingestion of foreign bodies or caustic substances
2. Penetrating trauma to the neck and thorax
3. Crushing chest wounds (rare)
4. Endoscopy (iatrogenic injury)
5. Boerhaave's syndrome

How is esophageal perforation diagnosed?

History, physical examination, chest radiograph, and esophagram with water-soluble contrast; esophagoscopy if the patient is unconscious

What are the findings on a chest radiograph following esophageal perforation?	Pneumomediastinitis, pneumothorax, pleural effusion, widened mediastinum, and subdiaphragmatic free air
What is the initial treatment for esophageal perforation?	Control of bleeding, broad-spectrum antibiotics, and a prompt surgical consult
What complication can occur as a result of esophageal perforation?	Mediastinitis (owing to the spread of acid and bacteria from the esophagus)
What mortality rate is associated with perforation of the esophagus:	
If surgery is performed within 24 hours?	5%
If surgery is delayed?	75%

ESOPHAGEAL VARICES

What are esophageal varices?	Engorgement of the esophageal venous plexus secondary to increased collateral blood flow from the portal system as a result of portal hypertension
In patients with known varices, how often are varices the source of their upper gastrointestinal tract bleeding?	About 50% of the time
What is necessary if standard treatment fails?	Emergent endoscopic sclerotherapy
List five options that are available if sclerotherapy fails to control the bleeding.	1. A vasopressin drip (with nitroglycerin to avoid myocardial infarction) or somatostatin 2. Repeat sclerotherapy 3. Gel foam embolization of the left gastric vein 4. Balloon tamponade of the bleeding vessels via a Sengstaken-Blakemore tube 5. Transjugular intrahepatic portacaval shunt (TIPS)

FOREIGN BODY INGESTION

Approximately how many people die each year as a result of foreign body ingestion?	1500
In what demographic groups is foreign body ingestion seen most often?	Children (80% of cases), edentulous adults, prisoners, and psychiatric patients

What objects tend to be ingested by:

Children?	Coins and small toys
Edentulous adults?	Bones and small pieces of meat
Prisoners and psychiatric patients?	Unusual items (e.g., razor blades, spoons)

Where do the objects tend to get caught in:

Children?	1. Proximal esophagus (specifically, at the cricopharyngeal narrowing at C6) 2. Thoracic inlet 3. Aortic arch 4. Tracheal bifurcation 5. Hiatal narrowing
Adults?	Distal esophagus (owing to underlying esophageal disease, such as strictures and webs)
List nine complications of esophageal foreign body.	1. Airway obstruction 2. Inability to clear secretions 3. Esophageal stricture 4. Esophageal perforation 5. Mediastinitis 6. Peritonitis 7. Cardiac tamponade 8. Paraesophageal abscess 9. Aorta–tracheoesophageal fistula
What symptoms characterize esophageal foreign body?	Anxiety, discomfort, retching, vomiting, dysphagia, choking, coughing, stridor, food refusal (children), retrosternal chest pain (adults)

Describe some of the possible physical examination findings.

Fever, palatal abrasions or erythema (rare), subcutaneous air in the neck

How is esophageal foreign body diagnosed?

The patient history usually provides the diagnosis, although a history may not be available for children. Radiographs will reveal radio-opaque objects. Fiberoptic endoscopy can be diagnostic as well as therapeutic.

What percentage of patients who have ingested coins are asymptomatic?

35%

What is the treatment for foreign body ingestion?

Treatment depends on what was ingested and where it is located in the gastrointestinal tract. In some cases (e.g., a smooth object located beyond the pylorus, an asymptomatic patient), observation may be all that is necessary. In these situations, many physicians monitor the progress of the object by performing repeat examinations and repeat abdominal films every 2–4 hours or by passing a metal detector over the body. In other situations (e.g., an irregular object, a symptomatic patient), endoscopic or surgical removal may be necessary.

What measures are necessary if the object is located in the esophagus?

Frequent suctioning of secretions is important to prevent aspiration.

List three situations that necessitate surgery.

1. The gastrointestinal tract is obstructed or perforated.
2. The object has toxic constituents.
3. The length, size, or shape of the object may prevent safe passage from the gastrointestinal tract (e.g., the object is longer than 5 centimeters and wider than 2 centimeters, or it has sharp edges).

Where does perforation occur following the passage of a sharp object beyond the stomach?

At the ileocecal valve

What is the treatment for food impaction?	Observation and sedation are often sufficient. Consider administering glucagon, which relaxes smooth muscle. Do not give the patient meat tenderizer.
Why should all adults with food impaction have upper endoscopy?	Most have a pathologic esophageal condition.
Why should button batteries be removed promptly?	Burns can occur in as few as 4 hours, and perforation can occur within 6 hours of ingestion.

MALLORY-WEISS SYNDROME

What is Mallory-Weiss syndrome?	A longitudinal laceration of the esophageal or gastric mucosa and submucosa that occurs following retching or emesis
Which site is more common—the stomach or the esophagus?	Mallory-Weiss tears usually occur in the gastric mucosa.
What causes the tear?	An increase in the intra-abdominal gastric pressure
With what conditions are Mallory-Weiss tears associated?	Hiatal hernia, alcoholism
What are the symptoms?	Post-emesis epigastric and thoracic pain, often accompanied by emesis and hematemesis
How is Mallory-Weiss syndrome diagnosed?	History, physical examination, and esophagogastroduodenoscopy (EGD)
What is the treatment for Mallory-Weiss syndrome?	In 90% of patients, a room-temperature water lavage will stop the bleeding. If lavage fails, electrocauterization, arterial embolization, or surgery may be necessary.

GASTROESOPHAGEAL REFLUX DISEASE (GERD) AND ESOPHAGEAL COLIC

Why is it important for the emergency department (ED) physician to be knowledgeable about these conditions?	Because the symptoms of esophageal colic and GERD often mimic chest pain of cardiac origin, these conditions are part of the differential diagnosis of chest pain.

Gastroesophageal reflux disease (GERD)

What causes GERD?

GERD is most often caused by an incompetent lower esophageal sphincter. It may also be caused by decreased or abnormal esophageal motility, gastric outlet obstruction, or a hiatal hernia.

What are the symptoms of GERD?

Heartburn (i.e., substernal discomfort after meals that is usually worse with exertion or recumbency)

What are the other esophageal causes of heartburn?

Esophageal spasm, achalasia, and esophagitis

Why is it difficult to differentiate the esophageal causes of heartburn from one another in the ED setting?

Administration of an antacid or the "pink cocktail" (a compound usually containing some combination of lidocaine, belladonna, and an antacid) will relieve symptoms caused by all of the esophageal causes of heartburn (except maybe achalasia); thus, if an oral remedy works, it is difficult to differentiate without esophagoscopy and manometry (and diagnosis is not essential).

How is GERD diagnosed:

In the ED?

By taking a careful patient history

In the outpatient setting?

Upper gastrointestinal tract contrast studies, endoscopy, esophageal manometry, pH monitoring, and the Bernstein acid perfusion test

What is the treatment for GERD?

Oral antacids, frequent small meals, elevation of the head of the bed 30° or more while sleeping, histamine-2 (H_2) blockers or omeprazole, and cisapride

Esophageal colic

What is esophageal colic?

Phasic, nonpropulsive contractions of the esophagus

What are the symptoms?

Acute, agonizing, spasmodic or crescendo-like substernal pain that may radiate to the back and may last seconds to hours

What other thoracic conditions can mimic the intense pain of esophageal colic?

Cardiac ischemia and mediastinitis

Why is it difficult to differentiate esophageal colic from cardiac ischemia?

Both can produce ST abnormalities on an electrocardiogram (EKG), and sublingual nitroglycerin can provide symptomatic relief in both esophageal colic (7–10 minutes) and cardiac ischemia (2–3 minutes).

What is the treatment for esophageal colic?

The pain usually resolves with antacids, repeated swallowing, or sublingual nitroglycerin. Avoid nonsteroidal anti-inflammatory drugs (NSAIDs) for treatment; narcotics may be used as a last resort.

FOOD POISONING

What is food poisoning?

An illness typically caused by the improper cooking or handling of food; often characterized by the sudden, severe onset of nausea, vomiting, diarrhea, and/or crampy abdominal pain

What is the defining characteristic of food poisoning?

A high attack rate (i.e., many people who shared the same meal should become ill)

Describe the two mechanisms by which food poisoning can occur.

1. Ingestion of a preformed toxin (*Bacillus cereus, Clostridium botulinum, Staphylococcus aureus*)
2. Ingestion of viable infectious agents (*B. cereus, Clostridium perfringens, Salmonella, Shigella*)

Describe the two forms of *B. cereus* poisoning.

The **emetic form** is caused by ingestion of a heat-stable enterotoxin (classically found in rewarmed fried rice).
The **diarrheal form** is caused by ingestion of a heat-labile enterotoxin (classically found in meat, poultry, or vegetables).

What foods are classically associated with:

   S. *aureus* poisoning?

Mayonnaise- or egg-based dishes that have been left at room temperature for prolonged periods of time (e.g., potato salad, custards)

   C. *perfringens* poisoning?

Beef or poultry

What are the onset and duration of symptoms in:

   S. *aureus* poisoning?

Onset of symptoms occurs 3–6 hours after ingestion, and symptoms last for less than 12 hours

   Emetic B. *cereus* poisoning?

Onset of symptoms occurs 2–4 hours after ingestion, and symptoms last for 20–36 hours

   Diarrheal B. *cereus* poisoning?

Onset of symptoms occurs 8–12 hours after ingestion, and symptoms last for 24 hours

   C. *perfringens* poisoning?

Onset of symptoms occurs 8–16 hours after ingestion, and symptoms last for 24 hours

What is the treatment for food poisoning characterized by vomiting and diarrhea?

Usually, supportive therapy is all that is required.

SCOMBROID

What is scombroid?

A food-borne illness characterized by histamine intoxication

What foods are implicated in scombroid?

Seafood, specifically tuna, mahi-mahi, and bluefish

What symptoms are associated with scombroid?

Typically, patients experience a histamine-like reaction characterized by flushing, pruritus, diarrhea, nausea, vomiting, urticaria, xerostomia, and headache within 30 minutes of ingesting contaminated fish.

What is the differential diagnosis for scombroid?

Acute allergic response

What is the treatment?	Although the disease is self-limited, antihistamines may be administered.

DIARRHEA

What is diarrhea?	Increased frequency and fluidity of bowel movements (stools are classically described as conforming to the shape of their container)
What causes diarrhea?	1. Infectious agents (i.e., viruses, bacteria, parasites, fungi) 2. Toxins 3. Drugs 4. Diet (e.g., juice can cause functional diarrhea in children)
What is the natural history of diarrhea?	Most cases are caused by viruses, are self-limited, and resolve spontaneously.
Is diarrhea a common presenting problem in the ED?	Yes, diarrhea accounts for as many as 5% of all ED visits.
How do patients with diarrhea who present to the ED vary from ambulatory patients with diarrhea?	Patients presenting to the ED are "sicker," and the cause of the diarrhea is more likely to be bacterial.
When is diarrhea considered chronic?	When it persists for longer than 3 weeks
What are the two kinds of acute diarrhea?	Invasive and noninvasive
What are the characteristics of:	
Invasive diarrhea?	1. Gradual onset 2. Patient may appear ill and have constitutional symptoms (e.g., fever) as well as abdominal pain and tenderness 3. Diarrhea may be accompanied by nausea and vomiting 4. Blood or mucus in the stool (positive results on guaiac testing) 5. Fecal leukocytes

Noninvasive diarrhea?

1. Sudden onset
2. Patient does not appear ill and has no fever, and the abdomen is nontender
3. Diarrhea may be accompanied by nausea and vomiting
4. The stools are profuse and watery, but do not contain blood or mucus (negative results on guaiac testing)
5. No fecal leukocytes

Why is it important to distinguish invasive diarrhea from noninvasive diarrhea?

Invasive diarrhea is treated differently than noninvasive diarrhea

List ten questions that should be asked while taking the history.

1. How long ago did the diarrhea begin?
2. What is the quantity and frequency of bowel movements?
3. Have you noted blood, pus, or mucus in the stools?
4. Have you experienced nausea or vomiting? Can you tolerate oral liquids?
5. Do you have any underlying illnesses, such as HIV?
6. Have you been in contact with anyone who has similar symptoms?
7. Have you traveled anywhere recently? If so, where?
8. Do you have any abdominal pain?
9. Have you eaten any raw seafood or eggs recently?
10. What prompted you to come to the hospital?

Why should a rectal examination be performed?

To look for fissures and impaction, and to guaiac the stool

What laboratory tests are indicated for a patient with acute diarrhea?

Usually, no laboratory tests are indicated. A fecal leukocyte test is indicated if invasive diarrhea is suspected. If the patient appears ill, dehydrated, or immunocompromised, consider a CBC with differential, a blood culture, and a serum chemistry panel.

When should a stool sample be sent for culture?

A stool sample should be sent for culture when:
1. Invasive diarrhea is suspected

2. The patient is ill or immunocompromised
3. There are public health concerns

NONINVASIVE DIARRHEA

What is the treatment of noninvasive diarrhea?

Treatment is supportive and centers around replacing lost fluids and electrolytes. Consider inpatient treatment for patients with very severe diarrhea, pediatric or geriatric patients, and patients who are unable to tolerate oral liquids. Antimotility agents (e.g., loperamide) or bismuth subsalicylate may also be administered to lessen and control symptoms.

What recommendations regarding diet should be given to the patient with noninvasive diarrhea?

Clear liquids (e.g., ginger ale, juice, broth) and bland solid foods (e.g., crackers, toast, rice, bananas) are best. Avoid milk and other dairy products, fatty foods, and caffeine.

What is a good recipe for an oral rehydration solution?

To 1.5 quarts of water, add 0.5–1 teaspoon salt, 4–8 teaspoons of sugar, and 1 teaspoon of baking soda.

Describe traveler's diarrhea.

It is usually caused by *Escherichia coli* and is mostly noninvasive.

What is the treatment for traveler's diarrhea?

Fluoroquinolone therapy is indicated if the diarrhea is moderate to severe. Trimethoprim–sulfamethoxazole may be used instead, but this drug is associated with high rates of bacterial resistance. Loperamide, an antimotility agent, can be given to control symptoms.

What is the dose of loperamide?

4 mg initially, followed by 2 mg after each loose bowel movement (to a maximum dose of 16 mg/day)

INVASIVE DIARRHEA

List five common causes of invasive diarrhea.

1. *Shigella* species
2. *Salmonella* species
3. *Campylobacter* species
4. *Yersinia enterocolitica*
5. *E. coli*

What cause of invasive diarrhea is most commonly isolated?	*Campylobacter*
Which organism can cause seizures?	*Shigella*
Which organism may cause symptoms similar to those of appendicitis?	*Y. enterocolitica*
Which organism is found in contaminated beef?	*E. coli,* serotype O157:H7
What systemic disorders are associated with *E. coli* infection?	Hemolytic-uremic syndrome (HUS) and thrombotic thrombocytopenic purpura (TTP)
Which organism is associated with contaminated poultry?	*Salmonella*
What diseases may mimic invasive diarrhea?	Crohn's disease, ulcerative colitis, intussusception, ischemic colitis, *Clostridium difficile* diarrhea
What laboratory studies may be appropriate for a patient with suspected invasive diarrhea?	CBC and a stool culture, with or without an ova and parasites (O&P) evaluation
What is the treatment for invasive diarrhea?	Patients with mild diarrhea require supportive treatment only. Patients with moderate or severe diarrhea and immunocompromised patients may require antibiotic therapy.
What is the best class of drugs for the treatment of invasive diarrhea?	Fluoroquinolones
What are the advantages of fluoroquinolones over other drugs in the treatment of patients with invasive diarrhea?	Fluoroquinolones have been proven to decrease symptoms and eliminate the carrier state, unlike the penicillins and trimethoprim-sulfamethoxazole.
What are the limitations of fluoroquinolones?	They are contraindicated in children and pregnant women.

What are the drawbacks associated with antibiotic therapy in general?

1. Possible side effects (e.g., allergic reactions, vaginal candidiasis, possibly even diarrhea)
2. Expense
3. Development of bacterial resistance

Why aren't antimotility agents indicated for patients with invasive diarrhea?

In patients with invasive diarrhea, antimotility agents can cause toxic megacolon and may prolong illness. CNS effects may develop in children.

CLOSTRIDIUM DIFFICILE COLITIS

What causes *C. difficile* colitis?

Toxins produced by *C. difficile,* a spore-forming, Gram-positive rod

What factors predispose to *C. difficile* colitis?

Antibiotic therapy and hospitalization

Which antibiotics are usually implicated?

Classically, clindamycin and the cephalosporins are implicated in cases of *C. difficile* colitis; however, any antibiotic may be responsible.

What are the symptoms?

Diarrhea, fever, and abdominal pain (may resemble invasive diarrhea)

List two ways the diagnosis can be made.

1. *C. difficile* toxin assay
2. Lower endoscopy (reveals friable mucosa with pseudomembranes)

How is *C. difficile* colitis treated?

If possible, therapy with the offending antibiotic should be terminated. Oral metronidazole or vancomycin can be administered if the patient appears ill.

What are the potential complications of *C. difficile* colitis?

Toxic megacolon and necrotizing colitis (mortality rate is high in severely affected patients)

PARASITIC DIARRHEA

When should parasites be suspected as the cause of a patient's diarrhea?

When the diarrhea is chronic or prolonged, the patient is immunocompromised, the patient has traveled recently, or standard treatments fail

Amebiasis

What is the prevalence of amebiasis (*Entamoeba histolytica* infection)?

10% of the world's population is infected with *E. histolytica*. Most people are asymptomatic carriers.

What symptoms are characteristic of amebiasis?

Acute inflammatory diarrhea or chronic intermittent diarrhea with foul-smelling, blood-tinged stools; flatulence; and abdominal cramps

List three ways the diagnosis can be made.

1. Isolation of trophozoites in the stool
2. Serology
3. Biopsy during colonoscopy

What is a potential complication of amebiasis?

Hepatic abscess

What drugs are used to treat amebiasis?

Metronidazole and iodoquinol

Giardiasis

What is giardiasis?

A water-borne diarrhea caused by *Giardia lamblia* that is common among campers and travelers

What are the symptoms of giardiasis?

Giardiasis is usually asymptomatic, although patients may have abdominal bloating; crampy abdominal pain; flatulence; and foul, loose stools. The diarrhea can become chronic.

List three ways of diagnosing giardiasis.

1. Microscopic examination of stool for trophozoites
2. Detection of *Giardia* antigen in stool
3. Biopsy
4. Duodenal aspiration
5. A positive "string" test (i.e., organisms found on a string inserted through the nose and into the small intestine)

What drug is used to treat giardiasis?

Metronidazole (alternatives are quinacrine or tinidazole)

What are the side effects of metronidazole?

Metronidazole can have a disulfiram-like reaction; therefore, the patient should be advised to avoid alcohol. Other side effects include nausea, vomiting,

headache, and a metallic taste in the
mouth.

INFLAMMATORY BOWEL DISEASE (IBD)

What is IBD?

Chronic inflammatory disease of
unknown etiology

**Which two conditions
constitute IBD?**

Ulcerative colitis (a premalignant
condition) and Crohn's disease

**List five epidemiologic
characteristics of IBD.**

1. More common in whites than in blacks
   and Asians
2. More common in Jewish people
3. Incidence the same in men and
   women
4. Peak incidence in patients between
   the ages of 15 and 35 years
5. Positive family history in fewer than
   15% of patients

**What are the extraintestinal
features of IBD?**

1. Joint disorders, ranging from
   arthralgia to acute arthritis (seen in
   25% of patients), typically migratory
   and nondeforming
2. Sacroiliitis or ankylosing spondylitis
3. Erythema nodosum
4. Pyoderma gangrenosum
5. Aphthous ulcers of the oral mucosa
6. Ocular findings, such as episcleritis,
   iritis, and uveitis (seen in 5% of
   patients)

**What is the differential
diagnosis of IBD?**

When rectal bleeding is present, a colonic
source [e.g., hemorrhoids, neoplasms,
colonic diverticula, arteriovenous malformation (AVM), radiation proctitis,
acute infectious colitis, and ischemic
colitis] must be ruled out.

**What are the pathogens
that cause infectious colitis?**

*Shigella, Salmonella, E. histolytica,
Y. enterocolitica, Campylobacter jejuni,
Chlamydia, Neisseria gonorrhoeae,
C. difficile, Mycobacterium tuberculosis,*
enteropathic *E. coli* 0157:H7, *Aeromonas
hydrophila, Plesiomonas shigelloides*

**What is the most common
cause of terminal ileitis?**

Y. enterocolitis causes 50%–80% of cases
of acute terminal ileitis.

What is the treatment for a patient with flares of IBD?	Supportive therapy entails fluid resuscitation and correction of electrolyte abnormalities, bowel rest, and nasogastric suction. Sulfasalazine or steroids may be administered, depending on the severity of the patient's illness. If these measures do not induce a remission, azathioprine or cyclosporine are sometimes added.

ULCERATIVE COLITIS

What is the pathology of ulcerative colitis?	Uniform and continuous inflammation of the colon, characterized by crypt abscesses, a "lead pipe" radiographic appearance, and pseudopolyps
Can ulcerative colitis affect the small bowel?	Yes. "Backwash ileitis" is involvement of the terminal ileum as well as the entire colon.
Describe the symptoms of a patient with ulcerative colitis who presents to the ED.	Bloody diarrhea and abdominal pain are typical. If the disease is severe, the patient may complain of frequent loose stools containing blood and pus, severe cramps, fever, weight loss, and signs of dehydration and anemia. If involvement is primarily rectal, constipation and tenesmus may be prominent.
What might physical examination reveal in a patient with ulcerative colitis?	Abdominal distention and tenderness; possibly extracolonic features as well (e.g., arthritis, skin changes, or liver disease)
What is the dreaded complication of severe ulcerative colitis?	Toxic megacolon
When should toxic megacolon be suspected?	When a patient with active ulcerative colitis experiences a marked decrease in the amount of stools
What radiographic findings suggest toxic megacolon?	Plain films of the abdomen show dilatation of the colon to greater than 6 centimeters, or free air if perforation has occurred
Describe the treatment for toxic megacolon.	Administration of a broad-spectrum antibiotic is indicated because of the high

risk of perforation. Colectomy may be necessary if the patient has not improved after 24–48 hours of medical therapy.

What is the mortality rate associated with toxic mega-colon?	The mortality rate approaches 50% in patients with toxic megacolon and perforation.
List two possible complications of a barium enema in an ill patient with ulcerative colitis.	1. Worsened inflammation of the bowel 2. Toxic megacolon

CROHN'S DISEASE

How can Crohn's disease be distinguished from ulcerative colitis on barium enema?	Usually "skip" lesions are present, or there may be rectal sparing
What are the pathologic features of Crohn's disease?	"Skip" lesions and strictures (more common than in ulcerative colitis)
What areas of the bowel can be involved in Crohn's disease?	**Small bowel only (regional enteritis):** About 30% of cases **Colon only:** About 30% of cases **Both small bowel and colon (usually the ileum and right colon):** About 40% of cases
What are the symptoms of Crohn's disease?	General symptoms include fever, abdominal pain, diarrhea, and fatigue. Diarrhea and pain are prominent when the colon is primarily involved. Right lower quadrant pain or colicky pain, anorexia, nausea, and vomiting are seen in patients with small bowel disease.
What is a possible complication of Crohn's disease?	Adhesions may develop, causing obstruction or mass.
Metronidazole appears to decrease the incidence of what complication in patients with Crohn's disease?	Fistula formation

HEPATITIS

What is hepatitis?	Inflammation of the hepatocytes, leading to necrosis
List four causes of hepatitis.	1. Infection (viral, bacterial, fungal, or parasitic) 2. Toxicity (e.g., as a result of alcohol and other hepatotoxins) 3. Immunologic mechanisms 4. Cholestasis
What symptoms are associated with hepatitis?	The clinical presentation ranges from a completely asymptomatic patient to a patient in fulminant hepatic failure. Characteristic symptoms include malaise, a low-grade fever, headache, jaundice, anorexia, nausea, vomiting, abdominal discomfort, and diarrhea.
What may be noted during the physical examination of a patient with hepatitis?	Elevated temperature, abdominal tenderness, hepatomegaly, possibly icterus
What is the differential diagnosis for hepatitis?	1. Infectious mononucleosis 2. Cholecystitis or ascending cholangitis 3. Sarcoidosis 4. Malignancies (e.g., lymphoma, liver metastasis, pancreatic or biliary tumors)
What laboratory tests are useful in the evaluation of a patient with suspected hepatitis?	CBC, serum biochemistry panel, LFTs, bilirubin level, and PT
What results on laboratory testing suggest a poor prognosis?	A persistent total bilirubin level greater than 20 mg/dl or a prolonged PT
What is the general treatment for hepatitis?	Supportive and symptomatic treatment
When should the patient with hepatitis be admitted to the hospital?	Patients who meet any of the following criteria require hospital admission: 1. Encephalopathy 2. Bleeding or a PT three times the normal value

3. Intractable vomiting
4. Hypoglycemia
5. Bilirubin level greater than 20 mg/dl
6. Age greater than 45 years
7. Immunosuppression

How is hepatitis managed on an outpatient basis?

Patients require rest and a proper diet. They should practice good personal hygiene and avoid hepatotoxins. Patients should be advised to return to the ED if the vomiting, fever, or jaundice worsens.

VIRAL HEPATITIS

What are the common causes of viral hepatitis?

1. Hepatitis A, B, C, D, and E viruses
2. Cytomegalovirus (CMV)
3. Herpes simplex virus (HSV)

Describe the mode of transmission for each of the following hepatitis viruses:

Hepatitis A virus

Fecal–oral route

Hepatitis B virus

Blood-borne (often sexually or parenterally transmitted)

Hepatitis C virus

Blood-borne (often transmitted through blood transfusions)

Hepatitis D virus

Blood-borne

Hepatitis E virus

Fecal–oral route (often transmitted through contaminated water sources)

Which types of hepatitis have carrier states?

Hepatitis B, C, and D

Describe the incubation period for each of the following hepatitis viruses:

Hepatitis A virus

15–50 days

Hepatitis B virus

45–160 days

Hepatitis C virus

15–160 days

Hepatitis D virus	30–180 days
Hepatitis E virus	15–60 days

Describe the epidemiology and course of each of the following types of viral hepatitis.

Hepatitis A

Children and adolescents are affected most often. The symptoms are abrupt in onset, but less severe than in other types of viral hepatitis. The mortality rate is low.

Hepatitis B

Hepatitis B is most common in adults. In 5%–10% of patients, a serum sickness–like syndrome precedes the hepatitis. Most patients are asymptomatic; symptoms, when present, are moderate to severe. The mortality rate is low.

Hepatitis C

In a typical patient, hepatitis C is associated with fewer symptoms than hepatitis B. The disease is of mild severity and is associated with a low mortality rate.

Hepatitis D

In a typical patient, hepatitis D superinfection in a hepatitis B carrier can lead to acute hepatic failure and is associated with a high mortality rate.

Hepatitis E

Sporadic water-borne outbreaks of hepatitis E have been reported in Asia, Africa, and Mexico.

What complications are associated with:

Hepatitis B?

Hepatocellular carcinoma

Hepatitis C?

Chronic hepatitis, cirrhosis, hepatocellular carcinoma

What would be the expected laboratory results in a patient with viral hepatitis?

Elevation of the aspartate aminotransferase (AST), alanine aminotransferase (ALT), γ-glutamyl transferase (GGT), alkaline phosphatase (AP), and bilirubin levels

In patients with viral hepatitis, what serologic markers should be assessed initially?	IgM-HAV, IgM-HBc, hepatitis B surface antigen (HBsAg), and anti-HCV

TOXIC HEPATITIS

List eight common hepatotoxins.	1. Acetaminophen 2. Carbon tetrachloride 3. Phosphorus 4. *Amanita phalloides* 5. Halothane 6. Methyldopa 7. Isoniazid 8. Phenytoin
What are the mechanisms of toxic hepatitis?	Primarily cytotoxic Primarily cholestatic Mixed (i.e., cytotoxic and cholestatic)
How can acetaminophen cause hepatotoxicity?	The toxicity is dose-related (overdose can occur as a result of an acute or chronic ingestion). Patients with alcoholism are more susceptible to acetaminophen hepatotoxicity because of chronic glutathione depletion.
What would the expected laboratory results be in a patient with toxic hepatitis?	The AST and ALT levels are often elevated to 2–10 times the normal values, with an AST:ALT ratio of more than 1.5.

CHOLESTATIC HEPATITIS

Describe two causes of cholestatic hepatitis.	1. Drugs (e.g., phenothiazines, anabolic steroids, oral contraceptives) 2. Idiopathic condition (seen in the third trimester of pregnancy)
What would the expected laboratory results be in a patient with cholestatic hepatitis?	Elevation of the AP level to more than 3 times normal is suggestive.

PANCREATITIS

What is pancreatitis?	Inflammation of the pancreas
Name the four types of pancreatitis.	1. Acute pancreatitis 2. Chronic pancreatitis

3. Hemorrhagic pancreatitis
4. Biliary (gallstone) pancreatitis

ACUTE PANCREATITIS

What are the three most common causes of acute pancreatitis in the United States?

1. Ethanol abuse (50% of cases)
2. Biliary disease (30% of cases)
3. Idiopathic (10% of cases)

What is the usual cause in:

Patients younger than 50 years?

Ethanol abuse

Patients older than 50 years?

Biliary disease

List nine other possible causes of acute pancreatitis.

1. Iatrogenic [e.g., following endoscopic retrograde cholangiopancreatography (ERCP)]
2. Trauma
3. Hyperlipidemia
4. Hypercalcemia
5. Familial pancreatitis
6. Infection
7. Vascular ischemia
8. Renal failure
9. Penetrating peptic ulcer

What spider bite can cause pancreatitis?

Scorpion

What worms can cause pancreatitis?

Ascaris and *Opisthorchis sinensis*

What medications can be associated with pancreatitis?

Metronidazole, ranitidine, cimetidine, furosemide, acetaminophen, tetracycline

What is the clinical course of acute pancreatitis?

Disease severity may range from mild to severe, complete with pancreatic necrosis

List eleven complications of acute pancreatitis.

1. Pseudocyst (i.e., a collection of fluid, tissue, pancreatic enzymes, and blood that is distinct from adjacent structures)
2. Phlegmon (i.e., pancreatic edema)
3. Abscess, infection, or sepsis

4. Pancreatic necrosis
5. Encephalopathy
6. Pancreatic ascites or pleural effusion
7. Severe hypocalcemia
8. Splenic, mesenteric, or portal vessel thrombosis or rupture
9. Diabetes
10. Acute respiratory distress syndrome (ARDS)
11. Disseminated intravascular coagulation (DIC)

What are the symptoms of acute pancreatitis?

1. Epigastric pain that frequently radiates to another quadrant of the abdomen and may be relieved by leaning forward
2. Back pain (classic)
3. Nausea and vomiting (common)

What are the signs of acute pancreatitis on physical examination?

1. Abdominal tenderness (usually mild and diffuse)
2. Hypoactive bowel sounds
3. Fever (variably present)
4. Dehydration and possibly shock

What is the differential diagnosis for acute pancreatitis?

1. Perforated viscus (e.g., as a result of peptic ulcer disease)
2. Gastritis
3. Acute appendicitis
4. Diverticulitis
5. Cholecystitis
6. Renal or biliary colic
7. Mesenteric ischemia or infarction
8. Ruptured abdominal aortic aneurysm
9. Referred thoracic pain (e.g., pneumonia, inferior myocardial infarction)

What laboratory tests are indicated when acute pancreatitis is suspected?

1. CBC
2. Serum biochemistry profile
3. LFTs
4. Amylase and lipase levels
5. Blood type and crossmatch
6. Coagulation studies
7. Serum calcium level
8. Serum lipid levels
9. Arterial blood gases (ABGs)

What results on laboratory studies suggest acute pancreatitis?

Elevated amylase and lipase levels (lipase is more sensitive, but less specific) and an elevated white blood cell (WBC) count

What imaging studies may be useful if the diagnosis is still in question?

Abdominal radiograph, ultrasound, or CT scan

What are the most common findings of acute pancreatitis on:

An abdominal radiograph?

1. Sentinel loop sign (i.e., air trapped in the small bowel near the inflamed pancreas; suggestive of a localized ileus)
2. Colon cut-off sign (i.e., gaseous distention of the colon with collapse of the distal colon; suggestive of an ileus)

Ultrasound?

Pseudocyst, phlegmon, abscess, cholelithiasis

CT?

Pseudocyst, phlegmon, abscess, necrosis

What is the treatment for acute pancreatitis?

1. The patient should have nothing by mouth. Insert a nasogastric tube and begin intravenous fluids and total parenteral nutrition.
2. Administer H_2 blockers and analgesics.
3. Correct any coagulopathies and electrolyte imbalances.

Which analgesics should not be used and why?

Morphine (may cause constriction of the sphincter of Oddi)

What percentage of patients with acute pancreatitis require surgery?

10%

Which patients should be admitted?

Patients with definitive evidence of pancreatitis (as determined by ultrasound or laboratory studies), dehydrated patients, and patients with abdominal pain when the cause cannot be determined

What are Ranson's criteria?   Prognostic indicators for patients with acute pancreatitis

What is the risk of mortality in patients who meet:

0–2 of Ranson's criteria?   Less than 5%

3–4 of Ranson's criteria?   Approximately 15%

5–6 of Ranson's criteria?   Approximately 40%

7–8 of Ranson's criteria?   Approximately 100%

List Ranson's criteria:

At presentation   Age > 55 years
WBC count > 16,000 cells/mm^3
Glucose level > 200 mg/dl
AST level > 250 U/L
Lactate dehydrogenase (LDH) level > 350 IU/L

At 48 hours   Base deficit > 4 mEq/L
BUN > 5 mg/dl
Fluid sequestration > 6 L
Serum calcium level < 8 mg/dl
A decrease in the hematocrit of 10% or more
PaO_2 < 60 mm Hg

BILIARY (GALLSTONE) PANCREATITIS

What is the cause of biliary pancreatitis?   Gallstones lodged in, or passing through, the ampulla of Vater

What percentage of patients with cholelithiasis develop gallstone pancreatitis?   4%–8%

What suggests biliary pancreatitis?   Cholelithiasis or choledocholithiasis in a patient with pancreatitis that cannot be attributed to another cause

What is the treatment for biliary pancreatitis?   Symptomatic treatment is the same as for acute pancreatitis (e.g., intravenous hydration, parenteral nutrition, H_2 blockers, analgesics). The gallstone should be removed via either cholecystectomy or intraoperative cholangiogram 3–5 days after the pancreatic inflammation has resolved.

HEMORRHAGIC PANCREATITIS

What is hemorrhagic pancreatitis?

Pancreatitis resulting from hemorrhage into the pancreatic parenchyma and the retroperitoneal structures

What is a possible complication of hemorrhagic pancreatitis?

Extensive pancreatic necrosis

What are the signs of hemorrhagic pancreatitis?

1. Abdominal pain, shock, and ARDS
2. Cullen's sign (i.e, bluish discoloration of the periumbilical area)
3. Grey-Turner's sign (i.e., flank discoloration)
4. Fox's sign (i.e., ecchymosis of the inguinal ligament)

What laboratory studies are appropriate for a patient with suspected hemorrhagic pancreatitis?

1. Amylase and lipase levels (will be elevated)
2. Hematocrit (will be decreased)
3. Serum calcium level (will be decreased)
4. CT of the abdomen with contrast

What is the treatment for hemorrhagic pancreatitis?

The treatment is the same as for acute pancreatitis. In addition, measures must be taken to stop the hemorrhage.

CHRONIC PANCREATITIS

What is chronic pancreatitis?

Chronic inflammation of the pancreas

What are the subtypes of chronic pancreatitis?

1. Chronic calcific pancreatitis (95% of cases)
2. Chronic obstructive pancreatitis (5% of cases)

What are the two most common causes of chronic pancreatitis?

1. Ethanol abuse (70% of cases)
2. Idiopathic (15% of cases)

List six other causes of chronic pancreatitis.

1. Iatrogenic (e.g., following ERCP)
2. Trauma
3. Familial pancreatitis
4. Hyperlipidemia
5. Hypercalcemia
6. Biliary disease

What are the consequences of chronic pancreatitis?

Destruction of the pancreatic parenchyma results in fibrosis and calcification and may cause loss of both endocrine and exocrine function.

What are the symptoms and signs of chronic pancreatitis?

The symptoms and signs are often similar to those of acute pancreatitis. In addition, weight loss, glucose intolerance, and steatorrhea may be present.

What is the treatment for chronic pancreatitis?

Patients should avoid ethanol in order to prevent progression of the disease. Pancreatic enzyme replacement, insulin therapy, analgesia, intravenous fluids, and correction of electrolyte imbalances may be necessary. Surgery is occasionally indicated.

6

Urologic and Nephrologic Emergencies

URINARY TRACT INFECTIONS (UTIS)

What are the signs and symptoms of a lower UTI?

Dysuria, urgent and frequent urination, nocturia, lower abdominal pain, suprapubic tenderness, and lower back pain

What are the signs and symptoms of an upper UTI?

The signs are similar to those of lower UTIs with fever, chills, malaise, nausea, vomiting, abdomen or flank pain, costovertebral tenderness, tachycardia, and sepsis.

What are the most common organisms that cause uncomplicated UTIs?

Escherichia coli, Proteus species, *Klebsiella* species, *Enterobacter* species

What are the differential diagnoses?

Mechanical or chemical urethritis
Urolithiasis
Vulvovaginitis
Cervicitis
Pelvic inflammatory disease (PID)
Prostatitis
Epididymoorchitis
Intraabdominal disease (e.g., appendicitis, cholecystitis, diverticulitis)

What is "honeymoon cystitis?"

A lower UTI that develops after a period of increased sexual activity

What measure can decrease the frequency of honeymoon cystitis?

Voiding after intercourse

How are UTIs diagnosed?

Bedside urine dipstick, urine culture

What are useful indicators on a bedside urine dipstick?

Nitrate, leukocyte esterase, presence of blood

What is considered a significant pyuria level in:

Women?

10 or more white blood cells (WBCs)/high-power field (HPF)

Men?

1–2 WBCs/HPF

What is considered a positive finding on urine Gram stain?

Any bacteria on uncentrifuged urine
More than 15 bacteria/HPF in a centrifuged specimen

What is considered a positive urine culture?

10^5 growth

List two causes of sterile pyuria.

Chlamydia trachomatis urethritis
Retrocecal infected appendix

What can cause false-positive results on a urine dipstick and microscopic analysis?

Myoglobinuria or contamination from fecal, vaginal, or skin sources

When is urine culture necessary?

When the patient has pyelonephritis, diabetes, a chronic indwelling catheter, recurrent UTIs, end-stage renal disease, or immunosuppression
When the patient is a child or male
When the patient is pregnant
When the patient has been admitted to the hospital

How effective is short-term therapy for an uncomplicated UTI?

Single-dose or brief-duration regimens have a high failure rate because of subclinical pyelonephritis. This is especially true in patients who present to the emergency department (ED), because these patients may have delayed seeking medical care and they may not return for follow-up.

What is the mortality rate associated with treated pyelonephritis in adults?

1%–3%

URINARY CALCULI

What are vesicular calculi?	Urinary calculi located in the bladder (rare)
What are renal calculi?	Urinary calculi located in the kidneys (nephrolithiasis)
Is nephrolithiasis more common in men or in women?	Men (3:1)
What percentage of adults with nephrolithiasis present with hematuria?	90%
What percentage of children with nephrolithiasis present with hematuria?	30%
What symptoms are associated with nephrolithiasis?	Unilateral flank pain radiating down the abdomen into the groin Back or suprapubic pain Nausea and vomiting
What is the primary symptom associated with vesicular stones?	Terminal stream hematuria (i.e., hematuria at the end of micturition)
What are the signs and symptoms of renal colic (i.e., pain from nephrolithiasis)?	Writhing in bed Abdominal tenderness Tachycardia Hypertension Hematuria Low-grade fever (occasionally)
What are the differential diagnoses of renal colic?	Abdominal aortic aneurysm rupture, pyelonephritis, renal infarction, papillary necrosis, ectopic pregnancy, appendicitis, biliary colic, diverticulitis, gonadal torsion
What percentage of urinary calculi are radiopaque on a kidney-ureter-bladder (KUB) radiograph?	90%
What are radiopaque stones usually composed of?	Calcium or phosphorus

What are radiolucent stones usually composed of?

Uric acid

What intravenous pyelography (IVP) findings are consistent with renal calculi?

Distention of the renal pelvis
Hydronephrosis
Calyceal distortion
Extravasation of dye
Ureter cut-off
Asymmetric progression of dye in the two kidneys and ureters

List four factors that can increase a patient's risk for radiocontrast nephrotoxicity.

1. Certain medical conditions [e.g., renal insufficiency, diabetes, hypertension, multiple myeloma, hyperuricemia, dehydration (may be manifested as hypovolemia or hypotension)]
2. Diuretic therapy (in a patient with cardiovascular disease)
3. A history of radiocontrast dye within 3 days
4. Age greater than 70 years

What is the treatment for kidney stones?

Fluids, nonsteroidal anti-inflammatory drugs (NSAIDs), narcotics

What size stones are likely to spontaneously pass?

Stones that are 5 mm or smaller in diameter may spontaneously pass, albeit with difficulty.

What size stones are unlikely to pass?

Stones that are 10 mm in diameter or larger

List six absolute indications for hospital admission.

1. High-grade obstruction from a large stone
2. Single functioning kidney
3. Pyelonephritis
4. Uncontrolled pain with oral medication
5. Uncontrolled emesis
6. Radiocontrast extravasation (a finding consistent with urinary perforation)

List six relative indications for hospital admission.

1. Proximal or bilateral stones
2. Large vesicular stones
3. Diabetes
4. Renal insufficiency
5. Severe underlying disease
6. Pregnancy

| What are the general discharge instructions for patients with urinary stones? | Fluid hydration
Oral pain medication
Close follow-up
Straining of all urine (collect any stones) |

URINARY RETENTION

What are the common causes of urinary retention?	Benign prostatic hyperplasia (BPH) Prostate cancer Stricture Thrombi (from tumors, or following surgery) Foreign bodies Bladder neck contracture (following surgery) Nephrolithiasis Posterior urethral valves Myopathic bladder Neuropathic bladder (as a result of spinal cord compression) Medications (anticholinergic drugs and antihistamines) Psychogenic causes (i.e., voluntary external ureteral spasm)
How is urinary retention diagnosed?	Medical history and physical examination
What is the treatment?	Bladder drainage with a Foley catheter
What is the treatment if a Foley catheter cannot be placed?	Suprapubic percutaneous catheter placement
What are the complications of obstruction relief?	Vasovagal-induced hypotension after bladder drainage, post-obstructive diuresis (> 200 ml/hr), and hemorrhage from bladder mucosal damage

RENAL FAILURE

| What metabolites are normally excreted from the kidney? | Urea, potassium, phosphate, sulfate, and creatinine |
| What signifies oliguric renal failure? | Passing less than 500 ml of urine per 24 hours |

What are the 3 categories of renal failure?

Prerenal, intrinsic (renal), and postrenal

What is prerenal kidney failure?

Renal failure resulting from inadequate perfusion of the kidneys (e.g., as a result of hypovolemia, excessive diuretic use, sepsis, or low cardiac output states)

What is intrinsic kidney failure?

Renal failure resulting from direct injury to the kidney

What is postrenal kidney failure?

Renal failure resulting from postrenal obstruction, such as that resulting from strictures

ACUTE RENAL FAILURE

What is acute renal failure?

An abrupt deterioration of renal function

List seven risk factors for acute renal failure.

1. Hypovolemia
2. Cardiac disease
3. Vascular, thrombotic, or embolic disorders
4. Glomerular or renal tubular disease
5. Anatomic anomalies of the genitourinary tract
6. Rhabdomyolysis
7. Nephrotoxic drug therapy

List seven nonrenal disorders that cause acute renal failure.

1. Vascular thrombosis resulting in ischemia [i.e., idiopathic thrombocytopenic purpura (ITP) and disseminated intravascular coagulation (DIC)]
2. Systemic lupus erythematosus (SLE)
3. Vasculitis
4. Endocarditis
5. HIV
6. Hemolytic-uremic syndrome
7. Nephrotoxic drugs

List a renal cause of acute renal failure.

Rapidly progressive glomerulonephritis (RPGN)

What signs and symptoms characterize RPGN?

Hematuria, azotemia, oliguria or anuria, proteinuria, edema, and hypertension

What are the causes of RPGN?

Poststreptococcal infection or idiopathic causes

What is Goodpasture's syndrome?

RPGN with pulmonary hemorrhage and hemoptysis

What are the late signs and symptoms of acute renal failure?

Volume overload [pulmonary edema and congestive heart failure (CHF)], hypertension, hyperphosphatemia, hyperkalemia (cardiac arrhythmias and arrest), mental status changes, nausea, and vomiting

What laboratory studies should be obtained for patients with acute renal failure?

Urinalysis (urine sodium, specific gravity, osmolality, and creatinine level)
Blood urea nitrogen (BUN) and serum creatinine levels
Serum electrolyte levels

What is the formula for the fractional excretion of sodium?

$FE_{Na} = [(U_{Na}/P_{Na})/(U_{Cr}/P_{Cr})] \times 100$

The following results suggest what diagnoses?

$U_{Na} < 20$ mEq/L and $FE_{Na} < 1\%$

Prerenal azotemia

$U_{Na} > 40$ mEq/L and $FE_{Na} > 1\%$

Acute tubular necrosis

What factors are associated with poor outcomes in patients with acute renal failure?

Multiple organ dysfunction
Concomitant severe chronic disease
Underlying medical conditions, such as diabetes, SLE, or scleroderma

What are indications for emergent dialysis?

AEIOU
Acidosis
Electrolyte imbalance
Intoxication
Overload (volume)
Uremia

CHRONIC RENAL FAILURE

What are the common causes of cardiac arrhythmias and arrest in patients with chronic renal failure?

Hyperkalemia, digoxin toxicity, and myocardial ischemia

What are the electrocardiogram (EKG) changes associated with hyperkalemia?	Tall, narrow T wave in the precordial leads (leads V_2–V_6) Flattening of the P wave Widening of the QRS complex Ventricular asystole
What is the treatment for hyperkalemia?	Calcium, insulin, albuterol, Kayexalate, diuresis, and dialysis

DIALYSIS-RELATED EMERGENCIES

What is a life-threatening complication of hemodialysis?	Systemic heparinization, which can cause major bleeding complications
Are patients undergoing dialysis at higher risk than others for intracranial hemorrhage or infection?	Yes.
What is dialysis disequilibrium syndrome?	A syndrome characterized by an increase in the intracranial pressure (ICP) within hours of hemodialysis
What causes dialysis disequilibrium syndrome?	A rapid osmotic shift of fluid from the plasma to the cerebrospinal fluid (CSF), which has relatively higher levels of urea
What symptoms are associated with dialysis disequilibrium syndrome?	Headache, nausea and vomiting, mental status changes
What organism is most commonly isolated following infection of a hemodialysis vascular access site?	*Staphylococcus aureus*
What complication can be associated with use of an artificial vascular graft to facilitate hemodialysis?	Thrombosis—grafts can become clotted, necessitating surgical balloon recanalization.
What is a common, life-threatening complication of peritoneal dialysis?	Peritonitis
What are the signs and symptoms of peritonitis?	Abdominal discomfort and tenderness, pain with the inflow of dialysate, and fever

What are the differential diagnoses for peritonitis?	Pneumonia, myocardial ischemia, and pulmonary embolus
What laboratory test is used to diagnose peritonitis?	Peritoneal fluid analysis (i.e., cell count, Gram stain, protein level, and culture)
What are the signs and symptoms of uremic peri-carditis?	Pleuritic retrosternal chest pain that is relieved by sitting up; tachycardia; transient pericardial rub; arrhythmias
What is dialysis-induced ischemic cardiac injury?	Ischemia resulting from episodes of hypotension and hypoxemia that occur during hemodialysis

MALE GENITOURINARY DISORDERS

DISORDERS OF THE SCROTUM

What is the differential diagnosis for scrotal pain?	Testicular or testicular appendage torsion Epididymitis Inguinal hernia (incarcerated or strangulated) Testicular tumor (rapidly growing) Scrotal abscess Renal colic
What is the differential diagnosis for a painless scrotal mass?	Testicular tumor Inguinal hernia Hydrocele Spermatocele Varicocele Paratesticular tumor Scrotal edema

Testicular torsion

What is testicular torsion?	Twisting of the testis on the spermatic cord
What complication can occur if testicular torsion is not treated?	Testicular infarction
What age groups are most commonly affected?	Adolescents and infants
Can this condition occur during sleep?	Yes, half of all cases are reported to occur during sleep.

What are two possible risk factors associated with testicular torsion?

Undescended testes and preceding trauma

What are the signs and symptoms of testicular torsion?

A sudden onset of testicular pain and swelling, nausea and vomiting, and lower abdominal pain
Isolated abdominal or inguinal pain
Red and edematous scrotum
Very tender and edematous testis

What is the position of the affected testicle?

The testicle is high in the scrotum with a horizontal lie and a relatively anteriorly placed epididymis. The spermatic cord is often swollen on the affected side.

What is a "bell clapper" deformity?

A retracted testicle that lies in the horizontal plane as a result of twisting of the spermatic cord

Describe two tests that can be used to diagnose "bell clapper" deformity.

Doppler ultrasound or a radioisotope scan (both would demonstrate a lack of arterial flow)

Should surgical exploration be delayed until the results of diagnostic studies are available?

No; it is important to definitively diagnose the condition as soon as possible.

What is the treatment for "bell clapper" deformity?

Detorsion and orchiopexy

Describe the usual direction of detorsion.

Like "opening a book" in an anterior to lateral direction

What is the testicular survival rate if the testicle remains torsed for more than 12 hours?

20%

What finding suggests torsion of the testicular appendages?

Palpation of a small, tender lump on the testicle

Is torsion of the testicular appendages common?

Yes. Torsion of the testicular appendages is more common than testicular torsion.

How is torsion of the testicular appendages diagnosed?

The clinical manifestations of testicular appendage torsion are similar to those of testicular torsion. If the diagnosis is unclear from the patient history and physical examination, surgical exploration is necessary.

What is the treatment for testicular appendage torsion?

Most appendages calcify or degenerate in 10–14 days. Symptomatic management is usually sufficient in the interim. The pain subsides over the course of 1 week, and the scrotal swelling subsides within a few weeks.

What is the "blue dot" sign?

This sign is pathognomonic for testicular appendage torsion and is caused when the cyanotic, engorged testicular appendage shows through the thin skin of the scrotum

Testicular tumors

At what time in his life is a man most likely to be diagnosed with a testicular tumor?

Between the ages of 20 and 40 years

How does a testicular tumor present?

A painless, firm testicular mass may be palpated. Some patients complain of a dull ache in the lower abdomen, or a feeling of "heaviness" in the testicle. In 10% of patients, pain secondary to hemorrhage or necrosis from rapid tumor growth is the presenting feature.

What are the common signs and symptoms of metastatic testicular cancer?

Supraclavicular lymphadenopathy
Abdominal masses
A chronic nonproductive cough resistant to conventional therapy

Hydrocele

What is a hydrocele?

A fluid collection within the tunica vaginalis surrounding the testes

What are the causes of hydrocele?

Most cases are idiopathic; however, tumors, infection, torsion, or systemic disease all may present with acute hydroceles.

What percentage of testicular tumors present with reactive hydroceles?	10%
What is the patient profile for hydrocele?	Hydrocele occurs mostly in older patients, but is also common in infants.
How do hydroceles present?	Hydroceles are almost never symptomatic. A pear-shaped swelling of the scrotum anterior to the testes may be noted. Testicular palpation is often difficult.
How are hydroceles diagnosed?	The diagnosis is usually made on the basis of clinical findings. Transillumination studies (which reveal transillumination of the hydrocele in a darkened room) or ultrasound (which reveals a simple cystic structure) are rarely necessary.
What other scrotal lesion will transilluminate?	Inguinal hernia
What is the treatment for hydrocele?	Supportive therapy and referral to a urologist to evaluate the underlying pathology.

Scrotal infections

What are the sources of scrotal infection?	Skin and subcutaneous tissue, the bulbous urethra, the epididymis, and the testis

Scrotal abscess

What is a scrotal abscess?	A suppurative superficial infection resulting from the progressive swelling of a pustule
What are the signs and symptoms of scrotal abscesses?	Gradual onset of pain, erythema, indurated skin, and a local cellulitis
How do deep abscesses present?	With a painful scrotal mass or fixed testicle within the scrotum; fever and leukocytosis are occasionally seen
What is the differential diagnosis for a scrotal abscess?	Fournier's gangrene, torsion, epididymitis, inguinal hernia

(incarcerated or strangulated), testicular tumor (rapidly growing), renal colic

How is scrotal abscess diagnosed?

Ultrasonography is used if intrascrotal pathology is suspected. Retrograde urethrography is used if urethral irregularities are present.

Fournier's gangrene

What is Fournier's gangrene?

A rapidly progressing infection of the scrotum that develops into gangrene

What causes this infection?

Fournier's gangrene is polymicrobial— Gram-negative, Gram-positive, or anaerobic organisms may be isolated. The source of the infection is usually a urinary, perianal, abdominal, or retroperitoneal infection, or trauma.

What is the patient profile for Fournier's gangrene?

Patients are usually older than 50 years and have an underlying systemic illness. Middle-aged men with diabetes are at the highest risk.

Describe the disease course in Fournier's gangrene.

Over the course of a few hours, rapidly progressing infection and necrosis may lead to septic shock.

What are the signs and symptoms associated with Fournier's gangrene?

Fournier's gangrene presents with abrupt and severe pain of the penis, the entire scrotum, or the perineum. Perineal or scrotal erythema, induration, skin necrosis, and crepitus may be noted, but fluctuance is rare. Pain out of proportion to the examination is seen on physical examination early in the disease course. It may not be possible to palpate the scrotal contents because of edema.

What are the differential diagnoses for Fournier's gangrene?

Superficial scrotal abscess, cellulitis, scrotal edema, allergic reaction, testicular torsion, and epididymoorchitis

What tests are used to diagnose Fournier's gangrene?

Blood, urine, and wound cultures should be ordered. A radiograph of the pelvis may reveal subcutaneous air. Anoscopy and retrograde urethrography can help localize the source of the infection.

How is Fournier's gangrene managed acutely?	With broad-spectrum antibiotics and fluid resuscitation
What other treatments should be considered?	Immediate surgical débridement, meticulous wound care, antibiotics, and hyperbaric oxygen therapy should be considered. Exploratory laparotomy or diverting colostomy are required occasionally.
What mortality rate is associated with Fournier's gangrene?	The mortality rate can be as high as 50%.

Epididymitis

What is epididymitis?	Epididymal inflammation
What causes this disorder?	Trauma, reflux of sterile urine, or infection
What are the most common infectious agents?	C. trachomatis and N. gonorrhoeae in young, sexually active men; Enterobacteriaceae species and Pseudomonas species (i.e., the same organisms responsible for UTIs) in older men
What are the signs and symptoms of epididymitis?	Pain may follow severe physical exertion, periods of sexual excitement, or urinary tract instrumentation. Patients report the gradual onset of pain and swelling (i.e., over hours) in the groin or lower abdomen. The scrotum is enlarged and the overlying skin is erythematous. Fever may be present. In some patients, an inflammatory hydrocele develops following thickening and enlargement of the epididymis, testicle, and spermatic cord.
What is Prehn's sign?	Elevation of the scrotum to the pubic symphysis reduces the patient's pain in cases of epididymitis. (This sign is not specific.)
What condition is often misdiagnosed as epididymitis?	Testicular tumor
What does urinalysis reveal in a patient with epididymitis?	Leukocytes and bacteria (50% of patients)

What is the treatment for epididymitis?	Antibiotics, antipyretics, and NSAIDs Bed rest (necessary for 3–4 days to allow scrotal elevation and the application of ice) Application of heat (after 3 days) No physical exertion or sexual intercourse Urologic referral for adolescents and children
Which patients with epididymitis require hospital admission?	Febrile patients and patients requiring pain control

Orchitis

What is orchitis?	Inflammation of the testes
What is a risk factor associated with orchitis?	A previous case of epididymitis
What causes orchitis?	Viral infection (mumps) or syphilis; primary orchitis is rare

DISORDERS OF THE PENIS

Penile urethritis

What is penile urethritis?	Inflammation of the urethra
What can cause penile urethritis?	STDs: *C. trachomatis, N. gonorrhoeae,* and *Trichomonas* species UTIs (especially in elderly patients): *E. coli, Klebsiella, Proteus* species, *Enterobacter* species, and *Pseudomonas* species Foreign bodies Chemical irritation
What are the signs and symptoms of penile urethritis?	Mild dysuria to peritonitis, urinary frequency, penile discharge
How is penile urethritis diagnosed?	The diagnosis is usually made on a clinical basis. A *C. trachomatis* and *N. gonorrhoeae* DNA probe or a wet preparation (to search for flagellated organisms) may be necessary to guide antibiotic therapy.

Balanoposthitis

What is balanoposthitis?

Inflammation and infection of the glans (balanitis) and foreskin (posthitis)

What condition can be associated with balanoposthitis?

Phimosis (i.e., the inability to proximally retract the penile foreskin over the glans)

The inability to retract the foreskin is normal up to what age?

5 years

What are common causes of balanoposthitis?

Overgrowth of normal bacterial flora secondary to poor hygiene, STDs, and *Candida* infection

What are the signs and symptoms of balanoposthitis?

Pain, dysuria, and meatal edema are characteristic. Retraction of the foreskin reveals a purulent, malodorous, tender, edematous, erythematous, and occasionally excoriated glans and prepuce.

How is balanoposthitis treated?

By treating the underlying cause (e.g., with antibiotics) and practicing proper hygiene

When is urologic follow-up necessary?

Patients considering elective circumcision should see a urologist when the inflammation has subsided.

Phimosis and paraphimosis

What is phimosis?

Abnormal narrowing of the distal foreskin as a result of chronic infections or inflammation

Does phimosis occur in adults with a normal foreskin?

Rarely. Congenital adhesions may cause a phimosis in infants.

What is the differential diagnosis?

Balanitis, hair tourniquet, urticaria, and contact dermatitis

What is the treatment for phimosis?

Minor phimosis can be managed with hygiene after manual retraction. Poor hygiene with infection can lead to a more severe phimosis.

What complications can be associated with phimosis?

Balanitis, posthitis, paraphimosis, and penile carcinoma

What is paraphimosis?

The inability to distally reduce a retracted foreskin over the coronal sulcus

What are the associated symptoms?

Secondary swelling, pain, erythema, and venous engorgement

Is paraphimosis a true emergency?

Yes; increasing edema can result in arterial compromise with infection, ischemia, and gangrene of the glans.

How is paraphimosis treated?

Manual reduction should be attempted, after ensuring adequate pain control with intravenous medication. If manual reduction fails, a superficial vertical incision or a circumcision should be performed by a urologist.

Penile lesions

What are the causes of penile lesions?

STDs, dermatologic abnormalities, cancer

What are some STDs associated with penile lesions?

Genital warts [human papilloma virus (HPV) infection]
Syphilis (*Treponema pallidum* infection)
Herpes [herpes simplex virus (HSV) infection)
Chancroid (*Haemophilus ducreyi* infection)

Describe the lesions associated with each of the following STDs:

Primary syphilis

A single painless ulcer with indurated borders

Herpes

Clustered painful pustules and vesicles that eventually erupt into painful ulcers that are often accompanied by inguinal lymphadenopathy

Chancroid

A tender papule that enlarges and erupts into a painful purulent ulcer with irregular margins

HPV infection

Fleshy, warty lesions

At what age is penile cancer most common?

Penile cancers are uncommon and can occur at any age, but these cancers usually present in patients older than 60 years.

What factor may be associated with penile cancer?

Chronic inflammatory disease resulting from poor hygiene, venereal disease, or phimosis

Are there any preventative measures that can protect against penile cancer?

Circumcision is protective.

What are the most common types of penile cancer?

95% of cases are squamous cell carcinomas. Lymphatic carcinoma can occur in the sentinel lymph node located near the pubic tubercle.

How do penile carcinomas present?

With a painless nodular, ulcerative, necrotic, or fungating lesion, most often on the glans

Penile fracture

What is a penile fracture?

An acute tear in the tunica albuginea

How do penile fractures occur?

Trauma during sexual intercourse or blunt trauma during a state of tumescence

What are the signs and symptoms of penile fractures?

The patient may report hearing a "snapping" sound at the time the trauma occurred. The penis is swollen, discolored, tender, and often angulated. Urethral injury is possible.

How should patients with suspected penile fracture be managed?

Consultation with a urologist is necessary for exploration and clot evacuation. Retrograde urethrography and corpus cavernosography may be necessary to localize the injury.

Priapism

What is a priapism?

A pathologic, painful erection that generally involves only the corpora cavernosa and not the spongiosum; the priapism may last several days to weeks

What are the causes of priapism?

Idiopathic causes

Drug therapy (e.g., phenothiazine, antihypertensives, anticoagulants, papaverine)

Sickle cell disease and trait (a common cause in children)

Neoplastic diseases that obstruct the corporal outflow (leukemia is the second most common cause in children)

Trauma, leading to compression of venous drainage by a hematoma

What symptoms prompt patients to seek care?

Pain and urinary retention

What is a potential complications of priapism?

Impotence can occur in 50% of patients with priapism.

What is the treatment for priapism?

Treatment within 24–48 hours reduces the risk of impotence. Patients should receive a subcutaneous deltoid injection of terbutaline. Intravenous narcotics may be used as an adjunct. Consultation with a urologist is indicated.

What should be done if initial therapy fails?

Sedation, local aesthesia, and aspiration of blood through the glans will relieve the patient.

7

Obstetric and Gynecologic Emergencies

PREGNANCY

NORMAL PREGNANCY

What are some signs and symptoms of early pregnancy?
Late menses, nausea, vomiting, fatigue, breast tenderness, urinary frequency

What is Chadwick's sign?
A blue tint to the cervix, noted in early pregnancy

What is Hegar's sign?
The isthmus (i.e., the portion of the uterus between the cervix and fundus) feels soft on palpation.

What is the EDC?
The estimated date of confinement, or due date

What is Nägele's rule?
The EDC for a woman with 28-day menstrual cycles is 9 months and 7 days after the first day of the last menses.

Gestational milestones

When should the fetal heart beat be visible on:

    Transabdominal ultrasound?
8 weeks' gestation

    Transvaginal ultrasound?
6 weeks' gestation

When is the gestational sac visible on:

    Transvaginal ultrasound?
5–6 weeks after the last menstrual period

(LMP), or when the serum human chorionic gonadotropin (β-hCG) level is approximately 1500 mIU/ml or greater

Transabdominal ultrasound?

When the serum β-hCG level is approximately 6500 mIU/ml or greater

At what rate does the serum β-hCG level normally increase during early pregnancy?

It should double every 1–2 days.

When does the uterine fundus reach the umbilicus?

At approximately 20 weeks' gestation

After about 20 weeks' gestation, how can the gestational age be estimated?

By fundal height (i.e., the distance from the pubic symphysis to the top of the fundus in centimeters is approximately equal to the gestational age in weeks)

What is quickening?

The first feeling of fetal motion (may occur as early as 16 weeks' gestation, but usually occurs later in first pregnancies)

What is lightening?

A sensation caused by the descent of the uterus 2–3 weeks before the onset of labor

What are Braxton-Hicks contractions?

Irregular contractions during the third trimester that are felt as a sensation of pressure

Physiologic changes in pregnancy

How does cardiac output change in pregnancy?

It increases by approximately 40%.

What other cardiovascular changes occur during pregnancy?

Increased heart rate
Decreased blood pressure (during the first two trimesters; during the third trimester, the blood pressure gradually increases, returning to nonpregnant levels by term)

What may be noticed on cardiac examination of a pregnant woman?

A systolic murmur (owing to increased flow)

What respiratory changes occur during pregnancy?

The residual volume is decreased.

What implications does a decreased residual volume have in an emergency setting?

Hypoxia develops more rapidly.

What gastrointestinal changes occur during pregnancy?

Gastrointestinal motility is decreased.

What does decreased gastrointestinal motility place the patient at risk for?

Aspiration (e.g., following trauma)

What genitourinary changes occur during pregnancy?

The bladder is displaced and more likely to be injured.

How do the results of renal function studies change in pregnancy?

Both the creatinine and the serum blood urea nitrogen (BUN) levels decrease during pregnancy.

What happens to the maternal blood volume during pregnancy?

It increases by as much as 50%.

How does the white blood cell (WBC) count change in pregnancy?

Leukocytosis is present, especially in the third trimester. There may also be a slight left shift.

Describe the classifications of medication safety for pregnancy.

A: Safe in human studies
B: Safe in animal studies
C: Uncertain safety
D: Unsafe
X: Highly unsafe

COMPLICATIONS OF EARLY PREGNANCY

How many pregnant women experience first-trimester vaginal bleeding?

More than 25%

What are two pathologic causes of first-trimester vaginal bleeding?

Ectopic pregnancy and spontaneous abortion

Ectopic pregnancy

What is an ectopic preg-nancy?

Development of a fertilized ovum outside of the uterine cavity

What is the most common site of ectopic gestations?

The fallopian tubes

List four risk factors for ectopic pregnancy.

1. Previous fallopian tube injury [e.g., as a result of surgery, pelvic inflammatory disease (PID), adhesions, or structural abnormalities]
2. Previous ectopic pregnancies
3. Intrauterine device (IUD) use
4. Failed emergency contraception

List five presenting signs and symptoms of ectopic pregnancy.

1. Late menses
2. Pelvic or abdominal pain
3. Vaginal bleeding
4. Chest pain (caused by diaphragmatic irritation by blood)
5. Hypovolemic shock (in patients with a ruptured ectopic pregnancy)

List four differential diagnoses for ectopic pregnancy.

1. Appendicitis
2. Spontaneous abortion
3. Ovarian torsion
4. Corpus luteum cysts

Which findings may be present on pelvic examination in a patient with an ectopic pregnancy?

An adnexal mass or uterine enlargement

What sudies are useful when trying to diagnose an ectopic pregnancy?

1. Serum β-hCG testing
2. Ultrasound
3. Culdocentesis
4. Laparoscopy

Can patients have a negative urine pregnancy test in ectopic pregnancy?

Yes.

A single serum quantitative β-hCG level provides what information?

It predicts the likelihood of visualizing a fetal pole on ultrasound.

How are ectopic pregnancies treated?

Surgically, or medically with obstetrical consultation

Spontaneous abortion

Describe each type of spontaneous abortion:

Complete	All products of conception have been expelled from the uterus.
Incomplete	Some products of conception remain in the uterus.
Threatened	The patient has vaginal bleeding but the cervix is closed; the fetus is in the uterus.
Inevitable	The fetus is in the uterus and there is bleeding from a dilated cervix.
Missed	The fetus has died but has not been expelled from the uterus.

Hyperemesis gravidarum

What is hyperemesis gravidarum?

Extreme vomiting and nausea during pregnancy, to the point of dehydration

What are some diagnoses that should be considered in women with hyperemesis gravidarum?

Molar pregnancy (hydatidiform mole) and multiple gestations

Molar pregnancy (hydatidiform mole)

What is a molar pregnancy?

Abnormal growth of trophoblastic tissue

What presenting signs and symptoms are typical of a molar pregnancy?

Pre-eclampsia or bleeding early in pregnancy, uterus that is large for dates, hyperemesis gravidarum

What laboratory finding is often seen in molar pregnancy?

A high quantitative β-hCG level

COMPLICATIONS OF LATE PREGNANCY

Placenta previa

What is placenta previa?

Implantation of the placenta low in the uterus (i.e., near or over the internal os).

What is the classic presentation?

Painless vaginal bleeding in the third trimester

How is placenta previa definitively diagnosed?

Using ultrasound

What maneuver should be avoided in patients with suspected placenta previa?

Manual vaginal examination—this can cause a fatal hemorrhage!

Abruptio placentae

What is abruptio placentae?

Separation of the placenta from the uterine wall before the fetus is delivered.

What is the mechanism of abruptio placentae?

The inelastic placenta pulls away from the elastic uterus during stretch

List three risk factors for abruptio placentae.

1. Trauma
2. Maternal cocaine use
3. Maternal hypertension

How common is abruptio placentae after trauma?

1%–5% of cases of minor trauma result in abruptio placentae. Following major trauma, 20%–50% of patients will experience abruptio placentae.

How do many patients with abruptio placentae present?

With abdominal pain and vaginal bleeding

What signs may be present?

Shock, disseminated intravascular coagulation (DIC), fetal distress (evidenced by a change in fetal heart rate), uterine enlargement (owing to accumulation of blood), uterine contractions

How much blood can accumulate in the uterus?

As many as 2 liters of blood can accumulate in the uterus; therefore, the amount of vaginal bleeding cannot be used to estimate the total blood loss.

How is placentae abruptio diagnosed?

A high index of suspicion is necessary. Cardiotocographic monitoring may indicate fetal distress, which should increase suspicion for abruptio placentae. Ultrasound has a sensitivity of approximately 50%.

How should a patient with placentae abruptio be managed?

Resuscitation measures should be initiated; consider delivery.

In placentae abruptio, what is the:

Maternal mortality rate?   1%–2%

Fetal mortality rate?   As high as 35%

Pre-eclampsia and eclampsia

What is the incidence of pre-eclampsia?   7%

List five risk factors for pre-eclampsia.

1. Age greater than 35 years
2. First pregnancy
3. Multiple gestations
4. Family history of pregnancy-induced hypertension
5. Pre-existing diabetes mellitus, hypertension, or renal disease

When does pre-eclampsia typically occur?   After 20 weeks' gestation

When is pre-eclampsia seen early in pregnancy?   In patients with a molar pregnancy

What is the classic presentation of pre-eclampsia?   Hypertension (i.e., a blood pressure greater than 125/75 mm Hg), edema, and proteinuria

What are other clinical findings associated with pre-eclampsia?

1. Excessive weight gain
2. Visual disturbances
3. Headache
4. Abdominal pain
5. Decreased urine output
6. Hepatic dysfunction, renal dysfunction, or both
7. HELLP syndrome (i.e., hemolysis, elevated liver enzymes, and low platelet count)
8. Microangiopathic hemolytic anemia (MAHA)
9. Confusion
10. Coma
11. Hyperreflexia

What is eclampsia?   Seizures in a pre-eclamptic woman

What is the ultimate treatment for pre-eclampsia?   Delivery

What are other therapeutic measures?	Observation and fetal heart tone monitoring, seizure prophylaxis with magnesium, and antihypertensive therapy with hydralazine or labetalol

TRAUMA IN PREGNANCY

How do you transport a patient in late pregnancy?	In the left lateral decubitus position, or on a backboard that has been tilted 15°–20°
Why?	To prevent hypotension owing to occlusion of the vena cava by the enlarged and displaced uterus
How common is trauma during pregnancy?	6%–7% of pregnancies are complicated by trauma.
What are the 4 leading causes of trauma during pregnancy?	1. Motor vehicle collisions (MVCs) 2. Penetrating injury 3. Falls 4. Assault
What are the most common causes of maternal death following trauma?	Head and abdominal injuries
Are seatbelts harmful during pregnancy?	No. If used correctly, seatbelts can prevent maternal injury and decrease the risk of fetal injury.
What are the fetal and maternal mortality rates from serious automobile accidents?	15% and 7%, respectively
What are the most common problems associated with maternal pelvic fractures?	1. Hemorrhage (retroperitoneal or interperitoneal) 2. Fracture of the fetus' skull 3. Bladder laceration
What is the volume capacity of the retroperitoneum?	At least 4 liters
What are the most common intra-abdominal injuries sustained by pregnant women as a result of blunt trauma during pregnancy?	Splenic lacerations, liver lacerations, and renal injury

What injuries does blunt abdominal trauma place the fetus at risk for?	Skull fracture and intracranial hemorrhage
What are the most common causes of fetal death following blunt trauma in pregnancy?	1. Maternal death 2. Maternal shock 3. Abruptio placentae 4. Uterine rupture
How common is uterine rupture?	Fortunately, it is rare.
List 3 causes of uterine contractions following trauma.	1. Contusion of the myometrial and decidual cells, leading to the release of prostaglandins 2. Placental separation 3. Uterine rupture
Should tocolytics be administered to a patient who is having post-traumatic uterine contractions?	No. In 90% of cases, the contractions stop spontaneously. In addition, tocolytics are contraindicated for patients with abruptio placentae.
What is the fetal mortality rate associated with maternal shock?	80%

Evaluation of the pregnant trauma patient

Kleihauer-Betke assay

What is the Kleihauer-Betke assay used for?	To quantitate fetomaternal hemorrhage
What is fetomaternal hemorrhage?	A condition in which fetal blood is found in the maternal circulation
Is this normal?	Yes, a small amount of fetal blood in the maternal circulation can be normal. The incidence and volume of fetomaternal hemorrhage are increased after even minor trauma.
Describe how the Kleihauer-Betke assay is performed.	In this test, potassium hydroxide (KOH) is added to a sample of maternal blood. This basic substance causes the maternal blood cells to rupture and become lighter in color than the fetal blood cells, which are resistant to changes in pH and remain

intact. The ratio of maternal blood cells (light) to fetal blood cells (dark) is calculated by assessing the sample microscopically and counting the cells. After calculating the maternal blood volume, this ratio is used to determine the total amount of fetomaternal hemorrhage.

Why is it important to be aware of fetomaternal hemorrhage?

Because Rh-negative women must be protected from isoimmunization.

How can isoimmunization be prevented?

By administering Rh immune globulin or RhoGAM

What is the typical dose of RhoGAM?

300 μg (this dose is sufficient when 30 ml or less of fetal blood has passed into the maternal circulation; a higher dose may be necessary if the hemorrhage is more severe)

How much blood does a 16-week fetus have?

30 ml; therefore, the Kleihauer-Betke assay is not necessary before 16 weeks' gestation.

Peritoneal lavage

Is diagnostic peritoneal lavage safe during pregnancy?

Yes, if it is performed using an open technique above the uterus.

Radiographic evaluation

When evaluating a pregnant trauma patient, should x-ray studies be performed?

Necessary studies should be performed with fetal shielding.

What are the potential effects of exposing the fetus to radiation?

Congenital malformations, mental retardation, early childhood neoplasia, growth retardation, and death

When is the fetus at highest risk for radiation-induced defects?

When organogenesis is occurring (i.e., during weeks 1–8)

What is an acceptable amount of radiation?

No significant increase in congenital malformations has been demonstrated following exposure to less than 5–10 rads.

What is the radiation dose associated with a typical:

Cervical spine x-ray?

Less than 0.5 millirad

Chest x-ray?

1 millirad

Abdominal computed tomography (CT) scan?

3–9 rads

Resuscitation and care of the pregnant trauma patient

What is the best form of fetal resuscitation?

Maternal resuscitation

What is the best way of predicting fetal outcome?

Fetal monitoring

When is cardiotocographic monitoring appropriate?

In the presence of a viable fetus (i.e., after 24 weeks' gestation) and after the mother is stabilized

How long is monitoring necessary?

For at least 4 hours

If monitoring is normal for 4 hours, how will the pregnancy progress?

Usually normally

What are signs of fetal distress?

Fetal bradycardia, fetal tachycardia, or a loss of normal fetal beat-to-beat variability

When is a postmortem cesarean section indicated?

When the fetus is viable but efforts at maternal resuscitation, including early thoracotomy, have failed

What special considerations must you be aware of when performing a thoracotomy in a pregnant patient?

Do not cross-clamp the aorta!

What is the rate of fetal survival following a postmortem cesarean section?

The chances of fetal survival are better if the cesarean section is performed early: The survival rate is 70% if the fetus is delivered within 5 minutes; 13% if the fetus is delivered within 6–10 minutes, and less than 5% after 15 minutes.

PARTURITION AND THE POSTPARTUM PERIOD

NORMAL DELIVERY

Describe the three stages of labor.	**Stage 1:** Cervix dilates and effaces **Stage 2:** Begins when the cervix is completely dilated and ends when the baby is born **Stage 3:** Begins when the baby is born and ends with delivery of the placenta
What is a normal baseline fetal heart rate?	120–160 beats/min
What should you look for when assessing the fetal heart rate?	Reactivity and beat-to-beat variability
What are the three types of decelerations and their causes?	**Early:** Head compression with contractions **Late:** Uteroplacental insufficiency **Variable:** Compression of the umbilical cord
What is the Apgar scoring system?	A standardized means of assessing and communicating the status of a newborn
How is the Apgar score obtained?	Points (0–2) are awarded in the following categories: Heart rate (present, less than 100 beats/min, greater than 100 beats/min) Respiratory effort (effort, crying) Muscle tone Reflex irritability Skin color
When is an Apgar score performed?	At 1 and 5 minutes after delivery, and every 5 minutes thereafter until the score is greater than 7
What is lochia?	A uterine discharge that occurs for 1–2 weeks after delivery but may last as long as 4 weeks
Does lochia have an odor?	No. Malodorous lochia suggests infection.

COMPLICATIONS OF DELIVERY

Premature labor and premature rupture of membranes

What is premature labor?

The onset of labor between 20 and 37 weeks' gestation

List seven risk factors for premature labor.

1. Young maternal age
2. Low socioeconomic group
3. Smoking
4. Cocaine use
5. Pyelonephritis
6. Chorioamnionitis
7. Multiple gestations

Describe the symptoms of premature labor.

Back pain, contractions, a sensation of pressure, vaginal bleeding or a change in discharge

What is the treatment for premature labor?

Bed rest and hydration may be sufficient. Some patients require tocolysis. Consider fetal monitoring.

What is amniotic sac rupture before the onset of labor?

Premature rupture of membranes

What maneuver can increase the risk of infection (chorioamnionitis) in patients with premature rupture of membranes?

Manual vaginal examination

How can amniotic fluid be differentiated from vaginal secretions?

1. If the secretion turns nitrazine paper blue, it is a basic substance (e.g., amniotic fluid, blood, cervical secretions, semen).
2. The appearance of a fern-like pattern ("ferning") when the fluid is dried on a slide is consistent with amniotic fluid.

Meconium aspiration syndrome

What is meconium?

Fetal stool

What is the consequence of meconium aspiration?

Chemical pneumonitis

When meconium is noted during a vaginal delivery, what action should be performed?	The nares, mouth, and pharynx should be suctioned following delivery of the infant's head, but before delivery of the body (i.e., at the perineum).

Umbilical cord prolapse

What is umbilical cord prolapse?	The umbilical cord lies in the lower part of the uterus (and may be seen in the vagina)
What complications are associated with umbilical cord prolapse?	Cord compression by the fetus or by uterine contractions can lead to decreased fetal blood flow.
What measures can be taken to manage these patients?	1. Administration of oxygen to the mother 2. Manual elevation of the fetus to relieve the pressure on the cord 3. Delivery of the fetus via cesarean section

Abnormal presentations

Identify the types of breech presentations in the figure below:

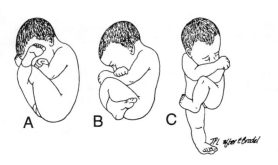

A = Frank (i.e., thighs flexed, legs extended)

B = Complete (i.e., thighs flexed, legs flexed)

C = Footling (i.e., baby presents with one or both feet or knees)

List 3 complications associated with a breech presentation.	1. Higher rate of prolapsed umbilical cord 2. Trauma during delivery, including difficulty delivering the head 3. Hypoxia
How are most breech babies delivered?	Via cesarean section
What is shoulder dystocia and when does it occur?	Shoulder dystocia is an inability to deliver the baby's shoulders. This problem is most common with large babies (i.e., large relative to the size of the mother). Dystocia is also associated with the way the baby presents (e.g., face first).

COMPLICATIONS OF THE POSTPARTUM PERIOD

List five causes of fever in the postpartum period.	1. Endometritis 2. Urinary tract infection (UTI) 3. Mastitis 4. Septic thrombophlebitis 5. Wound infections (following a cesarean section)
What is mastitis?	Infection of the mammary glands
What is the most common bacterial cause of mastitis?	*Staphylococcus aureus*
What is the treatment for mastitis?	Antibiotic therapy and warm compresses; the mother should be advised to continue nursing
When does endometritis occur?	Endometritis occurs 2–3 days after delivery.
What are the symptoms associated with endometritis?	Lower abdominal pain, foul-smelling lochia, fever, malaise
What is the treatment for endometritis?	Admit the patient, administer IV antibiotics, and perform cervical cultures. An obstetrical consultation is needed to consider evaluation for retained products of conception.

INFECTIONS OF THE UPPER FEMALE GENITAL TRACT

CERVICITIS

What is cervicitis?

Cervical inflammation with a mucoid discharge, usually occurring secondary to infection

Which organisms are most commonly implicated in cervicitis?

Chlamydia trachomatis
Neisseria gonorrhoeae
Mycoplasma species
Ureaplasma species

How common is coinfection with *C. trachomatis* and *N. gonorrhoeae*?

Concurrent infection occurs in 50% of women with cervicitis.

What are the signs and symptoms of cervicitis?

Patients may be asymptomatic or complain of a vaginal discharge, vaginal spotting, or dysuria. Patients do not appear ill.

What physical examination findings are typical of cervicitis?

Pelvic examination reveals a discharge emanating from the os or lesions on the cervix. Additional symptoms, such as cervical motion and adnexal tenderness, suggest PID.

How is the cervical discharge of *C. trachomatis* infection distinguished from that of *N. gonorrhoeae* infection?

A clear mucoid discharge suggests *C. trachomatis* infection, while a copious, viscous, purulent discharge suggests *N. gonorrhoeae* infection.

Can the diagnosis be made on the basis of the physical examination findings alone?

No. Culture or a DNA probe study is necessary.

PELVIC INFLAMMATORY DISEASE (PID)

What is PID?

An ascending infection of the female genital tract that is seen in sexually active women

List six risk factors for PID.

1. Prior sexually transmitted disease (STD)
2. Unprotected sexual intercourse with multiple partners

3. Adolescence
4. IUD use
5. Vaginal douching
6. Instrumentation of the uterine cavity

What are some preventive measures?

1. Use of a barrier method for contraception
2. Use of a nonoxynol-9 spermicide
3. Use of oral contraceptives
4. Pregnancy (after 6 weeks' gestation)

What are the signs and symptoms of PID?

Patients may complain of abdominal pain and bilateral pelvic pain. Systemic complaints include anorexia, nausea, vomiting, and fever. Physical examination reveals cervicitis and signs of pelvic peritonitis, including cervical motion and adnexal tenderness. An inflammatory pelvic mass may be detected, either on physical examination or via ultrasound. In advanced disease, patients may present in septic shock.

What is the chandelier sign?

Peritoneal pain elicited with manual manipulation of the cervix (not specific to PID)

What three findings must be present on physical examination in order to diagnose PID?

Abdominal tenderness, cervical motion tenderness, and adnexal tenderness

What might laboratory studies reveal in a patient with PID?

Gram staining of the cervical discharge may reveal *N. gonorrhoeae*. Blood work may reveal a WBC count greater than 10,000 cells/mm^3. WBCs and bacteria may also be seen in the peritoneal fluid or cervical discharge.

List six common complications in patients with PID.

1. Infertility
2. Increased chance of ectopic pregnancy
3. Chronic pelvic pain
4. Dyspareunia
5. Pelvic abscess
6. Ovarian dysfunction

List eight conditions that warrant hospital admission for a patient with PID.

1. Uncertain diagnosis
2. Patient is unable to tolerate oral nutrition
3. Patient is pregnant
4. Patient has a pelvic mass or an IUD is in place
5. Patient is nulliparous and this is the initial episode of PID
6. Patient fails to respond to oral therapy within 48 hours
7. Patient has severe illness with systemic toxicity
8. Patient's ability or willingness to comply with therapy is in doubt

What follow-up is necessary for patients who are being treated for PID?

These patients should be referred to a gynecologist for syphilis, HIV, and hepatitis B testing.

FITZ-HUGH-CURTIS SYNDROME

What is Fitz-Hugh-Curtis syndrome?

Right upper quadrant pain and hepatitis caused by a discharge from the fallopian tubes around the liver

What organisms can cause Fitz-Hugh-Curtis syndrome?

C. trachomatis and *N. gonorrhoeae* are the most commonly implicated organisms, although *Escherichia coli* and anaerobes (e.g., *Bacteroides* species, *Peptococcus* species, *Peptostreptococcus* species) can also cause the salpingitis that leads to Fitz-Hugh-Curtis syndrome.

What are the differential diagnoses for Fitz-Hugh-Curtis syndrome?

1. Abdominal disorders (e.g., acute appendicitis, bowel ischemia, diverticulitis, intraperitoneal hemorrhage)
2. Gynecologic disorders (e.g., pelvic adhesions, ectopic pregnancy, ovarian torsion, endometriosis, corpus luteum cyst rupture)
3. Renal disorders (e.g., UTI, renal colic)
4. Cardiopulmonary disorders (e.g., lower lobe pneumonia, rupture or dissection of an abdominal aortic aneurysm)

INFECTIONS OF THE LOWER FEMALE GENITAL TRACT

VULVOVAGINITIS

What is vulvovaginitis?
Inflammation and irritation of the vagina and vulva

What are the signs and symptoms of vulvovaginitis?
Pruritus and burning
Increased discharge with an abnormal odor
Pain when urine contacts the skin (if there is vulvar irritation)
Dyspareunia, perineal irritation, and spotting

List five typical causes of vulvovaginitis.
1. Vaginal infection
2. Estrogen deficiency
3. Foreign bodies
4. Irritant
5. Traumatic inflammation

Does *C. trachomatis* cause vulvovaginitis?
No, but it can cause a vaginal discharge.

What are the most common infectious causes of vulvovaginitis?
1. *Candida albicans*
2. *Trichomonas vaginalis*
3. *Gardnerella vaginalis*

What approach should be taken when a patient presents with suspected vulvovaginitis?
The clinical findings may suggest the specific cause of the vulvovaginitis. In addition, the vaginal discharge should be examined with saline and KOH preparations. The value of vaginal cultures is limited because many different species of bacteria comprise the normal vaginal bacterial flora.

Candidiasis

List five risk factors for *C. albicans* infection.
1. Use of systemic antibiotics or oral contraceptives
2. Diabetes
3. Immunocompromised status
4. Pregnancy or postmenopausal status
5. Unprotected intercourse

What physical examination findings are typical in a patient with candidiasis?
A white, cottage cheese-like discharge
Vulvar and vaginal edema and erythema

What does laboratory examination of the vaginal discharge reveal?	The discharge has a normal pH. A KOH smear reveals pseudohyphae.
What is the treatment for candidiasis?	Topical therapy with an antifungal agent (e.g., miconazole) for 3–14 days, depending on the agent

Trichomoniasis

What physical examination findings suggest a diagnosis of trichomoniasis?	A thin, greenish-grey, frothy, malodorous discharge. Vaginal erythema, possibly petechiae
What laboratory findings would be consistent with a diagnosis of trichomoniasis?	The discharge is acidic (i.e., the pH is greater than 4.5). Microscopic examination of a saline preparation reveals large numbers of WBCs and unicellular, pear-shaped, flagellated, mobile organisms.
What is the treatment for trichomoniasis?	Oral metronidazole (2 g orally, given once) has a 90% cure rate. Patients should be referred for HIV, syphilis, and hepatitis B testing.

Bacterial vaginosis

What is thought to cause bacterial vaginosis?	Bacterial vaginosis is thought be a symbiotic infection involving the anaerobes of the normal vaginal flora (e.g., *Bacteroides* species) and *Gardnerella vaginalis*
What physical examination findings are characteristic of bacterial vaginosis?	Thin, greyish white vaginal discharge Mild vaginal erythema Positive "whiff" test (i.e., mixing KOH with the vaginal discharge on a slide releases amines, which have a "fishy" odor)
What would be the expected findings on laboratory examination of the discharge?	The discharge is acidic, with a pH greater than 4.5. A saline preparation reveals clue cells.
What are clue cells?	Epithelial cells with clusters of bacilli adhering to most of the surface area

What is the treatment for bacterial vaginosis?	Oral metronidazole (2 g administered once, or 500 mg administered twice daily for 7 days) or topical metronidazole or clindamycin

GENITAL ULCER DISEASE AND GENITAL WARTS

Which STDs are characterized by genital ulcers or warts?	Genital herpes, chancroid, syphilis, and human papillomavirus (HPV) infection

Describe the lesions associated with each of the following disorders:

Primary syphilis	A single, painless ulcer with indurated borders
Genital herpes	Clustered, painful pustules and vesicles that eventually erupt into painful ulcers, often accompanied by inguinal lymphadenopathy
Chancroid	A tender papule that enlarges and erupts into a painful purulent ulcer with irregular margins
HPV	Fleshy warts on the external genitalia
What other diagnosis must be considered when a patient presents with a genital lesion?	Cancer
Describe the typical lesion associated with carcinoma.	A painless nodular, ulcerative, necrotic, or fungating lesion

OVARIAN DISORDERS

OVARIAN MASSES

What are the differential diagnoses of an ovarian mass?	1. Corpus luteum or follicular cyst 2. Dermoid cyst 3. Endometriosis 4. Neoplasm 5. Ectopic pregnancy 6. Abscess

What causes follicular cysts?   Follicular cysts result when a mature follicle fails to release its egg.

Are these cysts ever found in women with normal menstrual cycles?   Yes.

What are corpus luteum cysts?   Corpus luteum cysts persist after an egg erupts from its follicle. They are normal in pregnancy, but are abnormal and rare in non-pregnant women. Functional corpus luteum cysts may delay menstruation.

How do follicular and corpus luteum cysts present?   Enlargement, leakage, and subsequent rupture of the cyst causes poorly defined visceral pain followed by irritation of the peritoneum.

How are these cysts diagnosed?   Using ultrasound

What is the treatment?   Most cysts resolve spontaneously, but some ruptured cysts require surgical intervention.

What are dermoid cysts?   Teratoma germ cell neoplasms that may contain any type of tissue, including hair and teeth, and may cause a chemically induced peritonitis by secreting acidic or alkaline fluid

OVARIAN TORSION

What is ovarian torsion?   The twisting of the ovary on its pedicle

What is the danger of ovarian torsion?   Compromised blood supply, enlarged or abnormal ovaries

What are the signs and symptoms of ovarian torsion?   Severe, possibly intermittent, unilateral acute abdominal or pelvic pain that is often accompanied by diaphoresis, nausea, and vomiting

What is found in the history and on examination?   The medical history may reveal a similar milder episode. There is unilateral adnexal pain and occasionally a tender mass on pelvic examination.

What is the differential diagnosis for ovarian torsion?	Ectopic pregnancy
Will an ultrasound interpreted as normal rule out torsion?	No.
How is ovarian torsion treated?	Surgically

VAGINAL MASSES

What is the differential diagnosis of a vaginal mass?	1. Bartholin's gland abscess 2. Uterine prolapse 3. Cystocele 4. Rectocele 6. Leiomyoma, lipoma, and other soft tissue neoplasms

Bartholin's gland abscess

What causes a Bartholin's gland abscess?	A ductal obstruction, usually caused by trauma to the lower third of the vaginal introitus
What are the presenting features of a Bartholin's gland abscess?	A Bartholin's gland abscess presents with a painful mass on the labia majora and maximal fluctuance that extends toward the medial surface of the labia. Patients complain of dyspareunia.
What is the differential diagnosis for a Bartholin's gland abscess?	Epidermal inclusion cyst, sebaceous cyst, lipoma, vulvar hematoma, and vulvar neoplasm
What are the most common causative organisms?	A Bartholin's gland abscess is most often caused by mixed flora from vaginal and fecal sources. *N. gonorrhoeae* and *C. trachomatis* may be involved.
How is a Bartholin's gland abscess treated?	The abscess must be incised and drained in the emergency department (ED), after which sitz baths and local care are required. Recurrent abscesses require marsupialization by a gynecologist for definitive treatment.

Uterine prolapse

What is uterine prolapse?

Prolapse of the uterus through the pelvic floor

What are the signs and symptoms of uterine prolapse?

Patients report a sensation of inguinal pulling, lower back pain, urinary incontinence, and worsening of symptoms when a Valsalva maneuver is performed.

What is found on physical examination?

A vaginal mass

What is the treatment for uterine prolapse?

An exposed uterus requires manual reduction in the ED. Until the patient can be evaluated by a gynecologist, strict bed rest is necessary because of possible trauma and infection of the exposed tissues.

Cystocele

What is a cystocele?

A herniation of the posterior bladder wall into the vagina

What are the signs and symptoms?

Clinical features include vaginal fullness, urinary incontinence, incomplete bladder emptying, and possibly recurrent UTIs. Symptoms worsen when a Valsalva maneuver is performed.

What is found on physical examination?

A thin-walled bulge along the anterior vaginal wall

What is the treatment for cystocele?

Surgery performed by the obstetrician

Rectocele

What is a rectocele?

Herniation of the anterior rectal wall into the vagina posteriorly

What are the signs and symptoms?

Introital fullness, constipation, and incomplete rectal evacuation

What is found on physical examination?

Pelvic and rectal exams reveal a thin-walled bulge on the posterior vaginal wall.

What is the treatment for a rectocele?

Hydration, stool softeners, and laxatives (if needed)

Gynecologic follow-up

PELVIC PAIN

What is mittelschmerz?

A unilateral dull ache or pain in the lower quadrant that occurs with ovulation

Do any signs accompany the pain?

The patient may notice light vaginal spotting.

In the non-pregnant patient, what are the:

Gynecologic differential diagnoses for pelvic pain?

1. Ovarian cyst
2. Dysmenorrhea
3. Mittelschmerz
4. Endometriosis
5. Ovarian torsion
6. Uterine fibroids and neoplasms
7. Adnexal neoplasms
8. Pelvic floor relaxation
9. Foreign body
10. PID and cervicitis

Urologic differential diagnoses for pelvic pain?

1. UTI
2. Renal calculi
3. Hydronephrosis
4. Perinephric abscess

Gastrointestinal differential diagnoses for pelvic pain?

1. Constipation
2. Appendicitis
3. Bowel obstruction
4. Hernia
5. Adhesions
6. Gastroenteritis
7. Diverticulitis
8. Cholecystitis
9. Cholangitis
10. Peptic ulcer disease
11. Pancreatitis
12. Dietary intolerance
13. Inflammatory bowel disease

Orthopedic differential diagnoses for pelvic pain?

1. Herniated intervertebral disk
2. Pelvic fracture
3. Osteitis

What is endometriosis?	This disorder involves normal uterine endometrial tissue in ectopic locations (usually pelvic organs). The endometrium can proliferate, infiltrate, and spread to remote sites.
What are the signs and symptoms of endometriosis?	1. Cyclic pelvic pain, dysmenorrhea, and dyspareunia 2. Infertility 3. Severe abdominal pain (if the ectopic endometrium ruptures)
How is endometriosis diagnosed?	The medical history is suggestive, but surgery is definitive.
How is endometriosis treated?	Supportive therapy (i.e., pain medication) and gynecologic follow-up

DYSFUNCTIONAL UTERINE BLEEDING

What are common causes of dysfunctional uterine bleeding in premenopausal women?	An anovulatory cycle or pregnancy
What is a common cause of uterine bleeding in post-menopausal women?	Uterine fibroids or endometrial cancer
What can cause abnormal uterine bleeding in women of any age?	Trauma, infection, or a coagulopathy
What is the treatment for dysfunctional uterine bleeding?	Hormonal therapy and follow-up with a gynecologist
Describe the hormonal therapy used to treat uterine bleeding.	Hemodynamically unstable patients require intravenous estrogen. Stable patients can be treated with oral contraceptives.

SEXUAL ASSAULT

What is the physician's highest priority in the treatment of a rape victim?	To provide adequate medical treatment for the complications of the assault

What complications are common in rape victims?

Wounds from the assault; psychologic trauma; pregnancy, STDs, and tetanus (require preventive treatment); HIV (requires counseling)

What is the legal role an emergency physician may be asked to assume in the evaluation of a rape victim?

An emergency physician may be asked to collect physical evidence. Historical information about the assault is the responsibility of law enforcement personnel.

Should an emergency physician complete an evidence collection kit without prior communication with the pertinent law enforcement officials?

No.

8

Infectious Disease and Immunologic Emergencies

SKIN AND SOFT TISSUE INFECTIONS

CELLULITIS

What is cellulitis?
A bacterial infection of the skin and subcutaneous tissue seen most often in the face, legs, arms, and hands

What are the signs and symptoms of cellulitis?
1. Erythema
2. Warmth
3. Pain
4. Swelling
(Think "rubor, calor, dolor, tumor.")

List three epidemiologic characteristics of cellulitis.
1. More common in immunocompromised patients
2. More common in patients with vascular insufficiency
3. More common in patients who engage in high-risk behavior (e.g., intravenous drug abuse)

Which organisms are most commonly implicated in cellulitis?
1. *Staphylococcus aureus*
2. Group A β-hemolytic *Streptococcus*
3. *Haemophilus influenzae*

Which patients are at high risk for *Pseudomonas* infection (a rare cause of cellulitis)?
1. Patients who sustain a puncture wound of the foot through the sole of a shoe
2. Patients with diabetes
3. Patients who abuse intravenous drugs
4. Patients with vascular insufficiency

How is cellulitis diagnosed?
Clinically

What laboratory studies should be obtained in patients with suspected cellulitis?

Usually no laboratory studies are necessary; consider obtaining a complete blood count (CBC) with differential, blood urea nitrogen (BUN) and creatinine levels, and blood cultures in immunocompromised patients or patients who appear ill.

How effective is tissue culture for diagnosing cellulitis?

Needle aspiration of the leading edge of the infection has a low diagnostic yield.

When would a tissue culture be indicated?

For patient with refractory or recurrent cellulitis

What may an x-ray of the affected area reveal?

1. Subcutaneous gas
2. Foreign body
3. Osteomyelitis
4. Fracture

What is the treatment of cellulitis?

Immobilization, antibiotics (chosen according to the flora of the affected anatomic region), elevation, and analgesics

What are adjunctive therapies for cellulitis?

1. An intravenous dose of antibiotics may be administered in the emergency department (ED).
2. Local warm soaks and elevation of the affected area are indicated.
3. A follow-up wound check should be scheduled 24–48 hours after the initial treatment, if the patient is being treated on an outpatient basis.

What are the criteria for the inpatient management of cellulitis?

1. Systemic symptoms (e.g., fever, toxicity) in a patient with severe cellulitis
2. Immunosuppression or asplenia
3. Concurrent diabetes
4. History of intravenous drug abuse
5. History of peripheral vascular disease
6. History of alcoholism
7. History of steroid use
8. Infection of the face or hands

9. Failure of outpatient treatment
10. Concern that an alternative diagnosis exists or a more serious infection is present

What are the criteria for discharge from the ED?

1. Limited infection
2. Immunocompetent patient
3. No signs of systemic illness
4. Patient able to take oral drugs
5. Patient compliance and follow-up is likely

ERYSIPELAS (ST. ANTHONY'S FIRE)

What is erysipelas?

A superficial skin and soft tissue infection caused by group A β-hemolytic *Streptococcus*.

What are two epidemiologic characteristics of erysipelas?

1. More common in very young and very old patients
2. More common in immunocompromised patients

What are the signs and symptoms of erysipelas?

1. Rapidly evolving area of erythema with a distinct raised border
2. Warmth
3. Pain
4. "Peau d'orange" skin
5. Systemic symptoms (e.g., fever, general malaise, arthralgias, anorexia)

What parts of the body are usually affected by erysipelas?

1. The face and legs
2. Areas where trauma or a break in the skin has occurred

Why are facial erysipelas infections dangerous?

Infection can spread rapidly to the cavernous sinus and brain via the veins and lymphatics.

How is erysipelas diagnosed?

Clinically

What are the differential diagnoses for erysipelas?

1. Cellulitis
2. Contact dermatitis
3. Erysipeloid
4. Herpes zoster

How does erysipelas differ from cellulitis?

The individual with erysipelas is usually very young or very old, exhibits a sharply demarcated, very red rash on the face or legs, and has systemic symptoms.

What is the treatment for erysipelas?

1. **Outpatient:** Administration of oral penicillin for 10 days; erythromycin is prescribed for patients who are allergic to penicillin.
2. **Inpatient:** Administration of intravenous penicillin for 10 days.

ABSCESSES

What is an abscess?

A localized collection of pus in the tissue

What factors can precipitate the development of an abscess?

Abscesses may occur in anyone. They are usually precipitated by trauma or are secondary to plugging of a superficial exocrine gland.

What conditions or diseases predispose a patient to the development of abscesses?

1. Diabetes
2. Connective tissue diseases
3. Inflammatory bowel disease
4. Neoplasms
5. Immunosuppression (e.g., steroid use, HIV infection, organ transplantation)

Define the following types of abscesses:

Furuncle

A thin-walled abscess that evolves from superficial folliculitis

Carbuncle

Deep abscesses interconnected in subcutaneous tissue

Hidradenitis suppurative

A chronic, recurrent abscess of the apocrine glands in the axilla or groin

Bartholinian abscess

An abscess at the inferolateral margin of the vaginal introitus caused by obstruction of Bartholin's duct

Pilonidal abscess

An abscess over the gluteal fold near the coccyx; usually secondary to plugging of an epithelium-lined congenital "pit;" often recurrent

Perirectal abscess

An abscess originating from the anal

crypts and extending through fistula tracts into the surrounding deep tissue

How are abscesses diagnosed?

Clinically—look for a localized, fluctuant mass with evidence of erythema, warmth, pain, and swelling.

Are systemic symptoms common?

No, systemic symptoms suggest myonecrosis or fasciitis.

What studies are available as adjuncts to diagnosis?

1. **Needle aspiration:** Numb the skin and aspirate the abscess using a 20-gauge (or larger) needle. Even a drop of pus is an indication for incision and drainage.
2. **Radiography:** Look for gas, foreign bodies, or osteomyelitis.
3. **Ultrasound or computed tomography (CT):** Use these studies to help define the extent of the abscess.

Is the presence of gas or subcutaneous air a bad thing?

Yes! This finding represents a surgical emergency!

What laboratory studies should be ordered?

None are indicated for simple abscesses. If a patient will require surgery, then a CBC, serum chemistry panel, blood type and screen, prothrombin time (PT), and partial thromboplastin time (PTT) are required.

What are the most common pathogens associated with abscesses?

These infections are usually polymicrobial. *Staphylococcus* species and *Streptococcus* species are often isolated, and increased numbers of anaerobes are found in abscesses near the mouth or anus.

What is the standard treatment for abscesses?

Incision and drainage

When are antibiotics indicated during incision and drainage of an abscess?

Antibiotics are not usually indicated, but may be considered if:
1. The patient is at risk for endocarditis
2. There is evidence of concurrent cellulitis, or more extensive infection

3. The patient appears ill or is immunocompromised

What are the contraindications to performing incision and drainage in the ED?

Incision and drainage of an abscess should not be performed in patients who:
1. Appear ill or who have underlying systemic disease
2. Have extensive abscesses
3. Have an abscess located on the face, head, neck, hand, or orbit, or in a joint
4. Have an abscess in close proximity to an important neurovascular structure
5. Require general anesthesia

What types of anesthesia can be used during incision and drainage of an abscess in the ED?

Local anesthesia or parenteral analgesia/conscious sedation

Which is preferred?

Parenteral analgesia/conscious sedation—local anesthesia is associated with notoriously poor results, probably secondary to poor penetration and decreased effect of the anesthetic as a result of the low tissue pH.

What equipment should be assembled prior to incising and draining an abscess in the ED?

1. Povidone–iodine
2. Number 11 or number 15 scalpel blade
3. Scissors
4. Hemostat
5. Packing material (either zeroform or iodoform gauze)
6. Gauze sponges (4″ × 4″)
7. Normal saline

Describe the procedure for incising and draining an abscess in the ED.

1. Administer anesthesia (and antibiotics, when indicated).
2. Ensure a sterile field and sterilize the skin.
3. Incise the entire area of fluctuance.
4. Express pus and necrotic debris and irrigate.
5. Probe the cavity to break any loculations.
6. Generously irrigate the wound with normal saline, and pack it loosely.
7. Have the patient return in 24–48

hours for evaluation of the wound and removal of the packing.

What is the treatment for:

Hidradenitis suppurative?

Incision and drainage; surgical referral is usually necessary because of the recurrent nature of the disorder.

A bartholinian abscess?

Incision and drainage on the mucosal surface of the vaginal introitus, or marsupialization (i.e., eversion and suturing of the cyst wall to the mucosal surface)

A pilonidal abscess?

Incision and drainage, with surgical referral for recurrences; in addition, surgical excision of the congenital "pit" is required in most cases.

A perirectal abscess?

Well-circumscribed and noncomplicated abscesses may be incised and drained in the ED. Pain or fluctuance on rectal examination necessitates surgical consultation.

Other than hidradenitis suppurative and pilonidal abscess, which classically recur, list four common causes of recurrent abscesses.

1. Foreign body
2. Underlying systemic disorder (e.g., Crohn's disease)
3. Inadequate or improper prior incision and drainage
4. Fistula

How are recurrent abscesses managed?

Surgical referral

NECROTIZING FASCIITIS AND MYONECROSIS

What is necrotizing fasciitis?

Necrotizing fasciitis is a fulminant group A β-hemolytic *Streptococcus* infection that begins as severe or extensive cellulitis and spreads to involve the superficial and deep fasciae. Fascial involvement leads to thrombosis of the subcutaneous vessels and gangrene.

Necrotizing fasciitis is associated with which underlying illnesses?

Diabetes mellitus and other conditions associated with immunocompromise

What is myonecrosis?

Necrotizing fasciitis that involves the muscles as well

Which organisms are typically associated with necrotizing fasciitis and myonecrosis?

These infections are polymicrobial. Gram-positive, Gram-negative, and anaerobic bacteria may all be isolated.

Are necrotizing fasciitis and myonecrosis serious?

Yes! Both are associated with a high mortality rate (80%–90%).

What are common complications of necrotizing fasciitis and myonecrosis?

1. Sepsis
2. Metabolic abnormalities, especially hypocalcemia
3. Hemolysis with anemia
4. Disseminated intravascular coagulation (DIC)

How are fasciitis and myonecrosis diagnosed?

History: The infection may have started as a simple cellulitis infection.
Physical examination findings: Erythema without sharp margins, warmth, pain, and swelling are present. The pain may be severe and out of proportion to the physical findings. In the later stages, numbness replaces the pain. The swelling may also be significant, and necrotic areas may be noted. The patient looks ill (e.g., he is febrile, tachycardic, and, possibly, hypotensive). Crepitation may be noted, especially when *Clostridium difficile* is the causative organism.
Adjunctive studies: Radiographs may reveal subcutaneous air.

What laboratory studies should be considered in patients with suspected fasciitis or myonecrosis?

Consider obtaining fibrinogen, D-dimer, fibrin degeneration products, and hemoglobin levels; the hematocrit; the platelet count; and the PT and PTT to rule out DIC.

What is the initial ED treatment for necrotizing fasciitis and myonecrosis?	1. Resuscitation 2. Administration of a broad-spectrum antibiotic (**always** indicated) 3. Referral for emergency surgical exploration and débridement

BONE AND JOINT INFECTIONS

OSTEOMYELITIS

What is osteomyelitis?	Inflammation and infection of the bone marrow and adjacent bone
Which organisms are most likely to cause osteomyelitis in:	
Neonates?	*S. aureus*, Gram-negative organisms
Children?	*S. aureus, Haemophilus influenzae*
Otherwise healthy adults?	*S. aureus*
Immunocompromised patients or patients who abuse intravenous drugs?	Gram-negative organisms
Patients with sickle cell disease?	*Salmonella* species, *Staphylococcus* species
What are the signs and symptoms of osteomyelitis?	Tenderness, decreased movement, and swelling
What are the diagnostic steps?	1. Obtain the patient history and perform a physical examination. 2. Aspirate the joint to obtain fluid for analysis. 3. Order a CBC and erythrocyte sedimentation rate (ESR). 4. Order a bone scan.
How is osteomyelitis treated?	Antibiotics, possibly accompanied by surgical drainage
What is Marjolin's ulcer?	A squamous cell carcinoma that arises in a chronic sinus as a result of osteomyelitis

SEPTIC ARTHRITIS

What is septic arthritis?

Inflammation of a joint, beginning as synovitis and ending with destruction of the articular cartilage (if left untreated)

List the four risk factors for septic arthritis.

1. Previously injured joint
2. Recent trauma
3. Compromised immune system (e.g., as a result of diabetes, pharmacologic therapy, advanced age, or intravenous drug abuse)
4. Rheumatoid arthritis

List the six most common pathogens associated with septic arthritis.

1. *S. aureus*
2. Group A β-hemolytic *Streptococcus*
3. *H. influenzae* (most commonly introduced by trauma)
4. *Neisseria gonorrhoeae* (most common in young adults)
5. Gram-negative organisms (most common in immunocompromised patients)
6. *Mycoplasma* species (most common in immunosuppressed patients)

What are the signs and symptoms of septic arthritis?

1. Local erythema, heat, and swelling
2. Pain (even to passive motion)
3. Arthritis in the sternoclavicular and sacroiliac joints (in patients who abuse intravenous drugs)

Which diagnostic studies can be used to confirm a diagnosis of septic arthritis?

1. Joint aspiration (look for pus and submit the sample for culture, Gram stain, and joint fluid analysis)
2. Radiographic evaluation (e.g., plain film radiograph, bone scan)

What is the treatment for septic arthritis?

1. Aspiration to decompress the joint
2. Administration of intravenous antibiotics
3. Surgical incision, débridement, and drainage if the infection is in the hip, shoulder, or vertebral joints

PARASITIC INFECTIONS

Who is most susceptible to parasitic infections in the United States?

1. Children
2. Immigrants
3. Travelers

4. Immunosuppressed patients
5. Institutionalized patients

SCABIES

What is scabies?

A hypersensitivity reaction that occurs when the female mite, *Sarcoptes scabiei*, burrows into the skin and lays its eggs

How is scabies contracted?

Via close contact with an infected individual or that person's dirty bedding

When do symptoms appear?

Approximately 1 month after infestation

What is the hallmark clinical manifestation of scabies?

Pruritus (may be severe)

What areas of the body are most affected by scabies?

1. The interdiginous areas (i.e., between the fingers)
2. The wrists
3. The buttocks
4. The abdomen
5. The penis
6. The breasts (in women)

What areas of the body are spared from scabies?

The head and neck

How is scabies diagnosed?

Clinically, pruritus and skin lesions will be evident in typically affected areas. Microscopically, a scraping obtained from a skin burrow will reveal mites.

What is the treatment for scabies?

Application of permethrin 5% cream (contraindicated in pregnant women) and laundering of all clothes and linens in hot water

PEDICULOSIS

List the three types of lice.

1. Pediculosis corporis (body lice)
2. Pediculosis capitis (head lice)
3. Pediculosis pubis (pubic lice, "crabs")

Who is most likely to be affected by:

Pediculosis corporis?

People who live in overcrowded conditions or are homeless

Pediculosis capitis?   School-age children

Pediculosis pubis?   Adults with multiple sexual contacts

What is the hallmark clinical manifestation of pediculosis?   Pruritus (may be severe)

How is pediculosis diagnosed?   Clinically; lice eggs (i.e., nits) will be evident at the base of the hair shaft in affected areas.

What is the treatment for:

Pediculosis corporis?   All clothes and linens should be laundered in hot water. If nits are found in the body hair, then topical treatment with permethrin is recommended.

Pediculosis capitis and pediculosis pubis?   All clothes and linens should be laundered in hot water. A permethrin cream rinse is applied, allowed to remain on the affected area for 10 minutes, and then washed away. A solution of 8% formic acid is applied, left in for 10 minutes, and then washed out. The hair is then combed using a special comb for the removal of nits.

HELMINTHIC INFECTIONS

What is the hallmark of helminthiasis?   Eosinophilia. All helminth infections are characterized by eosinophilia, which is, unfortunately, a nonspecific finding.

Enterobius vermicularis infestation (pinworms)

What is *Enterobius vermicularis?*   A small, white intestinal nematode that averages 3–10 mm in length

Is pinworm infestation common?   Yes, it is the most common helminth infection in the United States.

How is *Enterobius vermicularis* transmitted?   By the fecal-oral route (i.e., ingestion or inhalation of eggs)

What is the classic symptom of pinworm infestation?   Intense pruritus in the anal region at night (pruritus ani)

What causes pruritus ani?

After the eggs hatch in the large intestine and appendix, the worms mature and another life cycle begins. Pruritus ani results when the pregnant females migrate to the anus (usually at night) and deposit new eggs on the perianal skin.

Name two ways pinworm infestation can be diagnosed.

1. **Cellophane tape test:** This test is best performed in the morning, before the patient has bathed or used the toilet. The patient should be asked to place the sticky side of the tape on the perianal area to obtain a sample. Examination of the tape under a microscope reveals eggs that resemble coffee beans.
2. **Flashlight test:** Adult worms may be visible in the perianal region at night.

What is the treatment for pinworm infestation?

Administration of a single dose of mebendazole, albendazole, or pyrantel pamoate is effective. All members of the patient's household should be treated for infestation, and all clothing and linens should be laundered in hot water to kill any remaining eggs.

Ascaris lumbricoides infestation (ascariasis)

What is *Ascaris lumbricoides*?

A large nematode (e.g., 200–300 mm long by 4–5 mm wide) that tends to take up residence in the ileum

How is *A. lumbricoides* transmitted?

Fecal–oral route

What is important to remember about the life cycle of *A. lumbricoides*?

The worms migrate from the gastrointestinal tract through the bloodstream, often to bizarre places.

What organs may be affected in ascariasis?

1. The biliary tree (associated with cholecystitis, ascending cholangitis, or pancreatitis)
2. The brain
3. The kidney
4. The eye
5. The lungs

What are the signs and symptoms of ascariasis?

Although infection is usually asymptomatic, pulmonary manifestations (e.g., cough, dyspnea, fever, hemoptysis), gastrointestinal manifestations (e.g., vague abdominal discomfort), or hematologic manifestations (e.g., fatigue as a result of anemia) may be noted.

How is acariasis diagnosed?   The large worms and their eggs are visible in the feces or vomitus.

What is the treatment for ascariasis?   Administration of albendazole, mebendazole, or pyrantel pamoate

What are the potential complications of ascariasis?

1. Worm migration to ectopic spots
2. Intestinal obstruction and volvulus
3. Growth retardation (as a result of malabsorption)

Ancylostoma species infestation (cutaneous larva migrans)

What is cutaneous larva migrans?   A localized skin infection caused by the burrowing larvae of *Ancylostoma caninum* (dog hookworm) or *Ancylostoma braziliense* (cat hookworm)

How are A. *caninum* and A. *braziliense* transmitted?   Through skin contact with contaminated soil

What is the clinical manifestation of cutaneous larva migrans?   A pruritic, serpiginous, creeping eruption, usually on the feet

What is the pharmacologic treatment for cutaneous larva migrans?   Albendazole or ivermectin

Strongyloides stercoralis infestation (strongyloidiasis)

What is *Strongyloides stercoralis?*   A threadworm with two life cycles (one that takes place within the human body and one that takes place in the soil)

Is strongyloidiasis common?   No. Sporadic cases have been reported in the Southeast region of the United States, and among immigrants.

What are the signs and symptoms of infestation with strongyloidiasis?   Infection is mostly asymptomatic, but patients may report pruritic dermatitis, diarrhea, weight loss, nausea, coughing, and hemoptysis.

What is the "hyperinfection syndrome?"

A flare-up of the *Strongyloides* infection owing to diminished host defenses (for example, as a result of steroids, chemotherapy, or malnutrition)

How is strongyloidiasis diagnosed?

A stool sample reveals ova and parasites. Serial specimens may be needed.

What is the treatment for strongyloidiasis?

Administration of ivermectin or thiabendazole

Trichinella spiralis infestation (trichinosis)

What is *Trichinella spiralis*?

A roundworm that burrows into the striated muscle

Is trichinosis common?

Yes, but a clinically apparent infection is rare in the United States.

How is trichinosis acquired?

By eating undercooked pork

What are the signs and symptoms of trichinosis?

1. **Early (1 week post-infection):** Diarrhea, nausea, vomiting, and crampy abdominal pain
2. **Later (1–2 months post-infection):** Myalgias and periorbital edema

List two laboratory studies that are useful for diagnosing trichinosis.

1. Eosinophil count
2. Creatine phosphokinase level

How is trichinosis definitively diagnosed?

Serologic tests [e.g., the bentonite flocculation test or enzyme-linked immunosorbent assay (ELISA)] become positive 3 weeks after infection. Histologic examination of a muscle biopsy sample may reveal larvae.

What is the treatment for trichinosis?

Mebendazole and prednisone can be administered. The mebendazole reduces the number of migrating larvae and kills encysting larvae, and the prednisone reduces the muscles' inflammatory response.

Tapeworm infestation

What is a tapeworm?

Tapeworms have a head (i.e., the scolex) and a flat, segmented body (the segments are called proglottids). Tapeworms attach to the intestinal wall via hooks or suckers on the scolex.

List the three most common types of tapeworms.

1. **Beef:** *Taenia saginata*
2. **Pork:** *Taenia solium*
3. **Fish:** *Diphyllobothrium latum*

How are tapeworms acquired?

By eating raw or undercooked meat or fish that contains the tapeworm larvae (cysticerci)

What is a complication of *Taenia solium* infestation?

Cysticercosis

What is cysticercosis?

Cysticercosis occurs when eggs hatch in the gastrointestinal tract and the embryos (i.e., oncospheres) burrow through the intestinal wall and into the blood vessels, where they are carried to distant locations such as the eyes and the brain. The oncospheres encyst in these distant locations to form cysticerci, a condition known as cysticercosis.

What is the most severe form of cysticercosis and what is its significance?

The larvae may go to the brain and cause neurocysticercosis, which is the primary cause of new-onset seizures in many parts of the world!

What are the signs and symptoms of tapeworm infestation?

Infection is usually asymptomatic, but the patient may complain of nausea and vague gastrointestinal complaints.

How are tapeworms diagnosed?

The tapeworm may be visible to the naked eye in the stool. Microscopic examination of a stool sample may reveal proglottids or eggs. ELISA is necessary to identify cysticercosis.

What drug is used to treat tapeworm infestation?

Praziquantel

MALARIA

What is malaria?

A mosquito-borne protozoan infection of the red blood cells (RBCs) caused by *Plasmodium* species

How is malaria transmitted?

Mosquitoes belonging to the genus *Anopheles* are the most common mode of transmission. Rarely, *Plasmodium* can be transmitted via blood transfusions, contaminated needles, or between a mother and a fetus.

Where is malaria endemic?

Latin America, Africa, Southeast Asia, East Asia, Oceania, and the Indian subcontinent

Has malaria ever been transmitted within the United States?

Yes, but very rarely (contained outbreaks have occurred).

List the four species of *Plasmodium* that can cause malaria.

1. *Plasmodium falciparum* (common)
2. *Plasmodium vivax* (common)
3. *Plasmodium ovale* (rare)
4. *Plasmodium malariae* (very rare)

Why is it important to diagnose the species of malaria?

P. falciparum is resistant to pharmacologic therapy and, as a result, is dangerous.

List the nine complications of untreated *P. falciparum* infection.

1. Severe anemia
2. Bleeding
3. Coagulopathy
4. Acidosis
5. Hypoglycemia
6. Coma
7. Seizures
8. Acute renal failure
9. Noncardiogenic pulmonary edema

What is important to remember about the life cycle of *Plasmodium vivax* and *Plasmodium ovale*?

P. vivax and *P. ovale* can lie dormant in the liver for many years and cause relapse.

What is the average incubation period following a bite from an infected mosquito?

12–15 days; longer for *P. malariae* infection

What are the pathognomonic symptoms of malaria?

There are none.

What are the symptoms of malaria?

Constitutional symptoms (e.g., fever, chills, malaise, fatigue, and myalgias) may be accompanied by nausea, vomiting, diarrhea, a sore throat, a cough, and abdominal or chest pain.

How common is the "classic" every-third-day cyclical fever?

Only one third of patients will have cyclical fever.

What else causes cyclical fevers?

Disorders such as relapsing fever (caused by *Borrelia recurrentis*), dengue fever (caused by an arbovirus), endocarditis, and brucellosis

What finding may be noted on physical examination?

Hepatosplenomegaly (sometimes)

What laboratory findings are associated with malaria?

Common nonspecific laboratory findings include a normochromic normocytic hemolytic anemia, an increased lactate dehydrogenase (LDH) level, a normal white blood cell (WBC) count with increased bands, and a low platelet count. Less common findings include increased levels of liver enzymes, high bilirubin levels, uremia, and hypoglycemia.

Is eosinophilia associated with malaria?

No.

Can the diagnosis of malaria be made on the basis of clinical findings?

No.

What test is necessary to definitively diagnose malaria?

Giemsa-staining of a blood smear

What is the sensitivity of this test?

95%–99%

What is the proper course of action if the first blood smear is negative?

Repeat the test with samples taken every 6 hours for 48 hours.

Is malaria curable?

Yes. If treated early, all cases of malaria should be 100% curable.

What is the treatment for malaria?

Nonresistant strains of *Plasmodium* are treated with chloroquinine. Other agents available for the treatment of malaria, depending on the clinical situation, include sulfadoxine-pyrimethamine, primaquine, mefloquine, and quinine, in various combinations. An infectious disease specialist should always be consulted, because the treatment approach depends on a variety of factors (e.g., the causative species, its drug resistance, the level of parasitemia and the degree of illness, whether the patient is pregnant, has a comorbid condition, or has allergies, and the patient's preexisting immunity).

Which patients require hospital admission for the treatment of malaria?

1. Patients who have been infected by *P. falciparum*
2. Patients who appear ill

List two methods of preventing malaria.

1. Patients should be advised to avoid mosquito bites when traveling to endemic areas by using a mosquito net and insect repellant.
2. Chemoprophylaxis can be prescribed; current recommendations for specific destinations can be obtained @ www.cdc.gov/travel.

TICK-BORNE DISEASE

List ten tick-borne diseases.

1. Lyme disease
2. Rocky mountain spotted fever (RMSF)
3. Ehrlichiosis
4. Tularemia
5. Ascending tick paralysis
6. Colorado tick fever
7. Relapsing fever
8. Babesiosis
9. Q Fever
10. Tick-borne encephalitis

How should ticks be removed from the skin?

By using forceps or tweezers

During which time of the year are tick bites most common?

April through September

LYME DISEASE

What organism causes Lyme disease?	*Borrelia burgdorferi* (a spirochete)
Which areas of the body are most often affected by Lyme disease?	The skin, brain, heart, and joints
Describe the epidemiology of Lyme disease.	Lyme disease is most common in those who live in the Northeast, Midwest, and Pacific regions of the United States. Men and children are affected more often than women because they are more likely to engage in activities that increase their exposure to ticks.
What proportion of people with Lyme disease remember being bitten by a tick?	Only one third of those bitten recall the bite!
What is the pathognomonic feature of the disease?	Erythema migrans (i.e., a painless, expanding annular erythematous lesion at the site of the tick bite that at its maximum, will be an average of 10 cm in diameter)
What percentage of people with Lyme disease have erythema migrans?	50%–80%
Describe the signs and symptoms of Lyme disease during:	
Stage I (1 week after the tick bite)	Erythema migrans, flu-like symptoms (e.g., fever, chills, general malaise, myalgias, and headache), secondary annular skin lesions similar to erythema migrans (seen in 50% of patients)
Stage II (weeks to months after the tick bite)	Systemic symptoms (e.g., general malaise, fatigue) are common. More severe neurologic manifestations (e.g., facial nerve palsy, meningoencephalitis, radiculopathy, neuropathy) and cardiac manifestations (e.g., conduction disturbances, myopericarditis) are much less common but may be seen.

Stage III (months to years after the tick bite)	Arthritis is very common—as many as 50% of all untreated patients develop arthritis that is usually monarticular and intermittent. The knee is the most commonly affected joint.
Can Bell's palsy be the initial presentation of Lyme disease?	Yes, and it may be bilateral!
List the diagnostic criteria for Lyme disease.	Either of the following findings are sufficient to diagnose Lyme disease: 1. Erythema migrans noted on a person living in an endemic area 2. Positive results on ELISA or IgM or IgG titers
When do serologic titers become positive?	It may take as many as 6 weeks for titers to become positive.
All equivocal and positive tests should be confirmed using what test?	A Western blot test
What is the treatment for:	
Stage I Lyme disease?	Administer doxycycline, 100 mg twice daily for 10–21 days (alternative drugs include amoxicillin, cefuroxime, and clarithromycin)
Stage II or III Lyme disease?	Administer intravenous ceftriaxone (or doxycycline, which recent studies suggest is probably as efficacious); temporary cardiac pacing may be necessary if the patient is experiencing conduction disturbances
Should patients with a history of a tick bite be started on doxycycline?	Probably not, even if they live in an endemic area

ROCKY MOUNTAIN SPOTTED FEVER (RMSF)

What is RMSF?	An acute, febrile tick-borne illness caused by *Rickettsia rickettsii*

In what region of the United States is RMSF most common?

Surprisingly, not the Rocky Mountains— RMSF occurs most commonly in the Southeast and mid-Atlantic regions of the United States.

How long does a tick need to be attached in order to transmit *R. rickettsii*?

Several hours

What is the incubation period for RMSF?

Approximately 1 week

What is the pathognomonic rash associated with RMSF?

There is none! The rash is nonspecific and may be confused with measles, viral exanthems, or meningococcemia.

What percentage of people do not develop a rash?

15%; some call the disease "Rocky Mountain spot*less* fever"

In patients who do develop a rash, when does the rash become apparent?

On day 4 of the illness, plus or minus 2 days

What is the appearance and progression of the typical rash?

The rash begins as a blanching macular rash at the wrists, palms, and ankles and spreads to involve the entire body in 6–12 hours. In approximately 4 days, the rash becomes petechial and may eventually coalesce and form large areas of purpura.

What are the other signs and symptoms of RMSF?

Patients generally appear ill, with an acute fever, headache, myalgias, nausea, and vomiting.

Can gastrointestinal symptoms be the most prominent?

Yes, but this would be uncommon.

How is RMSF diagnosed?

Clinically! No good diagnostic test for RMSF exists.

Is the clinical diagnosis difficult to make?

Yes, many of the clinical manifestations of RMSF are nonspecific. Therefore, RMSF should be on your differential list for any acute febrile illness.

What is the role of immunofluorescence skin biopsy in the diagnosis of RMSF?

Immunofluorescence skin biopsy may identify *R. rickettsii*. However, the rash must be biopsied and the sensitivity of this test is low.

What is the role of acute and convalescent antibody titers in the diagnosis of RMSF?

These titers are used to confirm the diagnosis only; they are not useful for making the initial diagnosis.

What laboratory findings are associated with RMSF?

Thrombocytopenia, left shift, and hyponatremia

What is the treatment for RMSF?

In patients with mild disease who do not appear to be ill, oral doxycycline is administered. Patients who appear ill require intravenous chloramphenicol.

Does early treatment affect patient outcome?

Yes! If untreated, RMSF can lead to organ damage and death; the mortality rate associated with untreated disease is approximately 35%.

What is the mortality rate associated with treated RMSF?

3%–6%

EHRLICHIOSIS

What is ehrlichiosis?

A rickettsial disease caused by *Ehrlichia chaffeensis* that is similar to RMSF, but without the rash

What is the difference between the two types of ehrlichiosis?

One type infects monocytes, and the other invades granulocytes.

Where in the United States is ehrlichiosis most prevalent?

The south-Central and south-Atlantic regions

What is the incubation period?

Approximately 10 days

What are the signs and symptoms of ehrlichiosis?

Patients experience the sudden onset of fever, chills, myalgias, nausea, vomiting, and headache.

What are the laboratory findings associated with ehrlichiosis?

Liver function tests are abnormal. The WBC and platelet counts are decreased.

How is ehrlichiosis diagnosed?

Polymerase chain reaction (PCR) has a sensitivity of 80%. A peripheral blood smear may also be diagnostic, although this test is much less sensitive.

How is the diagnosis of ehrlichiosis confirmed?

Acute and convalescent titers should be obtained to confirm the diagnosis.

How is ehrlichiosis treated?

With doxycycline or tetracycline (note, chloramphenicol should not be administered to these patients)

TULAREMIA

What organism causes tularemia?

The Gram-negative rod, *Francisella tularensis*

In which geographical location is tularemia prevalent?

It occurs most commonly in the Midwest region of the United States.

Is tularemia only spread by tick bites?

No, it is also spread via contact with rabbits, soil, fomites, flies, and mosquitoes.

Describe the three types of tularemia, and the clinical manifestations associated with each.

The clinical manifestations of tularemia depend on the bacterium's portal of entry into the body:
1. **Ulceroglandular tularemia** occurs in 85% of patients and is characterized by the development of a cutaneous ulcer approximately 4 days after the disease is contracted. Patients have regional lymphadenopathy and constitutional symptoms.
2. **Typhoidal tularemia** occurs in 10% of patients and is characterized by fever, chills, nausea, vomiting, gastrointestinal complaints, and fatigue.
3. **Pulmonary tularemia** is rare and characterized by symptoms similar to those of other bacterial pneumonias. The mortality rate associated with untreated pulmonary tularemia is as high as 30%.

How is tularemia diagnosed?

Usually, the diagnosis can be made on the basis of the clinical scenario. Blood cultures and acute and convalescent titers should be ordered.

What drug is used to treat tularemia?	Streptomycin

TICK PARALYSIS

What is tick paralysis?	An ascending paralysis, seen most often in children and domestic animals, that results from prolonged attachment (i.e., 4–7 days) of a female tick, usually of the species *Dermacentor andersoni,* and the subsequent elaboration of a neurotoxin
In what region is tick paralysis most common?	The Pacific Northwest (e.g., Oregon, British Columbia)
Can tick paralysis be fatal?	Yes, secondary to respiratory compromise
What disorder is a differential diagnosis for tick paralysis?	Guillain-Barré syndrome
What is the treatment for tick paralysis?	Removal of the tick should lead to resolution of the disorder.

HIV INFECTION AND AIDS

When should an HIV test be performed in the ED?	Probably never! By law, patients require proper counseling and follow-up. This type of follow-up is not feasible in an ED setting.
How many people in the United States are thought to be infected with HIV?	Approximately 1–1.5 million
What is the difference between "HIV-positive status" and "AIDS"?	A person with AIDS is infected with HIV and has an AIDS-defining illness, whereas a patient who is "HIV-positive" is infected with HIV but has not yet developed an AIDS-defining illness. The AIDS-defining illnesses are:

1. A CD4 count of less than 200 cells/μl
2. Candidiasis (esophageal, bronchial, tracheal, or pulmonary)
3. Disseminated coccidioidomycosis
4. Extrapulmonary cryptococcoses
5. Chronic cryptosporidiosis
6. Cytomegalovirus (CMV) infection

(except that involving the liver, spleen, or lymph nodes) or CMV retinitis

7. Central nervous system (CNS) toxoplasmosis
8. Chronic herpes simplex virus (HSV) infection (i.e., ulcers, bronchitis, pneumonitis, or esophagitis)
9. Disseminated histoplasmosis
10. Disseminated *Mycobacterium avium-intracellulare* (MAI) complex infection
11. Pulmonary tuberculosis
12. *Pneumocystis carinii* pneumonia (PCP)
13. Recurrent pneumonia
14. Isosporiasis
15. *Salmonella* sepsis
16. Kaposi's sarcoma
17. Lymphoma (primary lymphoma of the CNS, Burkitt's lymphoma, or large cell, immunoblastic lymphoma)
18. Invasive cervical cancer
19. HIV encephalopathy
20. Progressive multifocal leukoencephalopathy (PML)
21. AIDS wasting syndrome

What is the significance of a patient's CD4 count?

It may predict the risk a patient has for acquiring opportunistic infections.

What infections are common in patients with:

CD4 counts of 200–500 cells/µl?

1. Community-acquired pneumonia
2. Tuberculosis
3. Oral or vaginal candidiasis
4. Oral hairy leukoplakia
5. Varicella-zoster virus infection (herpes zoster)

CD4 counts of 50–200 cells/µl?

1. PCP
2. *Cryptosporidium* infection
3. *Microsporidia* infection
4. Disseminated HSV or varicella-zoster virus infection
5. Toxoplasmosis
6. *Cryptococcus* infection
7. Coccidiomycosis

CD4 counts of less than 50 cells/μl?	1. Primary lymphoma of the CNS 2. MAI complex infection 3. CMV retinitis
What is the most common bacterial infection in patients with AIDS?	MAI complex infection
What is a "viral load?"	The level of viral RNA in the blood
How is tracking the viral load helpful in the management of a patient with HIV?	Monitoring the viral load helps predict the rate of disease progression (a high viral load means a faster progression to AIDS) and assists the clinician in deciding when to initiate antiretroviral therapy.

What is considered a:

High viral load?	More than 30,000–50,000 copies/ml
Moderate viral load?	10,000–30,000 copies/ml
Low viral load?	10,000 or fewer copies/ml
What are the classes of antiretroviral agents?	1. Reverse transcriptase inhibitors (e.g., zidovudine, didanosine, lamivudine) 2. Protease inhibitors (e.g., indinavir, saquinavir, ritonavir)
When should antiretroviral therapy be considered?	When the viral load is in the moderate range (i.e., 10,000–30,000 copies/ml)
When should antiretroviral therapy be initiated?	1. When a qualified infectious disease specialist gives a recommendation 2. Usually when the patient's CD4 count is less than 500 cells/μl, and certainly when it is less than 200 cells/μl 3. When the viral load is greater than 30,000 copies/ml
What is the risk of contracting HIV from a needle-stick injury?	Approximately 1 in 250 healthcare workers will become infected with HIV following a needle-stick injury.
List four needle-stick injuries that would be considered high risk.	1. Injury caused by a large-bore needle 2. Injury with a grossly contaminated needle or one previously used for intravenous access

3. Injury that results in a deep penetrating wound
4. Injury with a needle contaminated by a patient with a known high viral load

What constitutes a moderate-risk exposure?

1. Injury caused by a small-bore or solid core needle
2. Injury that results in a superficial wound

Who should receive post-exposure prophylaxis?

All people who have experienced a high- or moderate-risk exposure are candidates for post-exposure prophylaxis. However, prophylaxis should be offered to anyone who has been percutaneously exposed to body fluids (except urine).

What is the treatment for occupational exposure to HIV?

Generally, patients receive reverse transcriptase inhibitors (zidovudine and lamivudine), but a protease inhibitor (e.g., saquinavir, ritonavir, indinavir) may also be administered if the patient has had a high-risk exposure.

List three common causes of fever in HIV-positive patients.

1. Body's response to initial infection with HIV
2. Opportunistic infection
3. Neoplasia

What evaluations should be considered in a febrile patient who is known to be infected by HIV?

1. History (including the patient's CD4 count) and physical examination
2. Chest x-ray, possibly sinus imaging
3. Laboratory studies, including a CBC with differential, a serum biochemistry panel, liver function tests, urinalysis, and a serum cryptococcal antigen level
4. Blood, urine, and cerebrospinal fluid (CSF) cultures

List the criteria for discharging an HIV patient with a fever.

1. No serious cause for the fever is discovered.
2. The patient is ambulatory and able to tolerate oral medication.
3. The patient is compliant and reliable, and follow-up is planned.

Why is diarrhea a significant occurrence in patients with HIV infection?

In as many as 90% of patients, diarrhea is a significant factor contributing to morbidity and AIDS wasting syndrome.

Which agents typically cause diarrhea in HIV-infected patients?

The usual organisms (i.e., *Salmonella* species, *Shigella* species, *Campylobacter* species, *Escherichia coli, Giardia lamblia, Entamoeba histolytica,* viruses), are often implicated, as well as opportunistic infections (e.g., *Cryptosporidium* species, *Microsporida* species, *Isospora* species) and HIV itself.

What is the significance of diarrhea caused by *Cryptosporidium* species?

The prolonged, watery diarrhea caused by *Cryptosporidium* species is very common and may lead to AIDS wasting syndrome because currently, there is no effective therapy.

What laboratory studies are important when evaluating an HIV-infected patient with diarrhea?

1. Fecal leukocytes or stool guaiac testing
2. Fecal testing for ova and parasites (O&P)
3. Stool culture
4. Serum chemistry and electrolytes (in patients with significant diarrhea)

How should an HIV-infected patient with diarrhea be managed in the ED?

1. Determine the need for hospital admission, which is based on the patient's hydration status, her ability to take oral drugs, and the likelihood that she will comply with follow-up examinations.
2. Initiate fluid and electrolyte replacement, if necessary.
3. Initiate empiric antibiotic therapy with fluoroquinolone if the patient has inflammatory diarrhea.
4. Educate the patient about the need for follow-up for culture results and re-evaluation.

ASSOCIATED NEUROLOGIC DISORDERS

In an HIV-infected patient with neurologic signs or a fever of unknown origin, which CSF studies are indicated?

1. Routine cell count and protein and glucose levels
2. Culture to isolate aerobic and anaerobic organisms, *Mycobacterium* species, and fungi
3. Gram and acid-fast staining
4. Cryptococcal antigen serum

agglutination test or an India ink preparation
5. *Toxoplasma* antigen
6. Coccidiomycosis titer (in endemic areas)

What is the differential diagnosis of a ring-enhancing lesion on a head CT scan?

CNS toxoplasmosis versus CNS lymphoma

What are the CT characteristics of:

CNS toxoplasmosis?

1. Multiple, small (i.e., <2.5 cm in diameter) lesions
2. Predilection for basal ganglia

CNS lymphoma?

CNS lymphomas usually appear as a single, large (i.e., > 3 cm in diameter) lesion.

What is the best imaging modality for picking up multiple CNS lesions?

Magnetic resonance imaging (MRI)

What is the most common cause of CNS mass lesions in HIV-infected patients?

CNS toxoplasmosis

What is the second most common cause of a CNS mass lesion in HIV-infected patients?

CNS lymphoma

CNS toxoplasmosis

What is toxoplasmosis?

A disease caused by the ubiquitous protozoan *Toxoplasma gondii* that is transmitted to humans via contact with cat feces or undercooked meat

What are the clinical characteristics of CNS toxoplasmosis?

Signs and symptoms develop over several days and include fever, headache, seizures, and altered mental status.

How is CNS toxoplasmosis diagnosed?

CNS toxoplasmosis may be diagnosed presumptively (i.e., on the basis of the

patient's clinical presentation, results of
head CT scanning, and response to
empiric therapy) or via brain biopsy.
Brain biopsy is a last resort.

**Do serologic tests help make
this diagnosis?**

No.

**What is the indication for
treatment?**

Strong clinical suspicion of CNS
toxoplasmosis

**What is the treatment for
CNS toxoplasmosis?**

CNS toxoplasmosis is treated with the
administration of pyrimethamine, folic
acid, and sulfadiazine. Consider another
diagnosis if there is no response in 10–14
days.

**Is relapse of CNS toxoplas-
mosis likely?**

Yes, all treated patients must receive
ongoing prophylaxis to prevent relapse.

CNS lymphoma

**How is CNS lymphoma
diagnosed?**

CNS lymphoma is definitively diagnosed
by brain biopsy. Suggestive radiographic
characteristics and failure of empiric
therapy against infectious agents suggest
a need for biopsy.

**What is the treatment for
CNS lymphoma?**

Radiation therapy

AIDS dementia

What is AIDS dementia?

Impairment of cognitive, motor, and
behavioral function secondary to long-
term HIV infection

**How is AIDS dementia
diagnosed?**

AIDS dementia is a diagnosis of
exclusion! Reversible CNS problems
must be ruled out before making this
diagnosis.

Is AIDS dementia common?

Yes, it is the most common neurologic
problem in patients with AIDS.

**What findings are seen on
CT scans in patients with
AIDS dementia?**

1. Cortical atrophy
2. Large ventricles
3. Subcortical and diffuse parenchymal
   lesions

What is the treatment for AIDS dementia?	None, but antiretroviral therapy may delay the onset of dementia.

Cryptococcal meningitis

What is cryptococcal meningitis?	An opportunistic CNS infection that may be focal or diffuse and is seen in as many as 10% of AIDS patients
What are the signs and symptoms of cryptococcal meningitis?	Fever, headache, altered mental status, seizures, cranial nerve palsies
How is cryptococcal meningitis diagnosed?	Positive results on an India ink preparation, fungal culture, or cryptococcal antigen serum agglutination test
What is the treatment for cryptococcal meningitis?	Cryptococcal meningitis is treated with amphotericin B and, possibly, flucytosine. Lifelong prophylaxis is required.

ASSOCIATED OPHTHALMOLOGIC DISORDERS

What is the key to managing HIV-positive patients with visual or eye complaints?	All HIV-positive patients with visual or eye complaints should be referred to an ophthalmologist immediately.
What disease can cause rapid, permanent blindness?	CMV retinitis
How is CMV retinitis diagnosed?	Fundoscopy demonstrates fluffy exudates and perivascular hemorrhages.
What drug is used to treat CMV retinitis?	Ganciclovir
Is prophylaxis indicated for CMV retinitis?	Yes, all patients with a history of CMV retinitis should receive prophylactic therapy against recurrences.

ASSOCIATED GASTROINTESTINAL DISORDERS

Is oropharyngeal candidiasis (thrush) common?	Yes, as many as 80% of patients with HIV infection develop oropharyngeal candidiasis at some point.
Is oropharyngeal candidiasis an AIDS-defining illness?	No, oropharyngeal candidiasis is not an AIDS-defining illness, although other

forms of candidiasis (e.g., esophageal candidiasis) are. Oropharyngeal candidiasis indicates immunosuppression and possible progression to AIDS.

How is oropharyngeal candidiasis diagnosed?

Clinically; white plaques are visible in the oropharynx. A potassium hydroxide (KOH) preparation can be obtained if the diagnosis is in question.

What condition must be differentiated from oropharyngeal candidiasis?

Oral hairy leukoplakia (lesions are usually limited to the sides of the tongue)

What is the treatment for oropharyngeal candidiasis?

Administration of clotrimazole, fluconazole, or nystatin

What does oropharyngeal candidiasis accompanied by dysphagia suggest?

Esophageal candidiasis until proven otherwise

What are the clinical manifestations of esophageal candidiasis?

Dysphagia, oropharyngeal plaques, and a CD4 count of less than 100 cells/μl

What is the treatment for esophageal candidiasis?

Administration of oral fluconazole or ketoconazole

What alternative diagnosis should be considered if the treatment fails?

Herpes or CMV esophagitis

ASSOCIATED CUTANEOUS DISORDERS

What skin conditions are common in patients with AIDS?

1. Xerosis, which is characterized by dry skin with pruritus
2. Seborrheic dermatitis
3. Psoriasis and atopic dermatitis
4. Opportunistic infections, including bacillary angiomatosis, staphylococcal infections (e.g., folliculitis, impetigo, abscesses), molluscum contagiosum, varicella-zoster virus and HSV infections
5. Kaposi's sarcoma

Kaposi's sarcoma

What is Kaposi's sarcoma?

Kaposi's sarcoma, the most common malignancy in patients with AIDS, is characterized by purple, non-blanching, **painless** patches on the skin, viscera, and mucus membranes.

What causes Kaposi's sarcoma?

The development of Kaposi's sarcoma, which is most common among the homosexual population, may be associated with herpes virus coinfection.

What is the typical course of disease progression?

There is none.

When does Kaposi's sarcoma become a problem?

1. When it becomes a cosmetic issue
2. When it affects the viscera, such as the lungs (where it may cause hemothorax)

What is the treatment for Kaposi's sarcoma?

No treatment is indicated if the patient is asymptomatic or cosmetic concerns are not an issue. Local treatment is achieved through the administration of vinblastine and liquid nitrogen. Systemic chemotherapy is not very effective and may worsen the patient's immune status.

Varicella–zoster virus and herpes simplex virus (HSV) infections

Why are varicella-zoster virus and HSV infections significant in patients with HIV infection?

These infections are much more common and aggressive in patients with HIV infection, as opposed to the rest of the population.

What is the treatment for:

Mild varicella-zoster virus or HSV infection?

Oral acyclovir (or a similar antiviral agent)

Severe varicella-zoster virus or HSV infection?

Intravenous acyclovir

ASSOCIATED RESPIRATORY DISORDERS

Pneumocystis carinii pneumonia (PCP)

What is PCP?

A type of pneumonia caused by a fungus, PCP is the most common opportunistic infection in patients with AIDS.

What are the signs and symptoms of PCP?

1. Insidious onset of fever, dyspnea, and a nonproductive cough

	2. Systemic symptoms, such as fatigue, general malaise, and weight loss
How is PCP diagnosed?	1. Patient history 2. Chest x-ray 3. Induced sputum or bronchoalveolar lavage 4. Laboratory studies, including an LDH level and a CD4 count 5. Arterial blood gases (ABGs)
What would be the expected findings on laboratory testing?	An elevated serum LDH level (i.e., greater than 450 U/L) and a depressed CD4 count (almost always less than 200 cells/μl)
What would be the expected ABG findings?	Severe hypoxemia (i.e., a PaO_2 of less than 70 mm Hg) and an elevated alveolar–arterial (A–a) gradient
What are the typical chest x-ray findings?	Bilateral diffuse interstitial infiltrates
What percentage of patients with PCP have a normal chest x-ray?	10%
Should empiric treatment for PCP be started in the ED?	Yes, especially if the infection is severe.
Is it important to establish a definitive diagnosis?	Yes, because the treatment for PCP may have serious side effects.
What is the treatment for PCP?	Trimethoprim-sulfamethoxazole is the drug of choice. For patients who are allergic to trimethoprim-sulfamethoxazole, pentamidine or atovaquone may be used instead. Intravenous administration may be necessary.
When are steroids indicated?	Patients with severe disease and an arterial oxygen tension (PaO_2) of less than 70 mm Hg should receive steroids.
What are the indications for initiating prophylactic therapy?	1. A CD4 count of less than 200 cells/μl 2. A history of PCP

What drugs are used for prophylaxis?	1. Trimethoprim-sulfamethoxazole
	2. Dapsone or pentamidine (for patients who are allergic to trimethoprim-sulfamethoxazole)

Community–acquired pneumonia

Is the incidence of community-acquired pneumonia increased in patients with HIV?	Yes.
What are the signs and symptoms of community-acquired pneumonia?	Patients complain of fever, chills, a productive cough, dyspnea, fatigue, and general malaise. The onset of symptoms is usually more abrupt in patients with HIV infection, as opposed to the general population.
What findings would be expected on laboratory testing and imaging studies?	Leukocytosis with increased bands and an abnormal chest x-ray
What is the differential diagnosis for community-acquired pneumonia in an HIV-positive patient?	PCP and tuberculosis

Tuberculosis

What is tuberculosis?	An infectious disease caused by *Mycobacterium tuberculosis,* a hardy, acid-fast bacterium. Tuberculosis is quite common, even in mildly immuno-suppressed individuals.
Who is most likely to contract tuberculosis?	Although everyone is susceptible, tuberculosis is most common in HIV-positive patients with CD4 counts of less than 500 cells/μl, patients who are institutionalized, patients who abuse intravenous drugs, homeless patients, and close contacts of people with tuberculosis.
What are the signs and symptoms of tuberculosis?	The clinical presentation may vary, but fever, night sweats, weight loss, cough, hemoptysis, dyspnea, and fatigue are common symptoms.

What does the chest x-ray of a patient with tuberculosis reveal?	Typically, apical and cavitary infiltrates are seen, although the findings may be atypical, especially in people with low CD4 counts. In these patients, infiltrates may be seen in the lower lobes. Lesions may be disseminated or miliary.
How is tuberculosis diagnosed?	1. Gram or carbolfuchsin staining and culture of a sputum sample or a sample obtained during bronchoalveolar lavage 2. Blood cultures 3. Biopsy (if other test results are negative)
Why is a purified protein derivative (PPD) test for tuberculosis not always useful?	Anergic patients can exhibit false-negative results.
What is considered a positive PPD test result?	An area of induration 5 mm or more in diameter
What is the treatment for tuberculosis?	A four-drug therapeutic regimen (i.e., isoniazid, rifampin, ethambutol, and pyrazinamide) is used to treat multi-drug–resistant strains of *M. tuberculosis.*
What is the usual response to treatment?	The response is usually similar to that in a patient who does not have HIV infection.

Mycobacterium avium-intracellulare (MAI) complex

What is MAI complex?	An opportunistic infection caused by the robust and ubiquitous *Mycobacterium avium-intracellulare,* an organism found in soil and water.
Which patients with AIDS are most susceptible to MAI complex infection?	Those with CD4 counts of less than 100 cells/μl; these patients require prophylactic therapy
What are the signs and symptoms of MAI complex infection?	Clinical manifestations are nonspecific (e.g., wasting, fatigue, fever, chills, night sweats, diarrhea, ill-defined abdominal pain).
How is MAI complex infection diagnosed?	1. Blood cultures (quite sensitive if the disease is disseminated)

2. Biopsy (common sites include lymph nodes, bone marrow, and the liver)

What is the treatment for MAI complex infection?

The infection is treated by administering clarithromycin, ethambutol, and rifampin. Patients who have had an MAI complex infection require lifetime suppressive therapy.

ASSOCIATED SEXUALLY TRANSMITTED DISEASES (STDS)

Does the presentation of syphilis differ in patients with HIV infection, as opposed to those without?

Yes, the infection is more aggressive and the presentation may be atypical.

What test should be performed in all patients with HIV infection and syphilis?

A lumbar puncture, to rule out neurosyphilis

Why is syphilis difficult to treat in HIV-infected patients?

These patients experience a high rate of treatment failure and relapse.

How does the treatment differ in the patient with HIV infection?

Higher doses of drugs and longer treatment periods may be required; current recommendations should be checked.

ASSOCIATED HEMATOLOGIC DISORDERS

List three common hematologic findings in patients with HIV infection.

1. Anemia
2. Leukopenia
3. Thrombocytopenia

What are the causes of hematologic complications in patients with HIV?

The causes are multifactorial and include the drugs used to treat the HIV infection, opportunistic infections, malnutrition, and the virus itself.

How are hematologic problems managed in patients with HIV infection?

1. Withdraw the offending agent, if possible.
2. If possible, treat any underlying causes (e.g., infection, malnutrition).
3. Consider blood transfusion, or therapy with granulocyte colony-stimulating factor (G-CSF)

ALLERGIC REACTIONS

What is a hypersensitivity reaction?	An exaggerated immune response to presented antigens
Name the four types of hypersensitivity reactions and the defining characteristics of each.	1. **Type I:** IgE-mediated; common allergens include penicillin and insect venom 2. **Type II:** Complement-induced target cell lysis and phagocytosis by killer cells; examples include transfusion reactions and hemolytic disease of the newborn 3. **Type III:** Antigen-antibody complexes activate platelets and IgE to form aggregates; examples include serum sickness and systemic lupus erythematosus (SLE) 4. **Type IV:** T cell-mediated; examples include the reaction to PPD
What is an anaphylaxis?	A severe hypersensitivity response leading to cardiovascular collapse and respiratory compromise
What are the most common causes of fatal anaphylaxis?	Parenteral administration of penicillin and Hymenoptera stings (e.g., bee stings)
What are the signs and symptoms of anaphylaxis?	**Cutaneous:** Erythema, pruritus, progressive urticaria, and angioedema **Respiratory:** Tightening of the throat or hoarseness, stridor, wheezing, and shortness of breath **Gastrointestinal:** Nausea, vomiting, and cramps **Cardiovascular:** Lightheadedness, tachycardia, hypotension, and dysrhythmias
List five differential diagnoses for anaphylaxis.	1. Pulmonary embolism 2. Myocardial infarction 3. Airway obstruction 4. Tension pneumothorax 5. Acute asthma
What is the treatment for hypersensitivity reactions and anaphylaxis?	1. Airway control 2. Administration of epinephrine 3. Establishment of intravenous access

4. Administration of intravenous fluids (colloid better than crystalloid)
5. Administration of glucocorticoids
6. Administration of antihistamines (H_1 and H_2 blockers)

When is hospital admission required?

Patients with significant hypersensitivity reactions or anaphylaxis (e.g., manifested by respiratory compromise or hypotension) require hospital admission.

What is the treatment if the patient is discharged to home?

Outpatient therapy entails the administration of antihistamines and glucocorticoids for 72 hours, and follow-up with the patient's primary healthcare provider within 24–48 hours.

What is an anaphylactoid reaction?

A nonimmunologically mediated reaction that manifests similarly to anaphylaxis

What is the most common cause of an anaphylactoid reaction?

Radiographic contrast media

What is the treatment for an anaphylactoid reaction?

The treatment is the same as that for anaphylaxis.

RHEUMATOLOGIC DISORDERS

ARTHRITIS

Why is joint aspiration a valuable diagnostic tool?

It permits one to accurately diagnose the cause of a patient's arthritis.

What are the relative contraindications to joint aspiration?

Cellulitis at the aspiration site, septicemia, and coagulopathy

Why is it important not to inject lidocaine into a joint?

It inhibits bacterial growth in the culture, which hampers diagnosis of the type of arthritis.

Crystal–induced synovitis (gout and pseudogout)

What is crystal-induced synovitis?

Inflammation of joint synovia caused by uric acid crystals (gout) or calcium pyrophosphate crystals (pseudogout)

In which patients is crystal-induced synovitis likely to be seen?

Crystal-induced synovitis is most common in middle-aged and elderly adults.

What are the risk factors for crystal-induced synovitis?

1. Stress
2. Trauma
3. Infection
4. Alcohol consumption
5. Starvation
6. Hyperalimentation
7. Some types of pharmacologic therapy

What are the signs and symptoms of crystal-induced synovitis?

Patients complain of extreme pain in a joint, occurring over hours (in gout) or days (in pseudogout). The joint is swollen, inflamed, erythematous, warm, and tender to palpation.

What are tophi?

Lumpy deformities near the joint caused by the accumulation of urate crystals in patients with gout

Which joint is classically involved in crystal-induced synovitis?

The first metatarsophalangeal joint (however, any joint may be involved)

What condition must be differentiated from crystal-induced synovitis?

Septic arthritis

How is crystal-induced synovitis diagnosed?

By joint aspiration; crystals must be seen in WBCs in order to make the diagnosis

What do uric acid crystals look like when they are perpendicular to polarized light?

Needle-shaped and blue

What do calcium pyrophosphate crystals look like on light microscopy?

Rhomboid

Is a serum uric acid level helpful in making the diagnosis?

No, because high serum uric acid levels do not necessarily mean the arthritis is crystal induced, and conversely, if the uric acid level is normal, a crystal-induced arthritis is still possible.

What is the treatment for crystal-induced synovitis?	Crystal-induced synovitis is treated with nonsteroidal anti-inflammatory drugs (NSAIDs) and colchicine. If therapy does not result in improvement, reconsider a diagnosis of septic arthritis.

Rheumatoid arthritis

What are the risk factors for rheumatoid arthritis?

1. Native American race
2. Female gender
3. Family history of the disease
4. Age between 30 and 60 years

Which joints are most often affected in rheumatoid arthritis?

1. Metacarpophalangeal joints
2. Wrists
3. Knees
4. Elbow

What are the signs and symptoms of rheumatoid arthritis?

1. Joint swelling
2. Joint pain on passive motion
3. Morning stiffness that persists for more than 1 hour
4. Fatigue, depression, and malaise
5. 3+ symmetric joints
6. Subcutaneous rheumatoid nodules

How is rheumatoid arthritis diagnosed?

Diagnosis is mostly clinical, but supported by radiographic and laboratory studies.

What condition must be ruled out before a diagnosis of rheumatoid arthritis is made?

Septic arthritis

Which laboratory findings are commonly associated with rheumatoid arthritis?

A CBC commonly reveals anemia, and the ESR is increased.

What findings are typical on joint fluid analysis?

Those consistent with an inflammatory arthritis: a WBC count of 10,000–100,000 cells/mm^3 and 50%–90% polymorphonuclear neutrophils (PMNs).

Are plain film radiographs helpful for making the diagnosis?

Radiography is not helpful in making the diagnosis, but it will rule out other causes of joint swelling if there is doubt.

What is the treatment for rheumatoid arthritis?

Initial therapy is with NSAIDs. Eventually, therapy with gold, anti-malarial agents, or immunosuppressive agents may be necessary, or surgery may be attempted.

What are emergent complications of rheumatoid arthritis?

Respiratory: Arthritic fixing of the cricoarytenoid cartilages in a closed position, pleurisy

Cardiovascular: Pericarditis, intervalvular rheumatoid nodules

Endocrine: Adrenal insufficiency crisis follow the sudden cessation of chronic steroid medications

Ocular: Scleritis (painful, purple, poor vision), episcleritis (painless, pink, perfect vision)

Musculoskeletal: Atlantoaxial subluxation secondary to pannus formation and destruction of the supporting ligaments (an atlantodental distance of more than 3.5 mm on a lateral view suggests cervical spine instability)

What is pannus?

An inflammatory invasive exudate that attacks the underlying joint synovia and is often seen in patients with rheumatoid arthritis

What is Lhermitte's sign?

A lightning-like sensation that radiates down the back on neck extension, indicating cervical spine instability

How is the airway managed in patients experiencing cervical spine instability or respiratory problems as a complication of rheumatoid arthritis?

In an emergency, all patients with a stiff or arthritic neck and a history of rheumatoid arthritis should be assumed to have atlantoaxial instability, which requires C spine immobilization during intubation. Patients with "frozen" cricoarytenoids require tracheostomy.

Osteoarthritis

What are the risk factors for osteoarthritis?

1. Obesity
2. Age > 50 years
3. Injury to joint
4. Prolonged stress (e.g., as a result of an occupation or participation in a sport)

Which joints are most likely to be affected in osteo-arthritis?	1. Distal interphalangeal joints 2. Proximal interphalangeal joints 3. Knees
What are the signs and symptoms of osteoarthritis?	1. Joint pain following use of the joint 2. "Gelling" (i.e., stiffness that persists for more than 15 minutes in the morning, or after sitting) 3. Decreased range of motion 4. Crepitation (seen in advanced disease) 5. Tenderness (may or may not be present)
What are Heberden's nodes?	Small, hard nodules that form at the distal interphalangeal joints in patients with interphalangeal osteoarthritis
What results are seen on joint fluid analysis in patients with osteoarthritis?	Noninflammatory results (i.e., a WBC count of 200–10,000 cells/mm^3, fewer than 25% PMNs)
What radiographic findings are typical in osteoarthritis?	1. Narrowed joint spaces 2. Osteophyte formation 3. Subchondral bony sclerosis and cysts
What is the treatment for osteoarthritis?	Physical therapy is indicated. Patients should be advised that weight loss (if they are overweight) and maintaining general fitness can help alleviate symptoms. The application of heat and the administration of acetaminophen and NSAIDs can provide immediate symptomatic relief.

SYSTEMIC LUPUS ERYTHEMATOSUS (SLE)

What is SLE?	An idiopathic, multisystemic autoimmune inflammatory condition
What are the risk factors for SLE?	1. Female gender (women are affected more than men, 10:1) 2. Black, Hispanic, Asian, or Native American race 3. Family history of the disease 4. Age between 30 and 50 years
What are the signs and symptoms of SLE?	1. Arthritis 2. Fever 3. Butterfly-shaped rash over the face (malar rash)

4. Oral ulcers
5. Malaise
6. Weight loss
7. Nausea, vomiting, and diarrhea
8. Chest pain
9. Shortness of breath
10. Psychosis or delirium

What emergent complications are associated with SLE?

Respiratory: Pleurisy, pulmonary hemorrhage

Cardiovascular: Pericarditis, hypertension secondary to renal failure

Renal: Nephritis, renal vein thrombosis

Hematologic: Thrombocytopenia ($<100,000$ platelets/mm^3), leukopenia (<4000 leukocytes/mm^3), hemolytic anemia, and lymphopenia (<1500 lymphocytes/mm^3)

What laboratory studies can help to make the diagnosis of SLE?

1. CBC
2. Serum antinuclear antibodies (ANA) level
3. ESR
4. Urinalysis
5. Creatinine level
6. Coombs' test

How can symptomatic relief of the arthritis in SLE be achieved?

Administration of NSAIDs

9

Hematologic, Oncologic, and Post-Transplant Emergencies

BLOOD TRANSFUSION AND COMPONENT THERAPY

How long does it take to get:

ABO group– and Rh type–specific blood?	10–15 minutes
Cross-matched blood?	30–60 minutes

What type of blood is used emergently?

Type O

What complications can be associated with blood transfusion and component therapy?

1. Infection
2. Hemolytic reaction
3. Hypervolemia
4. Hypothermia
5. Noncardiogenic pulmonary edema
6. Electrolyte imbalance
7. Graft-versus-host disease (GVHD)

BLOOD PRODUCTS

Whole blood

What is whole blood?

One unit is 435–500 ml of blood, including red blood cells (RBCs), platelets, plasma, and cryoprecipitate with a preservative/anticoagulant agent [citrate phosphate dextrose adenine (CPDA-1)].

What are the indications for using whole blood?

Whole blood is rarely used, but may have a very limited role in managing the patient who needs urgent volume in addition to RBCs. However, crystalloid and packed red blood cells (PRBCs) are preferred.

What are the advantages of using whole blood?

Whole blood provides volume and oxygen-carrying capacity with clotting factors.

What are the disadvantages of using whole blood?

1. Difficult to obtain (rarely available)
2. Low levels of clotting factors
3. Exposes patient to many antigens
4. Risk of volume overload prior to replenishing needed components

Packed red blood cells (PRBCs)

What are PRBCs?

PRBCs are obtained by centrifuging whole blood. One unit of PRBCs contains approximately 200 ml of RBCs suspended in 50–75 ml of plasma.

What is the shelf life of PRBCs?

35–42 days at 4°C, depending on which additives were used

How much should each unit of PRBCs raise the hemoglobin level (hematocrit)?

1 g/dl (3%)

What are the indications for using PRBCs?

Conditions characterized by an inadequate oxygen-carrying capacity (e.g., significant acute hemorrhage, surgical blood loss, chronic anemia)

What advantages are associated with the use of PRBCs?

1. Reduced risk of volume overload
2. Decreased risk of alloimmunization, owing to exposure to fewer antigens (as compared with the exposure when whole blood is used)
3. Rapid restoration of oxygen-carrying capacity

What are the indications for using:

Leukocyte-poor PRBCs?

1. Transfusion in a transplant recipient or candidate for transplant therapy
2. Transfusion in a patient with a history

of prior febrile nonhemolytic transfusion reaction

3. Prevention of immunization against leukocytes in transplant or potential transplant patients

Frozen PRBCs?

1. Transfusion in a patient with a rare blood type (the long storage life of frozen PRBCs increases their availability)
2. Autotransfusion (i.e., storing of a patient's own blood in preparation for elective surgery)

Washed PRBCs?

1. Transfusion in a patient at risk for experiencing a hypersensitivity reaction to plasma [usually seen in immunoglobulin A (IgA)-deficient patients]
2. Neonatal transfusions
3. Transfusion in a patient with paroxysmal nocturnal hemoglobinuria (to avoid precipitation of hemolytic episodes)

Platelets

What is the shelf life of stored platelets?

5 days at 20°C–24°C

How are platelets administered?

Patients receive six random donor units or one plateletpheresis pack at a time (250–350 ml containing 4×10^{11} platelets)

How much should the platelet count increase following the administration of platelets?

50,000–60,000 platelets/μl

How long should transfused platelets survive?

3–5 days

What are the indications for platelet transfusion?

1. Platelet dysfunction that is causing excessive bleeding
2. Platelet count less than 50,000 cells/μl in patients undergoing major surgery or with significant bleeding
3. Platelet count of 10,000–50,000

cells/µl in patients who have sustained trauma, are undergoing an invasive procedure, or are experiencing spontaneous bleeding

4. Platelet count less than 10,000 cells/µl (these patients are at high risk for spontaneous hemorrhage)

Which patients may be refractory to platelet trans-fusion?

1. Patients with a consumptive coagulopathy
2. Patients with antibodies against platelets

Which patients require:

Rh-negative platelets?

Rh-negative women of childbearing age

Irradiated platelets?

Immunosuppressed patients

Fresh frozen plasma (FFP)

What is FFP?

The acellular component of separated whole blood

What is the shelf life of FFP?

1 year at −18°C

What is in FFP?

Each bag contains 200–250 ml of FFP, with 1 unit of each coagulation factor per milliliter of FFP and 1–2 mg of fibrinogen per milliliter of FFP

What is the typical dose of FFP?

Four to six units are usually necessary to provide 30% or more of the coagulation factors needed for hemostasis, thereby significantly improving the coagulation profile

What are the indications for using FFP?

1. Active bleeding in a patient with coagulopathy owing to acquired factor deficiency
2. Planned invasive procedure in a patient with significant prolongation of the PT, PTT, or both (i.e., 1.5 times normal) or a specific coagulation factor assay less than 25% of normal
3. Congenital isolated factor deficiency (when virally safe replacement factors are unavailable)

4. Thrombotic thrombocytopenic purpura (TTP)
5. Liver disease with bleeding
6. Acute DIC
7. Massive transfusion-induced coagulopathy and active bleeding
8. Antithrombin III deficiency when antithrombin III is unavailable

Cryoprecipitate

What is cryoprecipitate?

The cold precipitable protein fraction from FFP maintained at a temperature of 1°C–6°C. It contains factor VIIIc (80–120 units), von Willebrand factor (vWF; 80 units), fibrinogen (200–300 mg), factor XIII (40–60 units), and fibronectin (variable levels).

What is the shelf life of cryoprecipitate?

1 year, frozen

What is the typical dose of cryoprecipitate?

Two to four bags per 10 kg (usually 10–20 bags at a time)

What are the indications for using cryoprecipitate?

1. Hypofibrinogenemia (< 100 mg/dl)
2. von Willebrand disease with active bleeding when desmopressin is unavailable or does not work and factor VIII concentrate containing vWF is unavailable
3. Hemophilia A when factor VIII is unavailable

Albumin

What is albumin?

The major plasma protein

Albumin constitutes what percentage of the body's circulating protein?

50%

What is the function of albumin?

Albumin serves as a transport protein and is responsible for creating plasma oncotic pressure (75% of the pressure results from the presence of albumin in the plasma).

What are the indications for administering albumin?

Albumin has limited applications in the emergency department (ED); but may be used for colloid replacement and for large volume paracentesis in patients with refractory ascites.

Immunoglobulins

What are the indications for administering intravenous immunoglobulins?

Immunoglobulins have limited use in the ED, but may be used in patients with primary or secondary immunodeficiency or in patients with immune or inflammatory disorders.

What are the potential complications of administering immunoglobulins?

1. Anaphylaxis
2. Transient positive serologies owing to the passive transfer of antibodies

Antithrombin III

What is antithrombin III?

A serum protein with inhibitory effects on coagulation factors, thrombin, and activated factors IX, X, XI and XII

What are indications for administering antithrombin III?

Hereditary antithrombin III deficiency with thromboembolism

TRANSFUSION COMPLICATIONS

Acute hemolytic transfusion reaction

What causes an acute hemolytic transfusion reaction?

Transfusion of incompatible RBCs, usually in the ABO blood group system, results in RBC destruction.

What are the signs and symptoms of an acute hemolytic transfusion reaction?

1. Fever
2. Chills
3. Low back pain
4. Dyspnea
5. Burning sensation at the infusion site
6. Hypotension
7. Bleeding
8. Respiratory failure
9. Acute tubular necrosis (ATN)

What findings are typical on laboratory studies?

Findings consistent with intravascular hemolysis (e.g., hemolysis, hemoglobinemia, hemoglobinuria)

How should a patient with an acute hemolytic transfusion reaction be managed?	1. Immediately discontinue the transfusion. 2. Monitor the patient for shock and bleeding. 3. Administer fluids to maintain diuresis at a rate of at least 100 ml/hour.

Febrile nonhemolytic transfusion reaction

What is a febrile nonhemolytic transfusion reaction?	An antigen–antibody reaction involving plasma, platelets, or white blood cells (WBCs) transfused with RBCs
What are the signs and symptoms of a febrile nonhemolytic transfusion reaction?	Temperature increase of at least 1°C and chills
How should a patient who is experiencing a febrile nonhemolytic transfusion reaction be managed?	Stop the transfusion and assess for an acute hemolytic transfusion reaction by repeat cross-matching and Coombs' tests.

Allergic transfusion reaction

What is an allergic transfusion reaction?	An allergic reaction caused by exposure to plasma proteins (seen primarily in IgA-deficient patients)
What are the signs and symptoms of an allergic transfusion reaction?	1. Erythema 2. Urticaria 3. Pruritus 4. Bronchospasm 5. Vasomotor instability 6. Anaphylaxis
How should a patient who is experiencing an allergic transfusion reaction be managed?	Stop the transfusion and administer diphenhydramine.

Infection

What is the estimated risk of acquiring each of the following infections from a blood transfusion?	
HIV?	1 in 700,000 units

Hepatitis C virus?	1 in 103,000 units
Hepatitis B virus?	1 in 63,000 units
Human T-cell leukemia/ lymphoma virus (HTLV), type I or II?	1 in 640,000 units
Which infections can be, but rarely are, transmitted through blood transfusions?	Epstein-Barr virus (EBV) infection (infectious mononucleosis), syphilis, malaria, babesiosis, toxoplasmosis, and trypanosomiasis

ANEMIA

What are the criteria for diagnosing anemia in:	
Women?	Hemoglobin level less than 12 g/dl (i.e., a hematocrit less than 36%)
Men?	Hemoglobin level less than 14 g/dl (i.e., a hematocrit less than 42%)
What are the general causes of anemia?	Blood loss, decreased production of RBCs, or increased destruction of RBCs (hemolytic anemia)
What are the signs and symptoms of anemia?	Fatigue, headache, pallor, dyspnea, lightheadedness, orthostasis, hypotension, angina, tachycardia, and hypoxemia
What is the mean corpuscular volume (MCV)?	A measure of the average volume of the RBCs (normal is 90 ± 9 fl)
What is the red blood cell distribution width (RDW)?	A parameter that reflects the variations in RBC size (i.e., the degree of anisocytosis)
What is the mean corpuscular hemoglobin (MCH)?	A measure of the amount of hemoglobin in each RBC (normal is 32 ± 2 pg)
What is the mean corpuscular hemoglobin concentration (MCHC)?	A measure of the concentration of hemoglobin in each RBC (normal is 34 ± 2 g/dl)
Why is it necessary to perform a reticulocyte count?	To measure bone marrow activity

What is the formula for calculating the corrected reticulocyte percentage (CRP)?

$$CRP = \text{reticulocyte \%} \times \frac{\text{patient hematocrit}}{45}$$

Why is the CRP calculated?   To evaluate bone marrow response to anemia

ANEMIAS RESULTING FROM DECREASED OR DEFECTIVE RED BLOOD CELL (RBC) PRODUCTION

Iron deficiency anemia

In which patients is iron deficiency the most common cause of anemia?   Women of childbearing age

What can cause iron deficiency anemia?
1. Dietary deficiency
2. Menstruation
3. Pregnancy
4. Malabsorption
5. Chronic inflammatory states
6. Chronic blood loss (varices, peptic ulcer disease, malignancy, hemolysis)
7. Hookworm infestation

What are the signs and symptoms of iron deficiency anemia?
1. Glossitis
2. Pharyngeal webs
3. Nail spooning
4. Pallor
5. Fatigue
6. Weakness
7. Pica
8. Dyspnea
9. Splenomegaly

What laboratory findings are associated with iron deficiency anemia?
1. Hypochromic, microcytic anemia
2. Low MCV
3. Low MCH
4. High RDW
5. Low serum ferritin level
6. Low serum iron level
7. Elevated total iron-binding capacity (TIBC)

What is the serum ferritin level used to evaluate?   The body's stores of iron

What is the serum iron level used to evaluate?	The amount of iron bound to transferrin
What is the TIBC used to evaluate?	The amount of iron that can be bound to transferrin
What is the treatment of iron deficiency anemia?	Iron replacement and treatment of the underlying disorder

Sideroblastic anemia

What is sideroblastic anemia?	Anemia characterized by an increased total body iron level, hypochromia, and ringed sideroblasts in bone marrow
What is the differential diagnosis for sideroblastic anemia?	1. Hereditary sideroblastic anemia 2. Idiopathic refractory sideroblastic anemia 3. Refractory anemia with ringed sideroblasts 4. Drug therapy (e.g., isoniazid, chloramphenicol, ethyl alcohol) 5. Toxins 6. Lead poisoning 7. Malignancy
What are the signs and symptoms of sideroblastic anemia?	Patients exhibit signs of iron overload (e.g., splenomegaly), diabetes, and altered cardiac function
What laboratory findings are associated with sidero-blastic anemia?	1. Normochromic or hypochromic microcytic anemia, poikilocytes, target cells, and Pappenheimer bodies (iron deposits) 2. Reticulocyte production index of less than 2 3. High serum iron levels 4. Normal or low TIBC 5. High ferritin levels
What is the treatment for sideroblastic anemia?	Pyridoxine, which is most effective when treating the hereditary form

Megaloblastic anemia

What are the most common cause of megaloblastic anemia?	Folate and vitamin B_{12} deficiencies

What are the signs and symptoms of folate and vitamin B$_{12}$ deficiency?

1. Lethargy
2. Weakness
3. Waxy or yellow pallor
4. Dyspepsia
5. Smooth, pale tongue
6. Weight loss

What laboratory findings are associated with megaloblastic anemia?

1. Oval macrocytes
2. Howell-Jolly bodies
3. Hypersegmented neutrophils
4. High lactate dehydrogenase (LDH) levels
5. High MCV
6. High MCH
7. Normal MCHC

Folate deficiency

What can cause folate deficiency?

1. Poor nutrition
2. Malabsorption of folic acid in the proximal jejunum
3. Increased dietary requirements without compensatory intake
4. Drug interference
5. Metabolic inhibition

What are nutritional sources of folate?

Green leafy vegetables and fruits

List four causes of malabsorption of folate.

1. Sprue
2. Lymphoma
3. Crohn's disease
4. Intestinal bypass

Name two factors that can increase a patient's folate requirement.

Pregnancy and dialysis

What drugs interfere with folate?

Anticonvulsants, cholestyramine, and oral contraceptives

What is the treatment of folate deficiency?

Administration of oral folate

Vitamin B$_{12}$ deficiency

What are the causes of vitamin B$_{12}$ deficiency?

1. Congenital defects (transcobalamin II deficiency)

2. Poor vitamin B_{12} intake (common in vegans)
3. Malabsorption of vitamin B_{12} [seen in patients with intrinsic factor deficiency, pernicious anemia, pancreatic insufficiency, Crohn's disease, sprue, lymphoma, fish tapeworm, ileal resection, Zollinger-Ellison syndrome, or AIDS]
4. Impaired utilization of vitamin B_{12} (for example, following nitrous oxide exposure)
5. Increased dietary requirements without compensatory intake

What is the most common cause of vitamin B_{12} deficiency?

Malabsorption of vitamin B_{12} (pernicious anemia)

What neurologic symptoms are associated with vitamin B_{12} deficiency?

1. Ataxia
2. Paresthesias
3. Confusion
4. Dementia
5. Decreased vibratory sensation
6. Decreased proprioception

What is the treatment of vitamin B_{12} deficiency?

Parenteral administration of vitamin B_{12}

Aplastic anemia

What can cause aplastic anemia?

1. Idiopathic condition
2. Pharmacologic therapy
3. Infections
4. Immunosuppression
5. Ionizing radiation
6. Stem cell abnormalities
7. Congenital defects

What drugs can cause aplastic anemia?

1. Antibiotics (e.g., chloramphenicol, penicillin, sulfonamides, cephalosporins)
2. Antidepressants [e.g., tricyclic antidepressants (TCAs), lithium]
3. Anticonvulsants (e.g., carbamazepine, valproate)
4. Anti-inflammatory drugs [e.g., phenylbutazone, nonsteroidal anti-inflammatory drugs (NSAIDs), gold]

5. Antiarrhythmics (e.g., lidocaine, quinidine, procainamide)
6. Diuretics (e.g., thiazides, pyrimethamine)
7. Antiuricemics (e.g., allopurinol, colchicine)
8. Insecticides
9. Hypoglycemics (e.g., tolbutamide)

What infections cause aplastic anemia?

1. Viral hepatitis
2. EBV infection
3. HIV infection
4. Rubella

What are the signs and symptoms of aplastic anemia?

1. Bleeding
2. Petechial and fundal hemorrhages
3. Infection (sometimes)

What laboratory findings are associated with aplastic anemia?

1. Normochromic, normocytic anemia
2. Pancytopenia

What is the treatment of aplastic anemia?

If possible, terminate exposure to the causative agent. Some patients may require transfusions, hematopoietic growth factors, or bone marrow transplantation.

ANEMIAS RESULTING FROM INCREASED RED BLOOD CELL (RBC) DESTRUCTION (HEMOLYTIC ANEMIAS)

What are the causes of hemolytic anemia?

1. **Hereditary:** Hemoglobinopathies, RBC enzyme deficiencies, RBC structural protein abnormalities
2. **Acquired:** Immune-mediated hemolytic anemia, drug-induced hemolytic anemia, paroxysmal nocturnal hemoglobinemia, microangiopathic hemolytic anemia (MAHA), trauma, hypersplenism, liver disease, toxins

What are the signs and symptoms of hemolytic anemia?

1. Jaundice
2. Hemoglobinuria
3. Gallstones
4. Pallor
5. Fatigue

What laboratory findings are associated with hemolytic anemia?

1. High LDH levels
2. High unconjugated bilirubin levels
3. High reticulocyte count
4. Low haptoglobin levels
5. Spherocytes or schistocytes (frequently)

What is the treatment of hemolytic anemia?

Treatment depends on the underlying cause. Supportive therapy is often indicated.

Where can hemolysis take place?

In the vessels (intravascular hemolysis), or in the spleen, liver, or bone marrow (extravascular hemolysis)

What are the causes of intravascular hemolysis?

1. **Complement activation:** Paroxysmal nocturnal hemoglobinuria, transfusion reactions
2. **RBC trauma:** MAHA, DIC, valvular abnormalities
3. **Hematologic abnormalities:** Protozoal infections (malaria), toxicity (venoms, arsine), bacterial infections

What organism can cause a profound intravascular hemolysis following acute cholecystitis, biliary surgery, abortion, or uterine infection?

Clostridium perfringens (*C. perfringens* septicemia resulting in intravascular hemolysis is associated with a mortality rate of more than 50%)

What can cause extravascular hemolysis?

1. Infections (e.g., malaria, *Mycoplasma* infection, EBV infection)
2. Drugs [e.g., doxorubicin, methylene blue, and primaquine in patients with glucose-6-phosphate dehydrogenase (G6PD) deficiency, autoimmune drug reaction]
3. Autoimmune hemolytic anemia
4. Hemoglobinopathies
5. Malignancy
6. Eclampsia
7. Hemolytic-uremic syndrome/thrombotic thrombocytopenic purpura (HUS/TTP)
8. RBC membrane defects

Hereditary hemolytic anemias

Sickle cell anemia

What is sickle cell anemia? An inherited hemoglobinopathy resulting from abnormal hemoglobin S (Hb S); structural changes in the RBC membrane result from the replacement of glutamic acid (in the sixth position of the β globin chain) by valine

What percentage of the African-American population in the United States carry the sickle cell gene? 8%

What percentage of the African-American population in the United States have abnormal Hb S? 0.25%

Sickle cell trait supposedly confers selective advantage over what disease? Malaria

What causes the RBCs to sickle in patients with sickle cell disease? Deoxygenated Hb S polymerizes with itself within the RBC, causing the cell to fold over and assume a crescent shape.

What causes the anemia in patients with sickle cell disease? Extravascular hemolysis of the aberrant RBCs

What factors increase sickling in patients with sickle cell disease?
1. Acidosis
2. Increased 2,3-diphosphoglycerate (DPG) levels
3. Vascular stasis
4. Dehydration
5. High Hb S levels
6. Low oxygen tension

What type of hemoglobin protects against sickling? Hemoglobin F (Hb F)

What is the average lifespan of:

    Sickled cells? 10–20 days

    Normal RBCs? 120 days

What laboratory findings are associated with sickle cell anemia?

1. Leukocytosis (12,000–18,000 cells/μl) with a normal differential
2. Decreased hemoglobin level (6–9 g/dl)
3. Reticulocytosis (reticulocyte count is 5%–15%)

What is the most common reason for ED visits among patients with sickle cell disease?

Painful vaso-occlusive crisis

What causes vaso-occlusive crisis?

Sludging in the microcirculation causes infarction

What are the most common manifestations of vaso-occlusive crisis?

Musculoskeletal pain (most common) and abdominal pain (second most common)

How are vaso-occlusive crises managed in the ED?

With hydration and analgesics; consider administering oxygen (if the patient is hypoxic) or antibiotics (infection can precipitate vaso-occlusive crisis)

In sickle cell disease, what are the:

Cardiovascular complications?

1. Congestive heart failure (CHF)
2. Cardiomegaly
3. Cor pulmonale

Pulmonary complications?

1. Acute chest syndrome
2. Decreased pulmonary function and reserve
3. Decreased arterial oxygen tension (PaO_2)

Gastrointestinal complications?

1. Right upper quadrant (RUQ) syndrome
2. Bilirubin gallstones (in 75% of patients)
3. Acute splenic sequestration

Genitourinary complications?

1. Isosthenuria (inability to concentrate urine)
2. Papillary necrosis
3. Gross hematuria
4. Priapism

Skeletal complications?

1. Bony infarcts
2. Biconcave "fish mouth" changes in vertebrae (pathognomonic sign)
3. Frontal bossing
4. Aseptic necrosis of the femoral and humeral heads
5. Dactylitis (hand-foot syndrome)
6. Osteomyelitis

Central nervous system (CNS) complications?

1. Cerebral infarctions
2. Cerebral hematomas
3. Seizures
4. Subdural and subarachnoid hemorrhages

Ophthalmologic complications?

Retinopathy and blindness

What is acute chest syndrome?

A life-threatening, febrile, pneumonia-like illness caused by either infection or thrombosis/embolism

What are the clinical manifestations of acute chest syndrome?

1. Chest pain
2. Hypoxia
3. Decreased pulmonary function
4. Infiltrates on chest x-ray

What is the treatment of acute chest syndrome?

Supportive care includes the administration of analgesics and supplemental oxygen. Transfusion therapy and antibiotic therapy are controversial.

What is RUQ syndrome?

The sudden onset of RUQ pain, progressive hepatomegaly, and extreme hyperbilirubinemia (> 50 mg/dl) as a result of intrahepatic cholestasis

What is acute splenic sequestration?

Acute splenic outflow obstruction leads to splenomegaly and hypovolemic shock

What is the treatment for acute splenic sequestration?

Transfusion

What is aplastic crisis?

Bone marrow erythropoiesis is slowed or stopped

What laboratory findings are associated with aplastic crisis?

Anemia and a low reticulocyte count

What is the treatment for aplastic crisis?

Although episodes are often self-limited, some patients may require transfusions.

Which organisms most commonly lead to overwhelming sepsis in patients with sickle cell disease?

Encapsulated organisms, including *Streptococcus pneumoniae* and *Haemophilus influenzae*

Which organisms most commonly cause osteomyelitis?

Salmonella typhimurium, Staphylococcus aureus, and *Escherichia coli*

How should a febrile patient with sickle cell disease be managed?

An unexplained temperature greater than 38°C (101°F) requires work-up for a bacterial source. The administration of broad-spectrum antibiotics may be indicated.

How is priapism managed?

Patients may require exchange transfusion and should be referred to a urologist. Initial management includes intravenous hydration and analgesics.

List five admission criteria for patients with sickle cell disease.

1. Pulmonary, neurologic, or infectious complications
2. Dehydration
3. Splenic sequestration or aplastic crisis
4. Uncontrolled pain
5. Unclear diagnosis

Thalassemia

What is thalassemia?

Thalassemia is an inherited defect in globin chain synthesis. Precipitation of the defective hemoglobin complexes leads to RBC membrane damage, causing the affected cells to lyse. RBC lysis leads to anemia.

Thalassemia is common among which populations?

African-American, Asian, and Mediterranean populations

What is thalassemia major?

Homozygous β-chain thalassemia

What are the signs and symptoms of thalassemia major?

Patients usually present before the age of 2 years with pallor, lethargy, and hepatosplenomegaly. Physical examination reveals signs of extramedullary hematopoiesis.

What laboratory findings are associated with thalassemia major?

1. Severe microcytic, hypochromic anemia with target cells, anisocytes, and poikilocytes
2. Normal to high serum iron and ferritin levels
3. Normal to low TIBC with high saturation

What complications of thalassemia major can lead to death?

Cardiac failure, tissue iron deposition, or infection

What is the treatment for thalassemia major?

Supportive care, including blood transfusions and iron-chelating therapy

What is thalassemia minor?

Heterozygous β-chain thalassemia

What are the signs and symptoms of thalassemia minor?

Patients are usually asymptomatic.

What laboratory findings are characteristic of thalassemia minor?

1. Mild microcytic, hypochromic anemia with target cells
3. Low MCV
4. Normal RDW
5. High hemoglobin A_2 (Hb A_2) levels

What is the treatment for thalassemia minor?

Usually, none is necessary.

What is α-thalassemia?

Thalassemia resulting from decreased α-chain synthesis

What are the signs and symptoms of α-thalassemia?

The clinical manifestations depend on the number of α gene mutations that are present, from one to four. Patients with one α gene mutation are asymptomatic carriers, whereas those with four α gene mutations usually die *in utero*.

What laboratory findings are associated with α-thalassemia?

1. Microcytic, hypochromic anemia with target cells and basophilic stippling
2. Normal iron studies

What is the treatment for α-thalassemia?

Treatment depends on the severity of clinical disease and ranges from no treatment to blood transfusions with iron-chelating therapy and splenectomy.

What is Hb S/β-thalassemia?	Inheritance of one sickle cell gene and one β-thalassemia gene
What are the signs and symptoms of Hb S/β-thalassemia?	Clinical manifestations vary, depending on the thalassemia gene. Patients may be asymptomatic or have moderately severe disease.
What laboratory findings are associated with Hb S/β-thalassemia?	Findings range from those of sickle cell anemia to those of heterozygous β-thalassemia (e.g., microcytic hypochromic anemia and a low MCV, MCHC, and MCH).

Acquired hemolytic anemias

Autoimmune hemolytic anemia

What does a positive direct Coombs' test indicate?	A positive test demonstrates immunoglobulin G (IgG) or complement (C3) on the RBC surface. This finding is indicative of an autoimmune hemolytic anemia.
What does a positive indirect Coombs' test indicate?	A positive test demonstrates isoimmunization or the presence of autoantibodies by detecting antibodies in the patient's serum.
List the two types of autoimmune hemolytic anemia.	1. Cold agglutin disease 2. Drug-induced hemolytic anemia
What infections are associated with cold agglutin disease?	*Mycoplasma pneumoniae* infection and EBV infection (i.e., infectious mononucleosis)
What drugs are most often associated with drug-induced hemolytic anemia?	1. α-Methyldopa 2. Procainamide 3. Thioridazine 4. Penicillins 5. Cephalosporins (some) 6. Sulfa-containing drugs

Microangiopathic hemolytic anemia (MAHA)

What is MAHA?	An anemia characterized by RBCs that fragment during passage through abnormal arterioles
What is seen on the peripheral blood smear?	Schistocytes

What MAHA syndrome occurs in pregnancy?	HELLP syndrome (hemolysis, elevated liver enzymes, and low platelets)
What is the treatment for HELLP syndrome?	Delivery of the infant
What malignancy is most frequently associated with MAHA?	Gastric adenocarcinoma

What is the pentad of TTP?

1. MAHA with schistocytes and reticulocytosis
2. Thrombocytopenia
3. Renal abnormalities (e.g., renal insufficiency, azotemia, proteinuria, or hematuria)
4. CNS abnormalities (e.g., headache, confusion, cranial nerve palsies, seizures, or coma)
5. Fever (90% of patients)

What is the treatment for TTP?

1. Steroids
2. Plasma exchange transfusion
3. Platelet therapy

What are the characteristics of HUS?

1. MAHA
2. Acute renal failure
3. Fever
4. Thrombocytopenia

What pathogens are associated with HUS?

1. *Escherichia coli* serotype O157:H7
2. *Shigella* species
3. *Yersinia* species
4. *Campylobacter* species
5. *Salmonella* species
6. *Streptococcus pneumoniae*
7. Varicella-zoster virus
8. Echovirus
9. Coxsackievirus A and B

THROMBOCYTOPENIA

What is the definition of thrombocytopenia?	Platelet count $< 100,000$ cells/mm^3
Spontaneous, severe hemorrhage may occur below what platelet count?	$20,000$ cells/mm^3

What are the causes of thrombocytopenia?	Increased destruction of platelets, decreased production of platelets, or splenic sequestration of platelets
What are the causes of increased destruction of platelets?	1. Idiopathic thrombocytopenic purpura (ITP) 2. HUS 3. TTP 4. DIC 5. Infection 6. Pharmacologic therapy with certain drugs
What are the signs and symptoms of thrombocytopenia?	1. Petechiae 2. Cutaneous ecchymosis 3. Epistaxis 4. Menorrhagia

COAGULATION DISORDERS

LABORATORY EVALUATION

What is the prothrombin time (PT) used to assess?	The extrinsic and common coagulation pathways
Does the administration of vitamin K affect the PT?	Yes.
What is the partial thromboplastin time (PTT) used to assess?	The intrinsic and common coagulation pathways
What is the bleeding time used to assess?	Platelet function and vascular integrity
Which does heparin affect—the PT, PTT, or bleeding time?	The PTT
Which does warfarin affect—the PT, PTT, or bleeding time?	The PT
Which does aspirin affect—the PT, PTT, or bleeding time?	The bleeding time

HEMOPHILIA

What coagulation factor is deficient in patients with:

Hemophilia A (classic hemophilia)?	Factor VIII
Hemophilia B (Christmas disease)?	Factor IX (Christmas disease)

What coagulation study is abnormal in a patient with hemophilia?

The activated partial thromboplastin time (aPTT), which evaluates the intrinsic pathway. The PT and thrombin clot time are normal.

What are the common bleeding manifestations of hemophilia?

1. Hemarthroses
2. Hematomas
3. Mucocutaneous bleeding (e.g., epistaxis, easy bruising, bleeding after dental extractions, menorrhagia, gastrointestinal bleeding)
4. CNS hemorrhage
5. Hematuria
6. Pseudotumor

What is the most common cause of bleeding death in patients with hemophilia?

Intracranial hemorrhage (associated with a 34% mortality rate)

What is the treatment for hemophilia A (factor VIII deficiency)?

Mild disease can be treated by administering factor VIII, cryoprecipitate, or desmopressin. Patients with moderate to severe disease require factor VIII concentrates or cryoprecipitate. If factor VIII inhibitor is present, patients can be administered factor VIII concentrates, prothrombin complex concentrates, activated prothrombin complex concentrates, or porcine factor VIII.

By what percentage does one unit of factor VIII increase the circulating levels?

2%

What is the treatment for hemophilia B (factor IX deficiency)?

The administration of factor IX concentrates or FFP is usually effective. If factor IX inhibitor is present, administration of factor IX concentrates, prothrombin complex concentrates, or activated prothrombin complex concentrates may be necessary.

By what percentage does one unit of coagulation factor IX increase the circulating levels?

1%

VON WILLEBRAND DISEASE

What is von Willebrand disease?

An inherited bleeding disorder caused by a deficiency of vWF, a glycoprotein that allows platelets to adhere to damaged endothelium and carries coagulation factor VIII in plasma

What coagulation study is abnormal in a patient with von Willebrand disease?

Bleeding time

What is the differential diagnosis for von Willebrand disease?

1. Myeloproliferative disorder
2. Dysproteinemia
3. Cardiopulmonary bypass
4. Uremia
5. Pharmacologic therapy with certain drugs (e.g., NSAIDs, ticlopidine, heparin, penicillin, dextran)
6. Alcohol

What are the signs and symptoms of von Willebrand disease?

Mucocutaneous bleeding (e.g., epistaxis, easy bruising, bleeding after dental extractions, menorrhagia, and gastrointestinal bleeding)

What is the treatment of von Willebrand disease?

Type I: Administration of desmopressin or cryoprecipitate

Types II and III: Administration of factor VIII concentrate or cryoprecipitate

ONCOLOGIC EMERGENCIES

What are the most common solid tumors in children?

1. Osteosarcoma
2. Ewing's sarcoma
3. Neuroblastoma
4. Retinoblastoma

    5. Brain tumor
    6. Rhabdomyosarcoma

What malignancies metastasize to bone?	1. Thyroid cancer 2. Breast cancer 3. Lung cancer 4. Ovarian cancer 5. Renal cancer 6. Testicular cancer
What malignancies metastasize to the brain?	1. Breast cancer 2. Renal cancer 3. Testicular cancer 4. Lung cancer 5. Colon cancer
What malignancies may invade the pericardium?	1. Hodgkin's disease 2. Non-Hodgkin's lymphoma 3. Leukemia 4. Breast cancer

COMPLICATIONS OF MALIGNANCY

Tumor lysis syndrome

What is tumor lysis syndrome?	A complication of chemotherapy, characterized by the triad of hyperuricemia, hyperkalemia, and hyperphosphatemia, that occurs when cells lyse, releasing their contents into the blood stream
Tumor lysis syndrome occurs most often following the treatment of what type of malignancies?	Malignancies characterized by a high growth fraction (e.g., hematologic malignancies, such as T-cell leukemia or lymphoma)
What are the potential complications of tumor lysis syndrome?	1. Renal failure 2. Arrhythmias 3. Neurologic changes 4. Sudden death
What is the treatment for tumor lysis syndrome?	Treatment entails aggressive hydration and alkalinization to promote diuresis and uric acid and phosphate excretion, and the administration of allopurinol to reduce uric acid formation. Very ill patients may require dialysis.

Infection in the neutropenic patient

What is a concern in a fe-brile patient with cancer?

Bacterial infection

How is the absolute neutro-phil count (ANC) calculated?

By multiplying the percent neutrophils by the WBC count

An ANC below what number suggests a significantly increased risk of invasive infection?

500 cells/μl

Neutropenic patients are at increased risk for infection by which pathogens?

S. aureus, Gram-negative organisms, and *Candida albicans*

Do neutropenic patients manifest infection in the same manner as immuno-competent patients?

No. The local inflammatory response is decreased, owing to the decreased WBC count.

What approach should be taken when managing a fe-brile, neutropenic patient?

1. Obtain a history and perform a physical examination.
2. Obtain a WBC count with differential, at least two sets of blood cultures, and a urine culture.
3. Order a chest x-ray.
4. Begin empiric intravenous antibiotic therapy.
5. Place the patient in protective isolation and admit her to the hospital.

Superior vena cava syndrome

What is superior vena cava syndrome?

Obstruction of the superior vena cava following compression, thrombosis, or infiltration by a mass

What malignancies are most often associated with super-ior vena cava syndrome?

Small cell cancer of the lung, testicular cancer, and breast cancer

What are the signs and symptoms of superior vena cava syndrome?

1. Facial swelling
2. Neck vein distention
3. Tachypnea
4. Shortness of breath
5. Cough
6. Headache
7. Cyanosis

Other complications

Hypercalcemia can occur with which malignancies?	1. Lung cancer 2. Ovarian cancer 3. Prostate cancer 4. Multiple myeloma 5. Leukemia 6. Thyroid cancer 7. Breast cancer 8. Renal cancer
Radiation therapy to the chest may cause what cardiac complication?	Pericarditis with possible effusion or tamponade

POST-TRANSPLANT EMERGENCIES

What is cell-mediated immunity?	Cell-mediated immunity is mediated by T-cell lymphocytes and requires human leukocyte antigen (HLA) presentation in order to be activated. Suppression of CMI increases the incidence of atypical and opportunistic infections.
What is humoral immunity?	Humoral immunity is mediated by B lymphocytes and is associated with the production of antibodies. Suppression of humoral immunity increases the incidence of infection by encapsulated organisms.
Immunosuppression affects which type of immunity?	Cell-mediated immunity, more than humoral immunity
List the four primary immunosuppressants.	1. Cyclosporine 2. Tacrolimus 3. Azathioprine 4. Corticosteroids
What is the mechanism of action of cyclosporine?	Cyclorsporine suppresses interleukin-2 (IL-2), resulting in potent helper T cell suppression; both cell-mediated and humoral immunity are affected.
What side effects are commonly associated with cyclosporine therapy?	1. Dose-related nephrotoxicity 2. Renal artery vasospasm 3. Systemic hypertension

4. Neurotoxicity (headache, seizure, coma)
5. Hyperglycemia

What is the mechanism of action of tacrolimus?

Tacrolimus is a strong inhibitor of cell-mediated immunity with a mechanism of action similar to that of cyclosporine.

What are common side effects of tacrolimus?

The side effects are the same as those of cyclosporine, but the risk of neurotoxicity is higher.

What is the mechanism of action of azathioprine?

Inhibition of DNA synthesis

What is the most common side effect of azathioprine?

Dose-related neutropenia

What is the mechanism of action of corticosteroids?

Profound suppression of cell-mediated immunity via inhibition of lymphocyte and leukocyte migration, lymphokine production and proliferation, and impaired inflammatory response

What are common side effects of corticosteroids?

1. Prolonged wound healing
2. Pseudotumor cerebri
3. Avascular necrosis
4. Osteoporosis
5. Cataracts
6. Gastrointestinal bleeding
7. Hyperglycemia
8. Adrenal suppression
9. Psychosis

List four common complications in transplant patients.

1. Primary organ failure (recurrence of original disease, rejection, and so on)
2. Infections
3. Medication side effects
4. Coexisting illness

INFECTION IN THE TRANSPLANT PATIENT

List three general ways transplant patients acquire infections.

1. Previous infection (either in the host or donor) prior to transplant (i.e., carrier state or latent infection)
2. Nosocomial infection (i.e., infection occurring during the transplant procedure)
3. Community-acquired infection

List three reasons infections are not diagnosed or are diagnosed late in transplant patients.

1. The signs and symptoms of infection are blunted by immunosuppression, making early diagnosis difficult.
2. Transplant patients are prone to infection by atypical organisms with unusual presentations.
3. Transplant patients often have comorbid disease.

What is an opportunistic infection?

Infection by an organism that normally is not pathogenic in an immunocompetent host but is able to produce clinically significant, and often severe, infection in an immunocompromised host

What fungal organisms are common opportunistic pathogens?

1. *Cryptococcus* species
2. *Coccidioides* species
3. *Blastomyces* species
4. *Histoplasma* species
5. *Aspergillus* species
6. *Candida* species

What bacterial organisms are common opportunistic pathogens?

Atypical bacteria, including *Listeria* species, *Nocardia* species, *Mycoplasma* species, *Mycobacterium* species, *Salmonella* species, *Staphylococcus epidermidis*, and *Streptococcus viridans*

What parasitic organisms are common opportunistic pathogens?

Pneumocystis, Toxoplasma, and *Strongyloides* species

What viruses are common opportunistic pathogens?

1. EBV
2. Cytomegalovirus (CMV)
3. Varicella-zoster virus
4. Herpes simplex virus (HSV)
5. Hepatitis B virus
6. Hepatitis C virus

Which infection is the most common, and the most serious, post-transplant infection?

CMV

Following transplant surgery, when do most fungal and viral infections occur?

1–6 months post-transplant

What laboratory studies are indicated for a transplant patient with a fever?

1. A CBC with a platelet count and differential
2. Serum electrolyte panel
3. Renal function studies and, often, liver function tests as well
4. Blood, urine, and sputum cultures, as well as cultures from any localizing source (e.g., the throat, joints)
5. Organ-specific studies (e.g., a creatine phosphokinase MB isoenzyme level in a patient who has undergone a heart transplant)
6. Chest radiograph
7. Additional studies, as necessary (per the patient's history and the severity of his symptoms)

What empiric therapy should be initiated in the ED for a transplant patient with a fever?

1. Broad-spectrum antibiotic therapy should be initiated. Fungal coverage, viral coverage, or both may be necessary if the patient does not respond to therapy within 24 hours.
2. Stress-dose steroids are often required in patients with significant changes in vital signs and a history of long-term steroid use.
3. Intravenous fluids should be administered. Be cautious in patients who have undergone renal or heart transplants, as volume overload can occur rapidly in these patients.

Bacterial infections

What is the most common bacterial gastrointestinal infection in transplant patients?

Diverticulosis

Why is diverticulosis often difficult to diagnose?

Lack of inflammation leads to an insidious onset of symptoms and subsequent perforation without peritoneal signs.

What two bacterial pathogens should be considered in transplant patients presenting with diarrhea and progression to sepsis or meningitis?

Salmonella species (nontyphoidal) and *Listeria* species

What is the likely pathogen in a transplant patient who presents with a history of productive sputum, pleurisy followed by seizures, and subcutaneous skin nodules?

Nocardia asteroides (the infection usually begins as a subacute pulmonary illness and then disseminates to the brain and skin)

Parasitic infections

Transplant patients require prophylaxis against which parasitic pathogen in order to avoid infection?

Pneumocystis carinii

What agent is used for long-term prophylaxis against *P. carinii* pneumonia (PCP)?

Trimethoprim–sulfamethoxazole

Which transplant patients are at increased risk for PCP?

1. Patients noncompliant with prophylaxis
2. Patients with concomitant CMV infection
3. Patients with a low CD4 count

What organism is responsible for hyperinfection syndrome?

Strongyloides stercoralis, an intestinal nematode

What complications are associated with hyperinfection syndrome?

Hemorrhagic pneumonia, disseminated strongyloidiasis, and bacterial sepsis

Viral infections

Which organ system is most commonly infected by CMV?

CMV infection is usually multisystemic, but the lungs are especially affected (pneumonitis is the most common manifestation).

Describe the clinical presentation of CMV infection.

The presentation is highly variable. Patients may present with fever, hepatitis, leukopenia, thrombocytopenia, gastrointestinal symptoms, and dyspnea.

How is the diagnosis of CMV infection made?

A high index of suspicion is necessary. Bronchoscopy can confirm the diagnosis.

How does CMV infection affect immunosuppression?	CMV infection induces further immunosuppression and simultaneously increases the incidence of rejection.
What is the treatment for CMV?	Administration of ganciclovir or foscarnet and CMV immunoglobulin
How does EBV infection present?	The clinical presentation is similar to that of CMV infection. There is a slow, insidious onset of symptoms, including malaise and pulmonary symptoms that escalate into multisystemic disease. Ultimately, multi-organ failure occurs.
EBV is associated with what other conditions?	CMV infection and lymphoproliferative interstitial pneumonitis
How is varicella-zoster virus infection acquired?	Reactivation of latent infection or primary infection
Which is more common?	Reactivation of latent infection
How does varicella-zoster virus infection present?	The clinical manifestation is herpes zoster. The infection rarely disseminates, except in patients who have undergone a bone marrow transplant.
What is the incidence of varicella-zoster virus infection in solid organ transplant recipients?	10% of solid organ transplant recipients develop varicella-zoster virus infection.
What is the treatment for varicella-zoster virus infection?	Administration of intravenous acyclovir hastens resolution of symptoms but does not lower the incidence of post-herpetic neuralgia.
When is prophylaxis necessary?	When a seronegative patient who has been infected with varicella-zoster virus has been exposed to an individual with chicken pox or herpes zoster
What is the prophylactic therapy against varicella-zoster virus?	Administration of high-dose varicella-zoster virus IgG
What is the presentation of HSV infection?	Ulcers are more common than vesicles.

What is the treatment of HSV infection?	Administration of acyclovir to prevent dissemination

COMPLICATIONS ASSOCIATED WITH KIDNEY TRANSPLANTS

Noninfectious complications

What are the noninfectious complications of renal transplant?

1. ATN, caused by an ischemic insult to the kidney
2. Cyclosporine nephrotoxicity
3. Arterial occlusion
4. Hemorrhage
5. Transplant artery stenosis (results in uncontrollable hypertension)
6. Thrombophlebitis
7. Lymphocele formation
8. Graft rejection

What are the three types of rejection?

Hyperacute, acute, and chronic

Which type of rejection presents within weeks to months of a transplant?

Acute rejection

What are the signs and symptoms of acute graft rejection?

Tenderness over the allograft, decreased urine output, rapid weight gain, low-grade fever, general malaise, worsening hypertension, and peripheral edema

What is the differential diagnosis?

Volume contraction and cyclosporine-induced nephrotoxicity

What laboratory tests are used to diagnose acute graft rejection?

1. Blood urea nitrogen (BUN) and creatinine levels
2. Serum electrolyte levels
3. Urinalysis (microscopic examination of sample)
4. Cyclosporine trough level

Does the serum creatinine level increase more in cases of acute graft rejection or in cases of cyclosporine toxicity?

Acute graft rejection (an increase of more than 50% is typical)

Is the rate at which the creatinine level increases faster with acute graft rejection or with cyclosporine toxicity?

Acute graft rejection

What imaging study is useful in the diagnosis of acute graft rejection?	Renal ultrasound (can identify obstruction, abscess, or perirenal fluid collection
What is the treatment for acute graft rejection?	Admission to the hospital for high-dose steroid pulses

Infectious complications

What infectious complications are associated with renal transplants?	1. Bacterial sepsis 2. Opportunistic infections 3. Pyelonephritis
What factors are responsible for the renal transplant patient's increased risk of infection?	Immunosuppression, leukopenia, hyperglycemia, and azotemia
What is the most common infection following kidney transplant?	Pyelonephritis secondary to infection by Gram-negative organisms from the gut and Gram-positive organisms from the wound
What percentage of renal transplant patients develop pyelonephritis within 4 months of the transplant?	35%
What drugs are used as standard prophylaxis against pyelonephritis?	Trimethoprim–sulfamethoxazole or ciprofloxacin
How is pyelonephritis in a renal transplant patient managed?	The patient should be admitted to the hospital for intravenous administration of antibiotics.

COMPLICATIONS ASSOCIATED WITH BONE MARROW TRANSPLANTS

List two general indications for bone marrow transplant.	1. Primary bone marrow disorder (e.g., aplastic anemia, leukemia) 2. Treatment of underlying disease that results in eradication of host bone marrow (e.g., x-ray therapy, chemotherapy)
What cell lines are transplanted in a complete bone marrow transplant?	1. Myeloid 2. Erythroid 3. Lymphoid 4. Megakaryocytic

How long does it take to regain immunocompetency following bone marrow transplant?

Months to years

What is an autologous bone marrow transplant?

The patient donates her own bone marrow prior to treatment.

Patients with which diseases may be candidates for an autologous bone marrow transplant?

Patients with Hodgkin's disease or non-Hodgkin's lymphoma, multiple myeloma, or small cell lung, breast, testicular, or ovarian cancer

What is the advantage of an autologous bone marrow transplant?

Once the cell lines are regenerated, the patient is no longer immunosuppressed and does not require immunosuppressive drugs.

What is the major drawback of an allograft bone marrow transplant?

The patient will always require some degree of immunosuppressive drug therapy to prevent rejection.

List the three phases that a patient passes through after undergoing a bone marrow transplant.

Phase I: Days 0–30
Phase II: Days 31–100
Phase III: Day 101 forward

During which phases do patients typically present to the ED with complications?

During phases II and III; complications that occur during phase I usually develop while the patient is still in the hospital following the original transplant surgery.

List the five possible complications of an allograft bone marrow transplant and the most likely phase of occurrence.

1. Graft rejection: Phase I
2. Infections: Phases I and III
3. GVHD: Phases II and III
4. Veno-occlusive disease: Phase I
5. Recurrence of underlying disease process: Phase III

When does graft rejection typically occur?

Within a few days of the transplant procedure

What is the typical result?

Aplastic anemia

What are the two most common causes of morbidity and mortality in patients who have undergone a bone marrow transplant?

Infection and GVHD

Infectious complications

What is the most important predictor of severity of infection in bone marrow transplant recipients?

The ANC

At what ANC level is the prognosis poor for the patient?

< 100 cells/μl

What percentage of bone marrow transplant patients experience a central line infection at some point?

40%

How is infection in a bone marrow transplant recipient treated?

1. Broad-spectrum antibiotics
2. Intravenous fluids
3. Stress-dose steroids
4. Isolation
5. Bone marrow stimulants
6. Immunoglobulin administration (if a specific cause is identified)
7. Supportive care

What percentage of bone marrow transplant patients will acquire symptomatic CMV infections?

50%

What is the incidence of reactivation of varicella-zoster virus infection in bone marrow allograft recipients who have had previous varicella-zoster virus infections?

35%

How long after an allograft does reactivation of a latent varicella-zoster virus infection typically occur?

5 months

What benefit is associated with the prophylactic administration of acyclovir?

The prophylactic administration of acyclovir prevents reactivation during treatment.

What are the two most common fungal infections following a bone marrow transplant?	Candidiasis and aspergillosis
Why are bone marrow transplant patients susceptible to aspergillosis?	The lung macrophages that normally ingest inhaled spores are no longer present and allow seeding of the lung.
When do candidiasis and aspergillosis infections typically occur?	6–8 weeks post-transplant
What is the mortality rate associated with fungal infections in bone marrow transplant patients?	85%

Graft-versus-host disease (GVHD)

What is GVHD?	A disease caused by the reaction of histoincompatible, immunocompetent donor T cells against the tissue of an immunocompromised host
What is the incidence of GVHD in transplants between HLA-matched siblings?	As many as 50% of patients who receive a transplant from an HLA-matched sibling develop GVHD.
GVHD typically occurs during what phase following a bone marrow transplant?	Phase II
What are the three most commonly affected sites and in what order are they affected?	1. Skin (symptoms range from a maculopapular eruption to epidermal necrosis) 2. Gastrointestinal system (symptoms include diarrhea and abdominal pain and distention) 3. Liver (liver enzyme levels are elevated as a result of hepatic injury)
What is the mortality rate associated with GVHD?	30%
What is the usual cause of death in patients who succumb to GVHD?	Infection (immune function is decreased and the risk for infection dramatically increases)

How is GVHD prevented?

By administering immunosuppressive drugs, including methotrexate, steroids, and cyclosporine

What is the incidence of chronic GVHD in patients who survive to phase III?

25%–50%

How is chronic GVHD different from acute GVHD?

1. It appears later (phase III instead of phase II).
2. Donor marrow (not just T cells) attacks the host tissues.
3. There is a higher incidence of bacterial infections secondary to decreased opsonizing antibody
4. Lack of IgA results in chronic sinopulmonary infections.

How are chronic and acute GVHD treated?

With the increased administration of immunosuppressive drugs

What is sicca syndrome?

A syndrome occasionally seen in patients with GVHD that is characterized by dry eyes (the lack of tears leads to keratoconjunctivitis) and a dry mouth (interference with swallowing leads to decreased nutrition)

What is the treatment for sicca syndrome?

Hydration, improved nutrition, and artificial tears

List eight causes of pulmonary infiltrates in bone marrow transplant patients.

1. Interstitial pneumonitis
2. Pneumonia
3. Atelectasis
4. Pulmonary edema
5. Toxic pulmonary effects from drugs or radiation
6. Malignancy
7. Pulmonary embolus
8. Alveolar hemorrhage secondary to thrombocytopenia

What is the most common cause of interstitial pneumonitis?

CMV infection

If a bone marrow transplant patient has a pulmonary infiltrate, what is the most likely etiology?

75% of pulmonary infiltrates in bone marrow transplant patients are secondary to GVHD or the immunosuppressive drugs used to counter GVHD.

10

Endocrinologic and Metabolic Emergencies

ENDOCRINOLOGIC EMERGENCIES

HYPERTHYROIDISM (THYROTOXICOSIS) AND THYROID STORM

List eight causes of hyper-thyroidism.

1. Graves' disease (most common)
2. Toxic multinodular goiter
3. Exogenous triiodothyronine (T_3) intake
4. Hashimoto's thyroiditis
5. Subacute granulomatous thyroiditis (de Quervain's thyroiditis)
6. Follicular carcinoma
7. Struma ovarii
8. Thyroid-stimulating hormone (TSH)-producing pituitary tumor

What are the signs and symptoms of hyperthyroid-ism?

1. Fever
2. Weight loss
3. Sinus tachycardia
4. Atrial fibrillation
5. Systolic hypertension
6. Anxiety
7. Agitation paranoia
8. Anorexia
9. Nausea and vomiting
10. Diarrhea and abdominal pain
11. Sweating
12. Congestive heart failure (CHF)

What antithyroid thiour-eylene drug is an alternative to propylthiouracil (PTU) for the treatment of hyper-thyroidism?

Methimazole

What is thyroid storm?

A life-threatening form of hyper-thyroidism that can be precipitated by various stressors

What stressors can cause a patient with hyperthyroid-ism to develop thyroid storm?

Stressors are nonspecific and include physiologic stress, infection, pulmonary embolus, and diabetic ketoacidosis (DKA) or hypoglycemia (in a diabetic patient)

What are the signs and symptoms of thyroid storm?

1. Delirium
2. Coma
3. Temperature greater than or equal to 105°F
4. Tachycardia
5. Restlessness

Are central nervous system (CNS) symptoms common in patients presenting with thyroid storm?

Yes, 90% of patients have CNS symptoms.

What is the difference be-tween apathetic thyrotoxi-cosis (a rare form of thyroid storm) and thyroid storm?

Apathetic thyrotoxicosis occurs more commonly among the elderly (i.e., patients older than 70 years), and is associated with increased weight loss, cardiovascular complications (e.g., CHF, atrial fibrillation), and CNS depression.

Do laboratory tests confirm the diagnosis of thyroid storm?

No, this is a clinical diagnosis. However, the thyroxine (T_4) level is elevated and the TSH level is depressed.

What is the treatment for thyroid storm?

1. Oxygen
2. Antipyretics (avoid aspirin); cooling blankets if the hyperthermia is severe
3. Digitalis and diuretics (to counteract CHF)
4. Dexamethasone (to counteract the increased glucocorticoid requirement)
5. PTU (to inhibit thyroid hormone synthesis)
6. Iodine (to prevent thyroid hormone release)
7. Propranolol (to block peripheral thyroid effects)

HYPOTHYROIDISM AND MYXEDEMA COMA

What is the difference between primary and secondary hypothyroidism?

Primary hypothyroidism results when the thyroid gland fails to respond to TSH. Secondary hypothyroidism results when the anterior pituitary gland fails to release TSH.

List four causes of primary hypothyroidism.

1. Autoimmune destruction
2. Surgical or radio-ablation of the thyroid gland
3. Antithyroid medication
4. Lithium therapy

List three causes of secondary hypothyroidism.

1. Pituitary tumors
2. Sheehan's syndrome (i.e., postpartum pituitary necrosis)
3. Sarcoidosis (infiltrating disease)

How is primary hypothyroidism distinguished from secondary hypothyroidism?

In primary hypothyroidism, the serum TSH level and the response to TSH are elevated.

What are the most common signs and symptoms of hypothyroidism?

1. Paresthesia
2. Cold intolerance
3. Weakness
4. Muscle pain
5. Menstrual changes
6. Hypothermia
7. Dry skin
8. Nonpitting facial and periorbital edema (myxedema)

What respiratory changes are associated with hypothyroidism?

Hypoventilation and upper airway obstruction

What are the cardiac manifestations of hypothyroidism?

Hypotension, bradycardia, and an enlarged cardiac silhouette on chest films

Should a normal body temperature in a patient with hypothyroidism be considered normal?

No, consider infection.

What is myxedema coma?

Myxedema coma is a life-threatening form of hypothyroidism.

Is myxedema coma common?	No, it occurs in 0.1% of all patients with hypothyroidism.
Which patient population most commonly is affected by myxedema coma and when does it usually occur?	Elderly women with hypothyroidism; winter months
What are the three most common precipitating factors of myxedema coma?	1. Exposure to cold environment 2. Infection 3. Heart failure
What are the signs and symptoms of myxedema coma?	1. Obvious hypothyroidism 2. Progressive stupor and coma 3. Seizures 4. Hyponatremia 5. Hypotension 6. Hypoglycemia 7. Hypoventilation with hypercapnia and respiratory acidosis
What electrolyte abnormality is associated with myxedema coma?	Hyponatremia
What is the treatment for myxedema coma?	1. Supportive therapy (without active rewarming) 2. Administration of thyroid replacement drugs (e.g., levothyroxine) 3. Administration of stress-dose hydrocortisone (possibly)

ADRENAL INSUFFICIENCY

What hormones are produced in the adrenal:	
Cortex?	Glucocorticoids (e.g., cortisol), mineralocorticoids (e.g., aldosterone), and androgens
Medulla?	Catecholamines, epinephrine, and norepinephrine
What is the role of cortisol?	Cortisol improves the body's response to stress by increasing glucose release and enhancing the response to catecholamines.

What is the role of aldosterone?	Aldosterone increases sodium reabsorption and potassium secretion in the distal tubules.
Increasing sodium reabsorption has what net effect, physiologically?	Increases extracellular fluid volume
What determines aldosterone secretion?	The renin-angiotensin system, the serum potassium level, and the serum adrenocorticotropic hormone level
What are the three types of adrenal insufficiency?	1. Primary insufficiency (failure of the adrenal glands) 2. Secondary insufficiency (pituitary failure) 3. Tertiary insufficiency (hypothalamic disorders)
List four causes of primary adrenal insufficiency.	1. Addison's disease, which may be idiopathic or caused by an autoimmune disease (e.g., Grave's disease, Hashimoto's thyroiditis, pernicious anemia, diabetes) 2. Infection (e.g., tuberculosis, fungal infections) 3. Infiltration (e.g., sarcoidosis, amyloidosis, hemochromatosis, metastatic disease) 4. Hemorrhage and sepsis from meningococcemia (Waterhouse-Friderichsen syndrome)
What are the signs and symptoms of primary adrenal insufficiency?	1. Lethargy 2. Weakness 3. Fatigue on exertion 4. Anorexia 5. Nausea and vomiting 6. Weight loss 7. Abdominal pain 8. Pigmentation of the face, hands, and other exposed areas 9. Lack of pubic hair (in women)
How would the patient presentation change if aldosterone production were also affected?	The patient would present with hypotension, postural syncope, and dehydration.

What is the most common cause of adrenal crisis?	Withdrawal of exogenous glucocorticoids
Are most cases of adrenal crisis the result of new adrenal failure or acute worsening of chronic adrenal insufficiency?	Acute worsening of chronic adrenal insufficiency
How do patients with adrenal crisis present?	1. Weakness 2. Confusion 3. Hypotension 4. Anorexia 5. Nausea and vomiting 6. Abdominal pain, which can mimic an acute abdomen
What abnormal laboratory values are associated with adrenal crisis?	Hypoglycemia, hyponatremia, hyperkalemia, and an elevated white blood cell (WBC) count
What is the treatment for adrenal crisis?	Administration of steroids; volume and electrolyte replacement therapy
Why is dexamethasone the steroid of choice?	Hydrocortisone will improve the patient's symptoms, yet not interfere with serum cortisol measurements (necessary to clarify the diagnosis).

METABOLIC DISORDERS

METABOLIC ACIDOSIS

What causes metabolic acidosis?	Anything that increases acid or decreases alkali
What is the primary effect of a metabolic acidosis?	Metabolic acidosis decreases serum bicarbonate.
How will the blood pH change following an acute change in the arterial carbon dioxide tension ($PaCO_2$)?	A 10-mm Hg increase in the $PaCO_2$ decreases the pH by 0.08.
If the pH change is greater or less than the calculated change, what does this suggest?	A mixed acidosis or alkalosis

What are the two types of metabolic acidosis?	Anion gap and nonanion gap
What is the formula for calculating the anion gap?	$(Na^+) - ([HCO_3^-] + [Cl^-])$
What is a normal anion gap?	12 ± 2 mEq/L
List the causes of anion gap acidosis.	**MUDPILES** **M**ethanol **U**remia **D**KA **P**araldehyde **I**ron and **I**soniazid **L**actic acidosis **E**thylene glycol **S**alicylates
What is the primary cause of anion gap acidosis in a patient with uremia?	Renal failure limits acid excretion
What are the two causes of lactic acidosis?	1. Poor oxygen delivery (e.g., as a result of hypoxia or hypoperfusion) 2. Production of lactic acid exceeds metabolism (e.g., as a result of sepsis, diabetes, or liver disease)
Does ethanol use cause a metabolic acidosis?	Yes, if the patient has alcoholic ketoacidosis
What is the osmolar gap?	The difference between the measured serum osmolality and the calculated serum osmolarity (used to help diagnose the cause of anion gap acidosis)
What is the normal serum osmolality?	285–295 mOsm/L
How is the serum osmolality calculated?	Calculated osmolarity (mOsm/L) = $2(Na+K) + (glucose/18) + (BUN/2.8)$
Which causes of anion gap acidosis are associated with elevated osmolar gaps?	Methanol, ethanol, and DKA
What two factors lead to a nonanion gap acidosis?	1. The inability to excrete hydrogen 2. Improper (i.e., excessive) bicarbonate loss

List five causes of a non-anion gap acidosis.	1. Chloride excess 2. Diarrhea 3. Therapy with carbonic anhydrase inhibitors 4. Renal insufficiency 5. Renal tubular acidosis
What is a possible treatment for metabolic acidosis?	Administration of sodium bicarbonate (if the pH is 7.0–7.2)
What complications can be associated with bicarbonate administration?	1. Alkalosis 2. Paradoxical cerebrospinal fluid (CSF) and intracellular acidosis 3. Hypokalemia 4. Hypocalcemia

DISORDERS OF GLUCOSE METABOLISM

What are the three major diabetes-related emergencies?	1. Hypoglycemia 2. DKA 3. Nonketotic hyperosmolar coma (NKHC)
What is the normal blood glucose range?	60–100 mg/dl, or a level at which the patient is asymptomatic level
What hormones elevate glucose levels?	Glucagon, epinephrine, growth hormone, and cortisol

Hypoglycemia

What neuroglycopenic symptoms are associated with hypoglycemia?	1. Dizziness 2. Headache 3. Confusion 4. Tiredness 5. Difficulty speaking 6. Inability to concentrate 7. Paralysis 8. Seizures 9. Coma
What autonomic symptoms are associated with hypoglycemia?	1. Sweating 2. Trembling 3. Warmth 4. Anxiety 5. Nausea
List six common causes of hypoglycemia.	1. Islet cell tumor of pancreas 2. Hepatic disease

3. Sepsis
4. Starvation
5. Exercise
6. Exogenous insulin administration

What is the Somogyi phenomenon?

Counter-regulatory, hormone-induced morning hyperglycemia following nighttime hypoglycemia induced by a dose of evening insulin that is too high

What drugs can cause hypoglycemia?

1. Ethanol
2. Acetaminophen
3. Amphetamines
4. Chloramphenicol
5. Lithium
6. Phenothiazines
7. Quinine
8. Sulfa drugs
9. Salicylates
10. Pentamidine
11. Didanosine
12. Haloperidol
13. Propoxyphene
14. Propranolol
15. Chlorpromazine
16. Monoamine oxidase inhibitors

Which drugs can potentiate the sulfonylureas?

1. Bishydroxycoumarin
2. Chloramphenicol
3. Clofibrate
4. Phenylbutazone
5. Ranitidine
6. Sulfonamides
7. Tricyclic antidepressants
8. Salicylates
9. Alcohol

What is the treatment for hypoglycemia?

Administration of oral glucose, intravenous dextrose, and intramuscular glucagon

Diabetic ketoacidosis (DKA)

What is the most common cause of death in pediatric patients with insulin-dependent diabetes mellitus (IDDM)?

DKA

What is the pathogenesis of DKA?	Insulin deficiency results in decreased tissue glucose utilization, increased lipolysis (which increases ketone production), and increased glucose production owing to gluconeogenesis.
Name the two ketone bodies found in ketoacidosis.	Acetoacetate and β-hydroxybutyrate
What are the possible signs and symptoms of DKA?	1. Polydipsia 2. Polyuria 3. Kussmaul's respirations 4. Abdominal pain 5. "Fruity breath" 6. Changes in mental status 7. Dehydration
What causes the dehydration associated with DKA?	Osmotic diuresis as a result of the hyperglycemia
Which four criteria must be present to diagnose DKA?	1. Hyperglycemia (glucose level > 200 mg/dl) 2. Metabolic acidosis (blood pH < 7.3 or a bicarbonate level < 15 mEq/L) 3. Hyperketonemia 4. Ketonuria
What laboratory findings can one anticipate in a patient with DKA?	1. Elevated blood urea nitrogen (BUN) and creatine levels 2. Hyperosmolality (i.e., 300–350 mOsm/kg) 3. Hyperlipidemia 4. Hypophosphatemia, hypomagnesemia, and pseudohyponatremia 5. Ketones and glucose on a urine dipstick test 6. Increased anion gap
What are the goals of therapy for DKA?	Reestablish circulating volume, reinitiate aerobic metabolism, replete electrolyte abnormalities
Should patients with DKA receive an isotonic fluid bolus?	Yes, to re-establish perfusion.
What is the recommended duration for replacing the fluid deficit in pediatric patients?	24–48 hours

Should insulin infusion be initiated immediately in the ED for a patient with DKA?

No, the serum glucose level will decrease with resuscitation.

Should bicarbonate be administered to a patient with DKA?

Only the most severely acidotic patients should be given bicarbonate.

What are some potential complications of DKA?

1. Cerebral edema
2. Persistent acidosis
3. Hypoglycemia
4. Hypokalemia

What are the signs of impending cerebral crisis?

1. Headache
2. Changes in mental status and vital signs
3. Papilledema and pupillary changes
4. Seizures
5. Vomiting and incontinence

When does cerebral edema typically occur?

Within 24 hours of initiating therapy for DKA.

Which groups of patients are at greatest risk for developing cerebral edema?

1. Patients with newly diagnosed diabetes
2. Children younger than 5 years
3. Patients with serum sodium levels greater than 140 mEq/L and a serum osmolality greater than 330 mOsm/L

What is the mortality rate associated with cerebral edema?

90%

How is cerebral edema treated?

1. Elevate the head of the bed.
2. Intubate, sedate, and mechanically ventilate the patient.
3. Administer mannitol.

How can cerebral edema be avoided?

By avoiding rapid rehydration

Nonketotic hyperosmolar coma (NKHC)

What is the basic difference between DKA and NKHC?

Patients with DKA have ketoacidosis.

Why does ketoacidosis not occur in patients with NKHC?

A small amount of insulin prevents lipolysis and gluconeogenesis.

What are the signs and symptoms of NKHC?

Dehydration and CNS changes

What two criteria are used to diagnose NKHC?

Hyperglycemia (glucose level of 500–2000 mg/dl) and a serum osmolarity of more than 350 mOsm/kg, with a normal blood pH

How is a patient with NKHC managed?

Administer fluids, insulin, and electrolytes. An effort should be made to determine the precipitating factor.

11 Neurologic Emergencies

INCREASED INTRACRANIAL PRESSURE (ICP)

What determines the ICP?
The amount of blood, brain tissue, cerebrospinal fluid (CSF), and extracellular fluid in relation to the fixed volume of the skull

What can increase cerebral blood flow?
Hypoxia, acidosis

What measures can be taken to decrease the ICP?
Decrease the intracranial blood volume, extracellular fluid volume, or CSF volume

What measures can be taken to decrease the:

Intracranial blood volume?
1. Control arterial flow via adequate oxygenation and ventilation.
2. Enhance venous drainage by elevating the head of the bed, keeping the head midline, and "sandbagging" the head instead of using a neck collar (the last two maneuvers decrease direct pressure on the jugular vein).

Extracellular fluid volume?
1. Remove fluid collections (via burr holes or transfontanel taps)
2. Administer steroids and mannitol to decrease cerebral edema

CSF volume?
Place a ventriculoperitoneal shunt or perform a lumbar or ventricular puncture.

How is the cerebral perfusion pressure (CPP) calculated?
$CPP = MAP - ICP$, where CPP = the cerebral perfusion pressure; MAP = the mean arterial pressure; and ICP = the intracranial pressure

What are the two supra-tentorial herniation syndromes?

Central and uncal

Describe the symptoms of:

Central herniation

Patients experience a subacute or chronic onset of decreased mental status. Pupillary activity is preserved until late in the course of the disorder. Cheyne-Stokes respirations are seen.

Uncal herniation

A fixed, dilated pupil (third nerve palsy) is seen following depression of conscious-ness, dilation of the contralateral pupil, and contralateral hemiparesis.

What are the symptoms of ventriculoperitoneal shunt malfunction?

Agitation, headache, emesis, persistent downward gaze, changes in coordination or cognition

What study is done to assess shunt function?

Head computed tomography (CT) scan

What study is done to assess shunt patency?

Plain radiographs of the entire shunt (including lateral skull and neck views and anterior–posterior chest and abdominal views)

What is the treatment for shunt malfunction?

Management of the ICP and consultation with a neurosurgeon

What are the features of normal pressure hydro-cephalus?

Dementia, gait disturbance, urinary incontinence

What is found on a head CT scan in a patient with normal pressure hydro-cephalus?

Communicating hydrocephalus

In a patient with normal pressure hydrocephalus, is the opening pressure (as measured with a lumbar puncture) normal or abnormal?

Normal

CEREBROVASCULAR DISEASE AND STROKE

How common is athero-sclerotic cerebrovascular disease?

Atherosclerotic cerebrovascular disease is the third leading cause of death (following heart disease and cancer).

List four risk factors associated with atherosclerotic cerebrovascular disease.

1. Hypertension
2. Hyperlipidemia
3. Diabetes mellitus
4. Smoking

Where does atherosclerosis tend to occur?

Where arteries bifurcate

What is the difference between a cerebrovascular accident (CVA), a transient ischemic attack (TIA), and a reversible ischemic neurologic deficit (RIND)?

CVA: Symptoms never reverse
TIA: Symptoms resolve within 24 hours
RIND: Symptoms resolve after 24 hours

What is a "stroke?"

The rapid onset of neurologic symptoms as a result of a regional blood flow disruption

What are the two types of strokes and which type is most common?

Ischemic strokes occur secondary to interruption of blood flow and account for 80% of all strokes. Hemorrhagic strokes result from bleeding into the brain parenchyma and account for 20% of all strokes.

What are the two causes of ischemic stroke?

1. Thrombosis following a series of TIAs or minor strokes
2. Embolism occurring abruptly without any prodromal symptoms

What is the most common source of emboli?

The heart

List seven common causes of emboli from the heart.

1. Atrial fibrillation
2. Recent myocardial infarction
3. Endocarditis
4. Valvular disease
5. Dilated cardiomyopathy
6. Left heart myxoma
7. Prosthetic valves

What is a paradoxical embolus?

An embolus that reaches the brain after passing through a patent foramen ovale or atrial septal defect.

List five typical distributions for an ischemic stroke.

1. Middle cerebral artery
2. Anterior cerebral artery
3. Posterior cerebral artery
4. Vertebrobasilar system
5. Penetrating branches from the middle cerebral artery

What are the signs and symptoms of a middle cerebral artery stroke?

1. Contralateral hemiplegia and hemianesthesia
2. Ipsilateral homonymous hemianopsia
3. Global aphasia (if the dominant hemisphere is affected)
4. Agnosia (if the nondominant hemisphere is affected)

What are the two types of aphasia?

Receptive and expressive

What are the signs and symptoms of an anterior cerebral artery stroke?

1. Paralysis of the contralateral leg
2. Sensory deficits paralleling paralysis
3. Gait apraxia (clumsiness)
4. Bowel and bladder incontinence
5. Altered mentation
6. Confusion
7. Impaired judgement
8. Frontal release signs (e.g., grasp and suck)

Are the arms affected more often in middle cerebral artery or anterior cerebral artery infarcts?

Middle cerebral artery infarcts

What are the signs and symptoms of a posterior cerebral artery stroke?

1. Homonymous hemianopsia or cortical blindness
2. Paralysis of the oculomotor nerve (cranial nerve III)
3. Visual agnosia (lack of recognition)
4. Alexia (inability to understand the written word)
5. Altered mental status
6. Impaired memory

Describe each of the following syndromes, which are often seen with posterior cerebral artery strokes:

Claude's syndrome?

Cranial nerve III palsy with contralateral ataxia

Weber's syndrome?	Cranial nerve III palsy with contralateral hemiplegia
What are the signs and symptoms of a vertebro- basilar stroke?	1. Vertigo 2. Nystagmus 3. Dysphagia 4. Facial numbness or paresthesias ("pins and needles") 5. Dysarthria 6. Contralateral loss of pain and temperature 7. Diplopia and visual field defects 8. Paralysis 9. Bilateral spasticity 10. Vomiting 11. Syncope 12. Coma
Where are deficits seen in vertebrobasilar stroke?	The ipsilateral face and contralateral body
What is a lacunar infarct?	A small infarct, typically located deep in the hemispheres or the pontomesen- cephalic region and resulting from involvement of the small penetrating branches of the middle cerebral artery
List four common sites of lacunar infarcts.	1. Basal ganglia 2. Thalamus 3. Pons 4. Internal capsule
What is a risk factor for primary intracerebral hemorrhage?	Hypertension
Hypertensive intracerebral hemorrhages occur in which four locations?	1. Cerebellum 2. Pons 3. Putamen 4. Thalamus
What are the classic pre- senting symptoms of a cerebellar hemorrhage?	Symptoms include repeated vomiting accompanied by an inability to walk or stand; occipital headache and vertigo may also occur. Symptoms often progress over hours.

How commonly do head-aches and vomiting occur in patients with hypertensive intracranial hemorrhages?

Vomiting is common and approximately 50% of patients experience headache.

Which classic ocular signs are seen in each of the following types of intracerebral hemorrhage:

Cerebellar hemorrhage?

Lateral eye deviation opposite the hemorrhage without paralysis

Putamen hemorrhage?

Lateral eye deviation opposite the hemorrhage with paralysis

Pontine hemorrhage?

Tiny, reactive pupils with impaired "doll's eye" examination

Thalamic hemorrhage?

Unreactive pupils with downward eye deviation

List four causes of lobar intracerebral hemorrhages.

1. Arteriovenous malformation
2. Bleeding into tumors (e.g., melanoma)
3. Bleeding diathesis (e.g., as a result of warfarin therapy)
4. Circle of Willis aneurysms

What laboratory tests should be ordered when evaluating a patient with a possible stroke?

1. Hematocrit
2. Coagulation studies
3. Electrocardiogram (EKG)
4. Pulse oximetry
5. Basic electrolyte panel (sodium, potassium, glucose)

What imaging study should be obtained for all acute stroke victims and why?

A head CT scan, to rule out intracerebral hemorrhage

What are the two goals of treatment in acute stroke?

Maximize perfusion to the brain and prevent progression of the stroke

What is the emergency department (ED) treatment for intracerebral hemorrhage?

Control of blood pressure and ICP

What is the definitive treatment of primary intracerebral hemorrhage?

Surgical decompression for cerebellar hemorrhage; surgery is not indicated for pontine and deep cerebral hemorrhage.

What is the differential diagnosis in a patient whose clinical condition is deteriorating following an ischemic stroke?	1. Cerebral edema 2. Continued emboli 3. Hemorrhage into an ischemic infarct 4. Heparin-induced thrombosis
What is the differential diagnosis for stroke in a young patient (i.e., a patient younger than 45 years)?	1. Drug abuse (especially cocaine) 2. Hypercoagulable state 3. Cardiogenic emboli 4. Vasculitis 5. Central nervous system (CNS) infection 6. Cancer
What is the criteria for admitting a stroke patient to the hospital?	Acute stroke or new-onset TIA

HEADACHE

When someone has a "headache," what anatomical structures hurt?	1. The skin, muscles, and blood vessels of the scalp 2. Parts of the dura and the dural arteries 3. The intracerebral arteries 4. Cranial nerves V, VI, and VII 5. The cervical nerves
What true emergencies may present as a headache?	1. **Infectious disorders:** Meningitis, sinusitis, mastoiditis, dental infections, and intracranial abscess 2. **Disorders that increase the ICP:** Tumors, pseudotumor cerebri, and intracranial bleeds 3. **Extracranial disorders:** Cranial neuralgias, glaucoma, optic neuritis, temporomandibular joint (TMJ) syndrome, and cervical spine disorders 4. **Inflammatory disorders:** Temporal arteritis and polyarteritis nodosa
How can migraine and tension headaches be differentiated from more malignant conditions?	Migraine and tension headaches tend to be recurrent and are similar from episode to episode.

MIGRAINE HEADACHE

What type of pain is associated with migraines?	Unilateral pain that starts as throbbing and progresses to a dull ache

What is the difference between a classic migraine and a common migraine?

Patients with classic migraines experience an aura during the prodromal stage, whereas patients with common migraines have vague prodromal symptoms (e.g., elation, depression, hunger, thirst) that may begin hours or days before the onset of pain.

What is an aura?

An ischemic phenomenon that is caused by vasoconstriction of the intracranial arteries

What are the symptoms of an aura?

1. Visual field defects (e.g., scintillating scotoma, scotoma, blindness)
2. Hemiplegia and ataxia
3. Nausea and vomiting
4. Loss of consciousness

What is a migraine equivalent?

A focal neurologic deficit without headache or vomiting; most common in older patients

What is an ophthalmoplegic migraine?

A dilated artery compresses cranial nerve III, leading to ophthalmoplegia and mydriasis

At what age do migraines typically start?

Puberty (they generally improve with age)

What are potential therapies for migraine headache?

Antiemetics, sumatriptan, ergotamines, analgesics, or nonsteroidal anti-inflammatory drugs (NSAIDs)

What are contraindications to the administration of ergotamine?

Pregnancy, hypertension, and coronary artery disease

What measures can be taken to prevent migraine headaches?

1. Avoidance of foods containing vaso-active amines (e.g., red wine, ripe cheese)
2. Maintenance of a regular sleep schedule
3. Reduction of stress
4. Pharmacologic therapy (e.g., with a time-release combination of ergotamine, belladonna, and phenobarbital, with or without propranolol; methysergide maleate; or amitriptyline)

What side effect is associated with the uninterrupted use of methysergide maleate?	Retroperitoneal and pulmonary fibrosis

TENSION HEADACHE

What causes a tension headache?	Sustained contraction of the deep neck muscles and muscles of mastication
What type of pain is associated with a tension headache?	A constant and nonthrobbing pain that worsens with muscle palpation; pain is often described as "squeezing" or "band-like"
What is the treatment of tension headache?	Analgesics and muscle relaxants; identification and treatment of the underlying cause

CLUSTER HEADACHE

Which patients are most susceptible to cluster headaches?	30- to 40-year-old men
Describe the typical pain patterns associated with cluster headaches.	One to three short episodes of periorbital pain per day for 4–8 weeks, followed by a lengthy pain-free interval (e.g., 1 year or more); nocturnal pain is common
What are the symptoms of cluster headaches?	1. A "burning" or "boring" pain, always on the same side of the face 2. Ipsilateral vasodilation 3. Flushing 4. Lacrimation 5. Rhinorrhea 6. Horner's syndrome (seen in one third of patients)
What is the treatment for cluster headaches?	1. 100% oxygen (improves symptoms for 90% of patients within 15 minutes) 2. Ergotamine 3. Methysergide maleate 4. Calcium channel-blockers 5. Corticosteroids 6. Lithium

TOXIC METABOLIC HEADACHE

What type of pain is associated with toxic metabolic headache?	Constant, occipital, nonpulsatile pain that is aggravated by head movement
What is the underlying cause of toxic metabolic headache?	Vasodilation
List nine causes of toxic metabolic headache.	1. Breakdown of ethanol to acetaldehyde (a vasodilator) 2. Withdrawal from a vasoconstrictor, such as caffeine 3. Hypoxia and hypercapnia 4. Hypoglycemia 5. Anemia 6. Carbon monoxide poisoning 7. Uremia 8. Water intoxication 9. Vitamin A toxicity

TRIGEMINAL NEURALGIA

What is another name for trigeminal neuralgia?	Tic douloureux
Why "tic?"	Because the pain can cause fasciculation of the facial muscles
Which patients are most often diagnosed with trigeminal neuralgia?	Women in their 40s
What are the symptoms of trigeminal neuralgia?	Unilateral paroxysms of cranial nerve V result in searing, "electrical" facial pain
What is the most common distribution of trigeminal neuralgia?	The third division of cranial nerve V (i.e., the mandibular division)
What are trigger zones?	Areas near the lips, gums, or nose that, when touched, evoke a trigeminal neuralgia attack
What is the treatment for trigeminal neuralgia?	Anticonvulsants

TEMPORAL ARTERITIS

What is the classic presentation of temporal arteritis?
Headache, fever, anemia, and an elevated erythrocyte sedimentation rate (ESR) in an elderly person

What is the typical age of onset for temporal arteritis?
Older than 60 years

What is the typical ESR in a patient with temporal arteritis?
> 50 mm/h

How is temporal arteritis diagnosed?
Temporal artery biopsy

What is the treatment for temporal arteritis?
Steroids

What is a feared complication of temporal arteritis?
Blindness

SUBARACHNOID HEMORRHAGE

What are the two most common causes of subarachnoid hemorrhage?
Trauma or rupture of a congenital aneurysm

What is a sentinel bleed?
A small leak from an intracranial aneurysm before it ruptures

What is the typical history in a patient with subarachnoid hemorrhage?
Patients typically complain of the sudden onset of "the worst headache of their lives," characterized by the sudden onset of pain that worsens with head motion

What percentage of patients with subarachnoid hemorrhage complain of a severe headache?
45%

What are the signs of a subarachnoid hemorrhage?
1. Neck stiffness
2. Projectile vomiting
3. Papilledema
4. Seizures
5. Focal neurologic deficits
6. Changes in the level of consciousness

What percentage of patients experience a sudden, brief loss of consciousness with a subarachnoid hemorrhage?	45%

Do patients who do not experience a loss of consciousness typically have neurologic deficits initially?	No.

What are the typical neurologic signs that can occur with a subarachnoid hemorrhage?	1. Sixth nerve palsy 2. Unilateral third nerve palsy 3. Hemineglect 4. Memory loss 5. Hemiparesis 6. Signs of increased ICP or a mass effect

How is subarachnoid hemorrhage diagnosed?	A lumbar puncture is needed to identify subarachnoid blood. An arteriogram identifies the origin of the bleeding.

Can a noncontrast CT scan diagnose all subarachnoid hemorrhages?	No.

What are the goals of therapy for subarachnoid hemorrhage, and how are these goals achieved in the ED?	1. **Minimize cerebral edema:** Intravenous steroids, hyperventilation, and osmotic diuresis 2. **Control vasospasm:** Isoproterenol, aminophylline, lidocaine, or calcium channel-blockers

CENTRAL NERVOUS SYSTEM (CNS) TUMORS

What types of primary CNS tumors can be associated with headache?	Astrocytomas (e.g., glioblastoma multiforme), oligodendrogliomas, meningiomas, schwannomas, lymphomas

What tumors commonly metastasize to the brain?	1. Breast tumors 2. Lung tumors 3. Melanoma 4. Ovarian tumors 5. Testicular tumors 6. Renal tumors

What type of pain is associated with a space-occupying lesion?	A nonthrobbing, constant, prolonged pain that occurs primarily in the morning
Contrast the headache of a supratentorial tumor with that of a posterior fossa tumor.	Headaches caused by supratentorial masses tend to localize to the side of the mass. Headaches caused by posterior fossa tumors may be occipital, retro-orbital, or retro-auricular.
What other symptoms may be associated with the headache?	Nausea and vomiting (as a result of the increased ICP), focal neurologic deficits, seizures
What are the most common causes of ring-enhancing lesions on a head CT scan?	Astrocytoma, metastasis (usually from the lung), abscess (toxoplasmosis or pyogenic)
What is the acute management of an intracerebral mass lesion?	Control of the ICP; steroids may be used to decrease edema

CENTRAL NERVOUS SYSTEM (CNS) INFECTIONS

MENINGITIS

What is meningitis?	Inflammation of the meninges, usually (but not always) caused by bacterial or viral infection
Name the two major types of meningitis.	1. Infectious (e.g., bacterial, viral, fungal, tuberculous) 2. Noninfectious (i.e., caused by neoplasm or connective tissue disease)
What is "aseptic" meningitis?	Meningitis not caused by bacteria; viruses (especially enteroviruses and the mumps virus) are the most common cause of aseptic meningitis
What are risk factors for meningitis?	1. Extremes of age (i.e., very young or very old) 2. Chronic disease 3. Immunocompromised state 4. Splenectomy 5. Alcoholism 6. Recent neurosurgical procedure 7. Infection (especially endocarditis, pneumonia, sinusitis, and otitis media)

Which two organisms are most commonly associated with bacterial meningitis?	*Streptococcus pneumoniae* and *Neisseria meningitidis*
Who is especially at risk for meningococcal meningitis?	Those who live in crowded conditions (e.g., residents of dormitories or military barracks) and those with complement deficiency
Who is especially at risk for meningitis caused by Gram-negative organisms and *Listeria monocytogenes*?	Elderly patients, immunocompromised patients, and patients with alcoholism
Which organisms are common causes of neonatal meningitis?	*Escherichia coli*, Group B *Streptococcus*, and *L. monocytogenes*
What are the signs and symptoms of meningitis?	Headache, fever, and nuchal rigidity
When are signs and symptoms not a reliable means of detecting meningitis?	Mostly in very young and very old patients
Which two signs suggest the presence of meningeal irritation?	Kernig's sign and Brudzinski's sign
What is Kernig's sign?	Pain in the hamstrings when the knees are extended with the hips flexed at 90° (Kernig = "kick leg")
What is Brudzinski's sign?	Flexion of the neck causes flexion of the knees and hips (Brudzinski = "bend neck")
Before performing a lumbar puncture, what two conditions must be ruled out?	An intracranial mass and a bleeding disorder
What is a common occurrence following a lumbar puncture?	Development of a post–lumbar puncture headache
How can a post–lumbar puncture headache be prevented?	Use a small-gauge needle and have the patient lie flat after the procedure.

What cerebrospinal fluid (CSF) findings suggest:

    Bacterial meningitis?

1. Neutrophilic [polymorphonuclear neutrophil (PMN)] pleocytosis (i.e., 200–5000 cells/μl)
2. High protein level ($>$ 50 mg/dl)
3. Low CSF glucose:serum glucose ratio ($<$ 0.6)
4. Positive Gram stain

    Viral meningitis?

1. Lymphocytic (mononuclear cell) pleocytosis (i.e., $<$ 1000 cells/μl)
2. High protein level
3. Normal CSF glucose:serum glucose ratio (0.6)

Should antibiotics be withheld until after the lumbar puncture is performed?

No!

Why is ampicillin used when treating infants?

To cover *L. monocytogenes*

Who should receive chemoprophylaxis against meningitis?

Close contacts of patients with either *Haemophilus influenzae* or meningococcal meningitis

ENCEPHALITIS

What is encephalitis?

A viral infection of the brain parenchyma

List seven viruses that cause encephalitis.

1. Herpes simplex virus (HSV)
2. Arboviruses
3. Rabies virus
4. Enteroviruses
5. Mumps virus
6. Epstein-Barr virus (EBV)
7. Lymphocytic choriomeningitis virus

What are the signs and symptoms of encephalitis?

Meningeal symptoms (e.g., fever, headache, nausea, vomiting) or neurologic findings (e.g., altered level of consciousness, seizures, focal neurologic deficits, new behavioral findings, or cognitive deficits)

How is encephalitis diagnosed?

MRI (especially useful for detecting HSV encephalitis) and serologies; the specific cause is often not identified

What is rabies?   A fatal viral encephalitis

**What is the annual inci-
dence of rabies:**

   In the United States?   Average of 2 cases

   Internationally?   Tens of thousands of cases

**How is rabies virus trans-
mitted?**
1. Animal bite (saliva exposure)
2. Inhalation (rare)
3. Corneal transplant (rare)

**Which animals are common
carriers of rabies?**
1. Dogs
2. Cats
3. Skunks
4. Bats
5. Raccoons
6. Horses
7. Cattle
8. Foxes

**Which animals are not
implicated as carriers of
rabies?**
1. Birds
2. Rodents (e.g., rats, mice, squirrels)
3. Reptiles
4. Lagomorphs (e.g., rabbits, hares)
5. Properly immunized animals

**What is the incubation
period for rabies?**
It averages 1–2 months, but can range
anywhere from 10 days to 2 years. The
length of the incubation period is directly
proportional to the proximity of the bite
to the CNS. For example, a bite to the
face would be associated with a shorter
incubation period than one to the hands
or feet.

**What are the signs and
symptoms of rabies?**
Prodrome: Nonspecific fever, chills,
   general malaise, and myalgias
Encephalitis: Altered mental status;
   rage; restlessness; spasms of the
   pharynx or larynx that lead to choking
   and gagging during attempts to drink
   (i.e., hydrophobia); and thick,
   tenacious saliva
Advanced disease: Autonomic and brain
   stem dysfunction, coma, and death

How can the diagnosis of rabies be confirmed?

Postmorten histologic examination of brain tissue may reveal Negri bodies (i.e., viral inclusions in neurons). Direct fluorescent antibody testing of brain tissue or nuchal skin may reveal the rabies virus antigen.

Is death from rabies inevitable?

No, post-exposure prophylaxis is 100% effective if therapy is started before symptoms of rabies begin.

What is the post-exposure prophylaxis regimen?

Passive immunity is achieved using human rabies immune globulin (HRIG). The total dose is 20 IU/kg; half is infiltrated locally around the wound, and the other half is administered intragluteally.

Active immunity is achieved using the human diploid cell vaccine (HDCV). One milliliter is injected into the deltoid muscle on days 0, 3, 7, 14, and 28.

What treatment is necessary after:

A bite from a captured healthy pet?

Observe for 10 days; no prophylaxis is necessary.

A bite from an escaped animal?

A full course of prophylaxis is necessary (because the animal cannot be recovered for testing).

A bite from a captured wild animal?

Begin prophylaxis; if the animal is not infected, prophylactic therapy can be terminated.

What are the side effects of prophylaxis?

Patients may experience a local reaction, a low-grade fever, general malaise, and headache. Some patients develop an allergic reaction, but this is rare.

Who should receive pre-exposure prophylaxis against rabies?

Animal handlers, veterinarians, and travelers to endemic areas

What treatment should be given to a person who has had pre-exposure prophylaxis after a potential exposure to rabies?

HDCV should be administered on days 0 and 3; do not give HRIG.

BRAIN ABSCESS

What is the clinical presentation of a brain abscess?

A subactue progression with headache, depressed level of consciousness, and seizures

What is the differential diagnosis for a brain abscess?

1. Brain tumor
2. Encephalitis
3. Chronic subdural hematoma
4. Chronic meningitis
5. Cerebral infarction
6. Migraine

What is the pathogenesis of a brain abscess?

Hematogenous or contiguous spread of infection

Which organisms are associated with brain abscess?

Mixed flora account for half of all brain abscesses; anaerobes are also often implicated.

Which organisms most often cause brain abscesses in immunocompromised patients?

Nocardia asteroides, Aspergillus fumigatus, Candida albicans, Cryptococcus neoformans, and *Toxoplasma gondii*

How is a brain abscess diagnosed?

CT scan, with and without contrast

What is the treatment for a brain abscess?

Surgical intervention and administration of antibiotics

SEIZURES

What clinical entities are often confused with seizures?

1. Syncope
2. Arrhythmias
3. Migraines
4. Narcolepsy
5. Vertigo
6. Hyperventilation
7. Tetanus

What are the two major types of seizures?	Generalized and partial
What is a generalized seizure?	A seizure that involves the entire cerebral cortex (loss of consciousness)
What are the two types of generalized seizures?	Tonic–clonic and absence
How long do absence seizures usually last?	Approximately 10 seconds
What is a partial seizure?	A seizure in a localized region of the cortex
Can a partial seizure become a generalized seizure?	Yes.
What is a complex partial seizure?	A focal seizure in which consciousness, mentation, or both is altered.
What is the origin of partial seizures?	The temporal lobes
What is the most important immediate therapy for the actively seizing patient?	Protection and maintenance of an adequate airway
Define status epilepticus:	A prolonged series of similar seizures without full recovery of consciousness between them; the episode usually lasts for longer than 30 minutes
What percentage of patients present in status epilepticus with no prior history of epilepsy?	Approximately 30%
What is the initial management of status epilepticus?	Establish and maintain the airway, breathing, and circulation (ABCs) and check the patient's glucose level.
What anticonvulsants are available for the management of seizures?	Benzodiazepines, phenytoin, and barbiturates
What complications can be associated with phenytoin loading?	Arrhythmias and hypotension

What is the incidence of febrile seizure in otherwise healthy children?	2%–5%
At what ages are children most susceptible to febrile seizures?	Between the ages of 6 months and 6 years
How long do febrile seizures last?	Less than 5 minutes
What is the recurrence rate of febrile seizures?	Approximately 30%
What is the minimum work-up in an adult with a first-time seizure?	1. Complete blood count (CBC) 2. Serum electrolytes (including calcium and magnesium), blood urea nitrogen (BUN) and creatine levels, and a serum glucose level 3. A head CT (usually warranted in the ED)
What is the risk of recurrent seizure after a first, unprovoked seizure?	50%
What is Todd's paralysis?	Transient postictal paralysis after a focal seizure

VERTIGO AND DIZZINESS

What is "dizziness?"	Dizziness may mean many things to many people, including "faintness," "light-headedness," vertigo, or "weakness."
What is on the differential diagnosis when a patient complains of being "dizzy?"	1. Cardiac disorder 2. Infection 3. Neurologic disorder 4. Gastrointestinal bleeding
What is vertigo?	The definite sensation that either one's own body or the environment is revolving
What is the essential distinction to be made in the vertiginous patient?	Is the vertigo peripheral or central?
What are the characteristics of peripheral vertigo?	1. Abrupt onset and related to position 2. Moderate to extreme vertigo

3. Nystagmus (but otherwise, the neurologic examination is normal)
4. Nausea and vomiting
5. Tinnitus and hearing loss

Describe the nystagmus of peripheral vertigo.

1. Rotatory or horizontal
2. Bilateral
3. Latency of onset (2–30 seconds)
4. Fatigable
5. Suppressed with gaze fixation

What are the characteristics of central vertigo?

1. Insidious onset and not related to position
2. Mild to moderate vertigo
3. Nystagmus
4. Neurologic deficits (especially cranial nerve deficits)
5. Nausea, vomiting, and hearing loss are uncommon

Describe the nystagmus of central vertigo.

1. Vertical, rotatory, or bizarre
2. Unilateral or bilateral
3. No onset latency
4. Nonfatigable
5. Not visually suppressed

What is the Hallpike maneuver?

Positional testing to differentiate peripheral from central vertigo

PERIPHERAL VERTIGO

List six causes of peripheral vertigo.

1. Benign paroxysmal positional vertigo (BPPV)
2. Acute labyrinthitis
3. Meniere's disease
4. Acoustic neuroma
5. Obstruction of the external auditory canal
6. Therapy with an ototoxic drug (e.g., furosemide, aminoglycosides, antimalarial agents)

What is the most common cause of peripheral vertigo?

BPPV

What are the symptoms of BPPV?

Repeated episodes of vertigo following rapid changes in position

What is the treatment for BPPV?	Administration of benzodiazepines, anticholinergics, or antihistamines with anticholinergic effects
What is the clinical triad of Meniere's disease?	Hearing loss, vertigo, and tinnitus
What are the typical symptoms of Meniere's disease?	Clustered episodes of vertigo lasting 1–2 hours and fluctuating, low-frequency hearing loss
Peripheral vertigo may be a presenting symptom of which demyelinating disease?	Multiple sclerosis

CENTRAL VERTIGO

What are causes of central vertigo?	1. Vertebrobasilar insufficiency 2. Acoustic neuroma 3. Cerebral concussion 4. Cerebellar hemorrhage 5. Posterior fossa tumor 6. Migraine headache
Describe the characteristics of a vertebrobasilar migraine.	A headache preceded by a prodrome of vertigo, ataxia, visual changes, and dysarthria
Why should gait be tested in patients with vertigo?	Gait is often abnormal with cerebellar hemorrhage.

MULTIPLE SCLEROSIS

What is multiple sclerosis?	A demyelinating disease of the CNS characterized by numerous episodes of neurologic deficiency and multiple areas of involvement within the CNS
What is the definition of clinical multiple sclerosis?	Two or more episodes, each lasting at least 24 hours and occurring at least 1 month apart (or in a progressive course over at least 6 months), and beginning between the ages of 10 and 50 years
What is the gender prevalence?	2:1 (female:male)

What is the typical age of onset?

35 years

Where are demyelinated plaques most often found?

The optic tracts, basal ganglia, spinal cord and brain stem

What are negative symptoms of multiple sclerosis?

Neurologic deficits owing to loss of action potential propagation

What are positive symptoms of multiple sclerosis?

Demyelinated axons may become hyperexcitable and generate action potentials with minimal stimuli (e.g., Lhermitte's sign).

What is Lhermitte's sign?

A momentary electric-like sensation in the legs evoked by flexion of the neck or coughing

In multiple sclerosis, what are the:

    Motor signs and symptoms?

1. Weakness in one or more limbs
2. Facial weakness (may mimic Bell's palsy)
3. Spasticity
4. Hyperreflexia
5. Loss of reflexes (e.g., Babinski's sign)

    Sensory signs and symptoms?

1. Paresthesias and hypesthesia (numbness), commonly starting in one foot and progressing proximally
2. Trigeminal neuralgia

    Cerebellar signs and symptoms?

1. Ataxia
2. Dysarthria
3. Intention tremor
4. Vertigo

    Autonomic signs and symptoms?

Bowel and bladder dysfunction

    Cognitive signs and symptoms?

1. Memory loss
2. Uncontrollable laughing or crying
3. Depression

    Visual signs and symptoms?

1. Optic neuritis
2. Internuclear ophthalmoplegia
3. Diplopia (owing to cranial nerve VI palsy)

What is optic neuritis?

Inflammation of the optic nerve head

What are the signs and symptoms of optic neuritis?

1. Pain on movement of the eye
2. Unilateral decreased visual acuity
3. Enlarged pupil
4. Scotoma
5. Papillitis and pallor of the optic disk with intact venous pulsations

How can optic neuritis be distinguished from papilledema?

Papilledema is typically bilateral and is not associated with loss of acuity or pain on movement of the eye. Fundoscopic examination reveals loss of venous pulsations.

What is internuclear ophthalmoplegia?

Injury to the medial longitudinal fasciculus causes paresis of the medial rectus muscle on conjugate lateral gaze to the uninvolved side, while convergence is preserved.

What does bilateral internuclear ophthalmoplegia suggest?

It is virtually diagnostic of multiple sclerosis.

What are common presenting symptoms in a patient with multiple sclerosis?

Weakness in one or more limbs, visual blurring, sensory disturbances, diplopia, and ataxia

Can new neurologic deficits in a patient with multiple sclerosis be assumed to be a result of their disease?

No; there are many causes of an acute neurologic deficit.

What is the differential diagnosis of an acute neurologic deficit?

1. Intracranial bleeding or mass
2. Brain abscess or meningitis
3. Embolism or thrombosis
4. Hypoglycemia or vitamin B_{12} deficiency
5. Migraine headache
6. Postseizure state

How is a diagnosis of multiple sclerosis established?

1. MRI
2. CSF analysis (reveals myelin basic protein and oligoclonal bands of immunoglobulin in the CSF, but a normal total protein level)

What is the clinical course of:

Relapsing multiple sclerosis?	Recurrent neurologic dysfunction, with complete, partial, or no recovery
Chronic progressive multiple sclerosis?	Gradual worsening without periods of stabilization or recovery
Inactive multiple sclerosis?	Fixed neurologic deficits

What is the treatment of an acute exacerbation of multiple sclerosis?　　Airway management, urinary drainage, skin care, and treatment of hyperthermia

NEUROPATHIES

HEAVY METAL INTOXICATIONS

Where is arsenic found?　　In insecticides, rat poisons, herbicides, and certain medical compounds

What does a low-dose arsenic intoxication cause?　　Polyneuritis

What does chronic exposure to small doses of lead cause?　　Peripheral motor neuropathy

GUILLAIN-BARRÉ SYNDROME

What is Guillain-Barré syndrome?　　An acute demyelinating motor polyneuropathy

What can precipitate Guillain-Barré syndrome?　　Infection, exposure to toxins, and collagen vascular disease

What is the typical age of patients most frequently affected by Guillain-Barré syndrome?　　30–40 years

What is the clinical presentation?　　An ascending transverse myelitis

What is the typical time course?　　The most severe symptoms develop within 1 week, with recovery taking weeks to months.

MONONEURITIS MULTIPLEX

What is mononeuritis multiplex?　　Multiple, isolated, peripheral nerve deficits in a random distribution

What is the pathophysiology of mononeuritis multiplex?	Arteritis causes infarction of the vasa vasorum that supply the arteries that supply the peripheral nerves
Which diseases are associated with mononeuritis multiplex?	Collagen vascular disease and diabetes mellitus

BELL'S PALSY

What is Bell's palsy?	An idiopathic mononeuritis of cranial nerve VII that results in a unilateral facial paralysis of sudden onset
What does facial examination of a patient with Bell's palsy reveal?	Unilateral facial weakness with forehead involvement
What symptom may be associated with the facial weakness?	Jaw or external ear pain
What is the treatment for Bell's palsy?	High-dose steroids and electrostimuation of the facial muscles
What are important diagnoses to consider in the patient with facial weakness?	1. Lesions of the middle ear 2. Cerebellopontine angle tumor 3. Lyme disease 4. Vascular disease

VOLKMANN'S ISCHEMIC PARALYSIS

What is Volkmann's ischemic paralysis?	Local paralysis as a result of impaired circulation
What is a common iatrogenic cause?	A tight-fitting cast

MYOPATHIES

ACQUIRED MYOPATHIES

Distinguish myopathy from neuropathy in terms of:	
The type of associated weakness	Neuropathy is associated with an ascending weakness, whereas the weakness associated with myopathy is diffuse and simultaneous.

Associated sensory deficits	Neuropathy has associated sensory deficits, but myopathy does not.
Associated loss of reflexes	In neuropathy, the reflexes are lost early in the course of the disease, whereas in myopathy, they are maintained until late in the disease course.
What is polymyositis?	An inflammatory myopathy characterized by weakness, muscle pain, and tenderness
What other clinical findings are associated with poly-myositis?	Arthralgia, fever, and Raynaud's phenomenon
What is the treatment for polymyositis?	Immunosuppression, usually with prednisone
What is alcoholic myopathy?	Severe muscle tenderness and swelling, muscle cramps, and weakness during prolonged periods of heavy alcohol intake
Describe the pathogenesis of alcoholic myopathy.	Alcohol causes acute necrosis of skeletal muscle fibers.
What are potentially serious complications of alcoholic myopathy?	Hyperkalemia, hypocalcemia, and myoglobinuria leading to renal failure
What is the treatment for alcoholic myopathy?	Supportive treatment to address electrolyte abnormalities and myoglobinuria

ACUTE PERIODIC PARALYSIS

What is acute periodic paralysis?	An autosomal dominant disorder characterized by recurring attacks of extreme weakness without pain; the attacks last 1–2 hours
What are the three types of acute periodic paralysis?	Hyperkalemic, hypokalemic, and normokalemic
Which is the predominant gender and age of patients with acute periodic paralysis?	Men between the ages of 7 and 21 years
List five factors that may provoke an attack.	1. Physical exertion 2. Cold weather

3. A large meal
4. Trauma
5. Surgery

DISORDERS OF NEUROMUSCULAR TRANSMISSION

TETANUS

What organism causes tetanus?	*Clostridium tetani*
How does *C. tetani* cause tetanus?	It produces tetanospasmin, an exotoxin that acts on the motor endplates of the skeletal muscles and on the spinal cord, brain, and sympathetic nervous system to prevent transmission at inhibitory interneurons in the CNS
What is the most common presenting symptom of tetanus?	Trismus
What is risus sardonicus?	A tight, rigid facial expression
How long after inoculation do symptoms of tetanus appear?	5–10 days
What is the treatment for tetanus?	Administration of antitoxin and supportive therapy (e.g., the administration of antibiotics and muscle relaxants; respiratory support)

BOTULISM

What is botulism?	A neurologic disease caused by the ingestion of a paralytic exotoxin elaborated by *Clostridium botulinum*
Describe the three types of botulism.	1. **Food-borne botulism** is seen in adults and older children and is caused by the ingestion of preformed toxin, most commonly found in contaminated home-canned foods or honey.
	2. **Infantile botulism** is seen in infants and is caused by the ingestion of *C. botulinum* spores, which then

proliferate in the infant's gastro-intestinal tract and release the toxin.

3. **Wound botulism** is rare. Anaerobic conditions at the wound site allow bacteria to grow and elaborate toxin.

How does the exotoxin produce signs and symptoms?

It inhibits the release of acetylcholine at the neuromuscular junction.

Which muscles does the exotoxin typically affect first?

Muscles innervated by the cranial nerves

What are the typical signs and symptoms of botulism?

Weakness, cranial nerve findings, descending paralysis, diplopia, xerostomia, dysarthria, and autonomic instability, all leading to frank respiratory failure

What is the typical presentation of botulism in an:

Adult?

Patients typically present with diplopia, which lasts for approximately 24 hours. Eventually, generalized weakness develops, possibly progressing rapidly to paralysis and respiratory failure.

Infant?

"Floppy baby," constipation, weak cry and poor feeding, decreased reflexes, and pooling of oral secretions

What is the differential diagnosis for botulism in an adult?

Myasthenia gravis; a high index of suspicion is necessary

How is botulism diagnosed?

Botulism can usually be diagnosed on the basis of the history and physical examination findings. If the diagnosis is in doubt, electromyography or a toxin assay may be useful.

What is the treatment for botulism?

Supportive therapy (i.e., respiratory care); possibly, administration of an antitoxin (made from horse serum)

What is the usual course of the disease?

The disease course may be as long as 3–6 months.

MYASTHENIA GRAVIS

What is myasthenia gravis?	An autoimmune disorder; antibodies are directed against the acetylcholine receptors on the muscles, leading to destruction of the receptors and weakness
Describe the typical patient with myasthenia gravis.	A woman in her mid-20s
What is the hallmark symptom of myasthenia gravis?	Muscle weakness that worsens with activity and improves with rest.
Which muscle group is most commonly affected by myasthenia gravis?	The extraocular muscles (patients experience recurring ptosis and diplopia)
What is the greatest threat to the patient with myasthenia gravis?	Unrecognized airway and ventilatory difficulty
What is the "Tensilon test?"	The patient is administered 1–2 mg of edrophonium bromide (Tensilon), an acetylcholinesterase inhibitor. A transient increase in muscle strength following the administration of edrophonium bromide suggests myasthenia gravis.
The "Tensilon test" can be used to differentiate which condition from myasthenia gravis?	Botulism
What is a "myasthenic crisis?"	Severe weakness in a patient with myasthenia gravis
List three factors that can precipitate a myasthenic crisis.	1. Poor compliance with medications 2. Drug interaction 3. Underlying infection
How is a myasthenic crisis managed in the ED?	With supportive care; consider plasmapheresis (after consulting with a neurologist)
What is a "cholinergic crisis?"	Overmedication with the cholinergic drugs used to treat myasthenia gravis

What are the symptoms of a cholinergic crisis?	1. **Muscarinic:** Miosis, sweating, salivation, gastrointestinal distress 2. **Nicotinic:** Fasciculations, muscle cramping
What is the treatment for cholinergic crisis?	Supportive therapy; atropine may be administered if the patient's symptoms are severe

EATON-LAMBERT SYNDROME

What is Eaton-Lambert syndrome?	A syndrome similar to myasthenia gravis that is associated with malignancies (especially small cell carcinoma of the lung)
What are the differences between myasthenia gravis and Eaton-Lambert syndrome?	1. Eaton-Lambert syndrome spares the cranial nerves. 2. There is less fluctuation of weakness with Eaton-Lambert. 3. Repeated activity will improve grip strength in patients with Eaton-Lambert syndrome. 4. The symptoms of myasthenia gravis will improve following the administration of edrophonium.
What are the signs and symptoms of Eaton-Lambert syndrome?	Xerostomia, vague sensory findings, and, occasionally, absent reflexes
What is the treatment for Eaton-Lambert syndrome?	There is no satisfactory therapy.

12

Psychiatric Emergencies

What psychiatric disorders are most commonly seen in the emergency department (ED)?	Substance abuse, affective disorders, anxiety disorders, antisocial personality disorder, severe cognitive disorders, and psychotic disorders
Name the three psychiatric emergencies.	Suicide, psychosis, and violent behavior
What is the standard reference used to diagnose psychiatric disorders?	The *Diagnostic and Statistical Manual of Mental Health Disorders* (DSM-IV), which provides diagnostic criteria based on the patient's signs and symptoms

EVALUATION OF THE PSYCHIATRIC PATIENT

What information should be noted in the history?	Suicidal or homicidal ideations Hallucinations Changes in behavior (discuss with family/friends) Involvement in substance abuse Past psychiatric history (including any episodes of violent behavior or suicide attempts) Current medications Review of systems
What should be included in the physical exam?	Vital signs and a thorough neurologic exam, including a mini-mental status exam
What is a mini-mental status exam?	A standardized exam that quickly tests the patient's cognitive function and screens for organic brain disorders, such as dementia and delirium
Describe the multiaxial categories of diagnosis.	**Axis I:** Clinical syndromes of mental disorders

Axis II: Personality disorders and developmental disorders

Axis III: General medical conditions

Axis IV: Psychosocial and environmental stressors

Axis V: Adaptive functioning

Name the differential diagnosis for psychiatric complaints.	Central nervous system (CNS) infection Intoxication Poisoning Withdrawal Hypoglycemia Hypoxia Hypertensive encephalopathy Intracranial hemorrhage Seizure disorder

VIOLENT BEHAVIOR

What cautions should you take when handling a violent patient?	1. Maintain distance between you and the patient. 2. Do not threaten the patient. 3. Do not allow the patient to get between you and the exit. 4. Allow the patient to verbalize his feelings. 5. Make neutral comments about the patient's situation and behavior. 6. Make sure that adequate force (e.g., security guards) is available and visible to the patient.
When are physical restraints used?	When the patient becomes violent or threatens violence
Who should place the restraints on the patient?	Security personnel or police (**not the ED staff**)
When are chemical restraints used?	When the patient continues to fight against the physical restraints, with the potential for injury
What medications can be used as chemical restraints?	Lorazepam is commonly used as a chemical restraint; however, if it is insufficient, haloperidol can be added.

SUICIDE

What is the prevalence of suicide?	Suicide is the second leading cause of death in people younger than 24 years; 1% of the population attempt suicide.
What is the ratio of attempted to completed suicide?	40:1
What gender is more likely to attempt suicide?	Women; they attempt suicide 2 to 3 times more than men
What factors contribute to attempted suicide?	Major depression, undesirable life events
What gender is more likely to complete suicide?	Men; particularly older men who live alone and are physically ill
What factors contribute to completed suicide?	Schizophrenia, major depression, substance abuse, violence, previous suicide attempt
What is the most common form of attempted suicide?	Drug overdose
What precautions are necessary for a suicidal patient?	Remove all dangerous objects from the room. Instruct staff members to watch the patient. Provide the patient with a hospital gown. Perform a weapons search.

COGNITIVE DISORDERS

DEMENTIA

What is dementia?	Cognitive impairment that reduces social functioning, but does not usually affect consciousness or alertness
Name the five types of cognitive functioning that may be affected by dementia.	1. Memory 2. Abstract thinking 3. Judgment 4. Personality 5. Language
What percentage of dementia cases are attributable to a reversible cause?	Approximately 15% (but only 3% of cases may fully resolve)

What are some reversible causes of dementia?	Subdural hematoma Normal pressure hydrocephalus Meningitis or encephalitis Metabolic or endocrine disorders Nutritional deficiencies Polypharmacy Pseudodementia
What is pseudodementia?	A depressive illness that often causes dementia, but is reversible; the patient complains of loss of cognitive skills
What is the time course for the onset of dementia?	Slow and gradual
How does a typical patient with dementia present to the ED?	With worsening memory loss, agitated or violent behavior; significant medical problems (e.g., fever, stroke, vomiting); the family may no longer be able to care for the patient
What is the differential diagnosis for acute dementia?	Medical condition or illness, adverse drug effect, environmental change
What are the complications of dementia?	Aggressive or violent behavior, wandering, psychosis, depression
What is the treatment for dementia?	Treat the reversible causes and any underlying medical illnesses.

DELIRIUM

What is delirium?	Global cognitive impairment with clouding of consciousness and sensory misperception, such as hallucinations
Who is at risk for delirium?	Elderly patients, postsurgical patients, intensive care unit patients, and patients with existing dementia
What are the causes of delirium?	Serious medical illness, drug intoxication or withdrawal
What is the typical time course for the onset of delirium?	Acute, with rapid deterioration

How does a typical patient with delirium present to the ED?

Patients may present with fractures, a systemic infection, or signs of drug abuse.

What is the treatment for delirium?

Treat the underlying cause or medical illness.

SUBSTANCE-INDUCED DISORDERS

What is substance abuse?

A maladaptive pattern of substance use leading to significant impairment and distress in at least 1 of the 4 following areas:
1. Occupation
2. Law
3. Relationships
4. Health

What is substance withdrawal?

Signs and symptoms associated with cessation of, or reduction in, substance use

What are the signs and symptoms of alcohol withdrawal that present at the following time periods?

    6–8 hours

Autonomic hyperactivity, evidenced by increased blood pressure, heart and respiratory rates, and temperature

    24 hours

Hallucinations

    24–48 hours

Major motor seizures

    3–5 days

Global confusion

What is the treatment for alcohol withdrawal?

Benzodiazepines, supportive care (including hydration and monitoring), nutritional supplementation, and anticonvulsants

A patient with a history of seizures presents to the ED experiencing alcohol withdrawal. Would inpatient therapy be required? Why or why not?

No. There is a low risk of seizure while receiving adequate supportive therapy.

PSYCHOTIC DISORDERS

What characterizes psychosis?	Hallucinations, delusions, disorganized thoughts and behavior
What are hallucinations?	False perceptions experienced in a sensory modality and occurring in clear consciousness
What are the 5 types of hallucinations (in decreasing prevalence)?	1. Auditory 2. Visual 3. Tactile 4. Olfactory 5. Gustatory
What are delusions?	Fixed false beliefs not shared by others of a similar culture; patients with delusions are not amenable to facts or arguments that contradict the delusion.
What is the most prevalent form of psychosis?	Schizophrenia
What are some of the characteristics of schizophrenia?	Deterioration in social or occupational functioning Presence of active-phase symptoms (e.g., delusions, hallucinations, disorganized speech and behavior) Catatonic behavior Negative symptoms, such as lack of volition, blunted emotions, anhedonia, or inattention Lack of insight
When is the typical onset of schizophrenia?	During late adolescence or early adulthood
How does a typical patient with schizophrenia present to the ED?	With worsening psychosis (owing to stress or noncompliance with medications), suicidal ideations or attempts, violent behavior, or extrapyramidal side effects from antipsychotic medications
What is the differential diagnosis for schizophrenia?	Substance abuse Intoxication from a prescribed medication Infection Metabolic or endocrine disorders

Brain tumor or mass lesion
Temporal lobe epilepsy
Other mental illness with psychotic
    features (e.g., schizoaffective disorder
    or mood disorder)

**What is the treatment for
schizophrenia?**

Antipsychotic medications and supportive
psychotherapy

AFFECTIVE DISORDERS

**What is the prevalence of
affective disorders?**

Approximately 10% to 15% of the general
population experience an affective
disorder during the course of life.

**What are the complications
of affective disorders?**

Suicide, substance abuse, marital or
occupational disruption

**What type of affective
disorder occurs more
frequently—depression or
mania?**

Depression

MAJOR DEPRESSION

What is major depression?

A persistent dysphoric mood and
pervasive loss of interest in usual activities
that lasts longer than 2 weeks

**What are the associated
symptoms?**

Guilt
Self-reproach
Feelings of worthlessness or hopelessness
Inability to experience pleasure
Recurrent thoughts of death or suicide
Loss of appetite or weight
Sleep disturbances
Fatigue
Inability to concentrate
Psychomotor agitation or retardation

**What gender is more likely
to have major depression?**

Women; particularly those with a medical
or psychiatric history or a family history of
depression or suicide

**How does a patient with
major depression typically
present to the ED?**

With suicidal thoughts or worsening of
depressive symptoms

What is the differential diagnosis for major depression?	Substance abuse Side effects of therapeutic medications (e.g., sedatives, tranquilizers, antihypertensive agents, oral contraceptives) Lupus Normal bereavement
What is the treatment for major depression?	Antidepressants and supportive psychotherapy; hospitalization may be indicated if the patient is actively suicidal

BIPOLAR DISORDER

What is bipolar disorder?	Manic depression
What are the associated symptoms?	Mood shifts from elation to irritation Inflated self-esteem Expansive, energetic, or precarious feelings Argumentative, hostile, or sarcastic demeanor Poor judgment (e.g., financial irresponsibility, excessive sexual behavior) Decreased need for sleep; increased activities; rapid, pressured speech; racing thoughts Possible lack of insight
What gender is more likely to have bipolar disorder?	Bipolar disorder is equally common among men and women.
What is the typical age of onset?	Bipolar disorder typically develops in people 20–30 years of age.
How does a patient with bipolar disorder typically present to the ED?	With depression, suicidal thoughts, a manic episode, or signs of poor judgment or psychosis
What is the differential diagnosis for bipolar disorder?	Substance abuse, schizophrenia
What is the treatment for bipolar disorder?	Lithium is the drug of choice; however, carbamazepine and valproate may also be used. Supportive psychotherapy is another aspect of the treatment.

What medications can be used to treat severe agitation?	Benzodiazepines or antipsychotics

PANIC DISORDER

What is panic disorder?	A disorder characterized by recurrent, unexpected panic attacks; patients develop anxiety about additional attacks, the consequences of attacks, or the development of significant changes in behavior.
What are panic attacks?	The sudden onset of at least 4 of the following symptoms: Palpitations Tachycardia Diaphoresis Tremor Shortness of breath Choking Chest pain Nausea Dizziness Derealization or depersonalization Fear of losing control Fear of dying Paresthesia Hot flashes
What is phobic avoidance?	Avoiding situations that seem to exacerbate panic attacks; this disorder can severely impair functioning
What gender is more likely to have panic disorder?	Women
How does a patient with panic disorder typically present to the ED?	With chest pain, shortness of breath, or palpitations—the ED is frequently the initial source of medical attention for these patients.
In a patient with previously undiagnosed panic disorder, what might the history reveal?	Domestic violence or sexual abuse or assault
What is the differential diagnosis for panic disorder?	Hyperthyroidism Hyperparathyroidism

Pheochromocytoma
Vestibulitis
Hypoglycemia
Supraventricular tachycardia
Angina
Myocardial infarction
Depression

What is the treatment for panic disorder?

Supportive psychotherapy and medications (e.g., antidepressants, β blockers, buspirone, and less commonly, benzodiazepines)

What medications may be used in the ED for acute attacks?

Benzodiazepines may be given as a one-time dose, with medical follow-up

CONVERSION DISORDER

What is conversion disorder?

Loss of function due to psychological, not physical, factors

How does a patient with conversion disorder typically present to the ED?

With neurologic complaints, such as paralysis, blindness, or numbness

How is conversion disorder diagnosed in the ED?

It is not wise to make this diagnosis in the ED; always arrange medical follow-up

What percentage of patients diagnosed with conversion disorder actually have an underlying medical condition?

25%

PERSONALITY DISORDERS

What is a personality disorder?

A long-term behavior or trait that causes significant impairment in social and occupational functioning or considerable stress; not limited to periods of illness

Which personality disorder is seen most frequently in the ED?

Antisocial personality disorder

What are the characteristics of antisocial personality disorder?

A continuous pattern of maladaptive behavior with disregard for others' rights

What are some examples of maladaptive behavior?	Criminal behavior Fighting Lying Abuse or neglect of dependents and spouse Financial irresponsibility Recklessness Inability to sustain enduring relationships with others
Name some of the other personality disorders.	Borderline, narcissistic, histrionic, paranoid, schizoid, schizotypal, avoidant, dependant, obsessive–compulsive
What are the complications of personality disorders?	Substance abuse, traumatic injury, accidental or violent death, poor medical compliance
What is the treatment for personality disorders?	Supportive psychotherapy can be used; however, patients rarely seek treatment and are usually resistant to it.
How should patients with personality disorders be managed in the ED?	Firmly limit behavior and focus on the chief complaint.

ANOREXIA NERVOSA AND BULIMIA

Who typically has it?	5%–10% of adolescent girls and young women and 0.1% of young men (across all racial and socioeconomic groups)
What is the typical age of onset for each disorder?	
Anorexia	12 years–the mid-30s
Bulimia	17–25 years
What is anorexia?	A starvation syndrome characterized by a disturbance in body image perception. Patients refuse to maintain a body weight over the minimum and have an intense fear of obesity, even when they are underweight.
What are the signs and symptoms of anorexia?	Unexplained growth retardation Amenorrhea—primary or secondary

(latter is evidenced by the absence of at least 3 consecutive menstrual cycles)

Weight loss of unknown origin

Hypercholesterolemia or carotenemia in a thin person

Exercise abuse

What is bulimia?

Bulimia is an eating disorder characterized by binge eating followed by vomiting or laxative abuse.

What are the signs and symptoms of bulimia?

Hypokalemia of unknown cause or complications of hypokalemia

Parotid or submandibular gland enlargement

Esophagitis

Esophageal bleeding or rupture

Large unexplained weight loss or fluctuations

Elevated serum amylase

Secondary amenorrhea

Loss of dental enamel or several new dental caries

Easy bruising due to the loss of bile salts and poor absorption of vitamin K

Scars on the knuckles of the hands from induced vomiting

Name three risk factors for an eating disorder.

1. Juvenile diabetes
2. Other disorders of impulse control, such as substance abuse or borderline personality disorder
3. High-risk vocation (e.g., model, ballet dancer, wrestler, gymnast)

What is the differential diagnosis for eating disorders?

Schizophrenia, with aversion to eating

Major depression with anorexia or hyperphagia

Obsessive–compulsive disorder

Superior mesenteric artery syndrome

Inflammatory bowel disease

Chronic hepatitis

Addison's disease

Diabetes

Hyperthyroidism

Hyperemesis gravidarum

Tuberculosis

Malignancy

HIV

PSYCHOTROPIC MEDICATIONS

ANTIPSYCHOTICS (NEUROLEPTICS)

What are the indications?

Psychotic behavior, agitation, potential to harm self or others

What are the contraindications?

Known allergy, pregnancy, and history of neuroleptic malignant syndrome

Name the seven classes of neuroleptics, along with at least one example of each.

1. **Phenothiazines:** Promethazine, prochlorperazine, chlorpromazine, thioridazine
2. **Thioxanthenes:** Thiothixene
3. **Butyrophenones:** Haloperidol, droperidol
4. **Dibenzoxazepines:** Loxapine
5. **Dihydroindolones:** Molindone
6. **Dibenzodiazepine:** Clozapine
7. **Benzisoxazoles:** Risperidone

Side effects

What are some common side effects?

Orthostatic hypotension (as a result of α blockade)
Anticholinergic symptoms
Akathisia
Acute dystonic reaction
Parkinsonian syndrome
Tardive dyskinesia
Neuroleptic malignant syndrome

Which neuroleptics are more likely to cause anticholinergic symptoms and α blockade?

Low-potency neuroleptics, such as chlorpromazine or thioridazine

Which neuroleptics are more likely to cause extrapyramidal (motor) side effects?

High-potency neuroleptics, such as haloperidol or droperidol

Orthostatic hypotension

What is the mechanism for orthostatic hypotension?

α-Adrenergic blockade

What is the treatment for orthostatic hypotension?

Initiate intravenous fluids and administer an α agonist (e.g., norepinephrine, phenylephrine, or metaraminol bitartrate). Avoid β agonists, which may worsen the hypotension.

Anticholinergic symptoms

Describe anticholinergic symptoms.

Delirium and sedation (mad as a hatter)
Dry mouth and skin, constipation, and urinary retention (dry as a bone)
Flushing (red as a beet)
Hyperthermia (hot as a poker)
Blurred vision and exacerbation of narrow-angle glaucoma (blind as a bat)
Cardiac arrhythmias

What is the treatment for anticholinergic symptoms?

Stop the neuroleptic agent and initiate supportive measures. If the symptoms are life-threatening, administer physostigmine.

Akathisia

What is akathisia?

Motor restlessness and anxiety, which often occur early in treatment

What is a common misdiagnosis for akathisia?

Worsening psychosis; this misdiagnosis may result in an increase in the drug dosage

What is the treatment for akathisia?

Decrease the dose of the neuroleptic or change to a different antipsychotic agent and administer benztropine.

Acute dystonic reaction

What is an acute dystonic reaction?

Muscle spasms usually occurring in the face and extremities; may sometimes include an oculogyric crisis or laryngospasm (although rarely life-threatening); occurs early in treatment and is caused by a dopaminergic blockade

What gender is more likely to have an acute dystonic reaction?

Men

What is the treatment for an acute dystonic reaction?

Diphenhydramine or benztropine

Parkinsonian syndrome

What are the symptoms of parkinsonian syndrome?

Bradykinesia, resting tremor, cogwheel rigidity, shuffling gait, masked faces

When does drug-induced parkinsonian syndrome occur most frequently?

In elderly patients during the first month of treatment

What is the treatment for parkinsonian syndrome?

Decrease the dose of neuroleptic and initiate therapy with anticholinergic agents.

What is tardive dyskinesia?

Abnormal involuntary movement, usually of the face and tongue

Which patients are more likely to develop tardive dyskinesia?

Elderly patients; more often women and patients with mood disorder

What is the treatment for tardive dyskinesia?

Tardive dyskinesia is usually untreatable and often irreversible. Decreasing the dose or stopping the neuroleptics may actually worsen symptoms; therefore, it is more effective to **add or increase antipsychotics and cholinergic stimulation.** Note that anticholinergics may worsen the symptoms and should be avoided.

Neuroleptic malignant syndrome (NMS)

Describe NMS.

Uncommon idiosyncratic reaction characterized by rigidity; altered mental status; hyperthermia; autonomic instability (e.g., labile blood pressure, tachycardia); increased creatine phosphokinase (CPK) and liver enzyme levels; and an increased white blood cell (WBC) count

What is the mortality rate?

4%–20%

What is the treatment for neuroleptic malignant syndrome?

Stop the neuroleptic agent and consider administering dantrolene or bromocriptine.

Atypical antipsychotics

What is clozapine? Name some of its side effects.

Clozapine is an atypical antipsychotic agent that is associated with few extrapyramidal side effects. Side effects include agranulocytosis, sedation, hypotension, anticholinergic symptoms, and decreased seizure threshold.

What is risperidone? Name some of its side effects.

Risperidone is an atypical antipsychotic agent that is associated with few extrapyramidal side effects. Side effects include sedation, insomnia, constipation, weight gain, tachycardia, hypotension, and prolonged QT interval

What is seen with risperidone overdose?

An overdose of risperidone is rarely fatal when taken alone; however, hypotension, anticholinergic symptoms, and extrapyramidal symptoms may be seen.

ANXIOLYTICS (BENZODIAZEPINES)

What are the indications?

Anxiety
Agitation
Acute pain reactions
Muscle relaxation and cooperation during painful procedures
Seizure control
Treatment of alcohol and sedative or hypnotic withdrawal

What are the contraindications?

Known hypersensitivity or acute narrow-angle glaucoma

What are the common side effects?

Potentiation of the effects of other CNS depressants, suppression of the hypoxic respiratory drive, sedation, and ataxia

What is seen with the paradoxical response?

Insomnia and agitation (common in elderly patients)

What is seen with overdose when combined with other CNS depressants?

Sedation, coma, and apnea

What is buspirone?

Buspirone is an atypical anxiolytic agent with a delayed onset of action (from days to weeks).

HETEROCYCLIC ANTIDEPRESSANTS (TRICYCLIC ANTIDEPRESSANTS)

How do they work?

Tricyclic antidepressants potentiate the action of norepinephrine, serotonin, or both by blocking their neuronal reuptake (and subsequent inactivation).

What are the indications?

Major depression
Dysthymic disorder
Panic disorder
Agoraphobia
Obsessive–compulsive disorder
Enuresis
School phobia

What are common side effects?

Anticholinergic symptoms are most common. Other side effects include:
Cardiotoxicity, including nonspecific T wave changes, prolongation of the QT interval, varying degrees of atrioventricular (AV) block, and atrial and ventricular arrhythmias
Orthostatic hypotension
Obstructive jaundice
Decreased seizure threshold

MONOAMINE OXIDASE INHIBITORS (MAOIS)

How do they work?

These drugs block the oxidation of biogenic amines (e.g., tyramine, serotonin, dopamine, norepinephrine), thereby increasing serotonin and norepinephrine levels.

What are the indications?

Atypical major depression (hyperphagia, hypersomnolence, emotional lability)
Heterocyclic antidepressant–resistant major depression
Panic disorder

What are common side effects?

Orthostatic hypotension
CNS irritability
Mild anticholinergic symptoms
Possible hypertensive crisis when combined with sympathomimetic amines (e.g., L-dopa, narcotics, heterocyclic antidepressants, tyramine-containing foods)

Name examples of tyramine-containing foods.	Aged cheese, beer, wine, pickled herring, yeast extracts, chopped liver, yogurt, sour cream, fava beans

SELECTIVE SEROTONIN REUPTAKE INHIBITORS (SSRIS)

How do they work?	SSRIs block the reuptake of serotonin.
What are the indications?	Major depression, panic disorder, obsessive–compulsive disorder
What are common side effects?	May initially increase suicidality May also cause headache, nausea, diarrhea, insomnia, agitation, and serotonin syndrome
What are the symptoms of serotonin syndrome?	CNS irritability, including restlessness, tremor, myoclonus, hyperreflexia, and seizures Gastrointestinal irritability, including nausea, vomiting, and diarrhea
When does serotonin syndrome most often occur?	When SSRIs are combined with other serotinergic medications, such as MAOIs

ATYPICAL SECOND GENERATION ANTIDEPRESSANTS

Bupropion

How does it work?	Unknown mechanism
What is the indication?	Major depression
What are the contraindications?	Known allergy; history of eating disorder; history of head trauma; predisposition toward seizures, including medications that decrease the seizure threshold
What are the common side effects?	Dry mouth Dizziness Headache Tremor Insomnia Psychomotor agitation May exacerbate psychotic episodes May exacerbate baseline hypertension Seizures, especially in bulimic patients

Venlafaxine

How does it work?

Venlafaxine is a potent inhibitor of neuronal serotonin and norepinephrine reuptake and a weak inhibitor of dopaminergic reuptake.

What is the indication?

Major depression

What are common side effects?

CNS effects: Asthenia, dizziness, anxiety, tremor, blurred vision, somnolence
Gastrointestinal effects: Nausea and vomiting, constipation, anorexia, dry mouth
Peripheral effects: Diaphoresis, abnormal ejaculation, impotence

Lithium

How does it work?

Unknown

What are the indications?

Acute mania
Maintenance therapy for bipolar disorder
Major depression
Self-mutilation

What are common side effects seen in the first few weeks (unrelated to levels)?

Gastrointestinal distress, dry mouth, excessive thirst, fine tremor, mild polyuria, peripheral edema

What are chronic side effects (unrelated to levels)?

Polyuria, nephrogenic diabetes insipidus, benign diffuse goiter, hypothyroidism, rash, psoriasis, leukocytosis

Name three risk factors that may predispose a person to lithium toxicity

1. Neurologic illness
2. Dehydration
3. Salt-restricted diet

What determines the severity of lithium toxicity?

The severity of toxicity is related to the CNS lithium level.

When can symptoms develop?

Up to 48 hours after acute ingestion

Name the signs that are present at each of the following stages of lithium toxicity:

    Early stage

Nausea, vomiting, dysarthria, lethargy, coarse hand tremor

Intermediate stage

Ataxia, myasthenia, incoordination, hyperreflexia, muscle fasciculations, blurred vision, scotomas

Late stage

Confusion, choreoathetosis, myoclonus, seizure, coma

At what serum lithium level should the patient be admitted to the hospital for treatment?

> 2 mEq/L or the patient is symptomatic

What signs would be expected when the lithium level exceeds 4 mEq/L?

Nonspecific T wave changes, hypotension, AV conduction defects, ventricular arrhythmias, cardiovascular collapse

What is the treatment for lithium toxicity?

Lithium toxicity is considered a medical emergency. Treatment includes electrolyte replacement and diuresis. Hemodialysis is also performed if the lithium level is greater than 4 mEq/L or if the patient's clinical condition is poor.

13 Toxicologic Emergencies

GENERAL MANAGEMENT OF THE POISONED PATIENT

What is the first step in the management of the poisoned patient?

Assess airway, breathing, and circulation (the ABCs).

Name three general ways to treat the poisoned patient.

1. Use supportive therapy.
2. Decrease the patient's exposure to the poison.
3. Administer a specific antidote.

How do antidotes work?

Antidotes reverse the effects of the poison and enhance its metabolism.

Name three general ways to decrease the patient's exposure to the poison.

1. Eliminate the environmental exposure.
2. Remove the chemical from the gastrointestinal tract (gastric decontamination).
3. Increase elimination of the absorbed toxin.

Name seven specific methods of minimizing toxicity in a poisoned patient.

1. Gastric emptying
2. Activated charcoal
3. Administration of cathartics
4. Whole-bowel irrigation
5. Dialysis
6. Hemoperfusion
7. Urinary alkalinization

What is the most effective means of gastric emptying?

Gastric lavage

What is the most common complication of gastric lavage?

Aspiration

When is gastric lavage completed?

When no particulate matter is seen in the lavage

What are contraindications to gastric lavage?

1. Ingestion of an alkaline substance or drug packets
2. Delayed presentation
3. A history of vomiting soon after the ingestion

How does activated charcoal work?

By decreasing absorption of the toxin or increasing elimination of the toxin

Activated charcoal increases the elimination of which toxins?

Digoxin, phenobarbitol, theophylline, amitriptyline, carbamazepine, and salicylates

What substances are not adsorbed to activated charcoal?

Lithium, iron, alcohols, lead, hydrocarbons, and caustics

What types of toxins respond to repeated doses of activated charcoal?

Those metabolized via enterohepatic recirculation and those with long half-lives

What are contraindications to the use of activated charcoal?

1. Ingestion of a caustic substance
2. Factors increasing the risk of aspiration (e.g., decreased mental status)

List three commonly used cathartics.

1. Sorbitol
2. Magnesium citrate
3. Magnesium sulfate

What are the contraindications to the use of cathartics?

1. Intestinal obstruction
2. Renal failure

Whole-bowel irrigation may be indicated for which ingestions?

Drug packets, sustained-release drugs, slowly dissolving toxins

Hemodialysis is effective for treating which intoxications?

Ethanol, ethylene glycol, lithium, methanol, salicylates

What occurs during hemoperfusion?

Blood is perfused against activated charcoal.

What types of materials can be removed by hemoperfusion but not by hemodialysis?	Those that are protein bound
Hemoperfusion is useful in the treatment of what intoxications?	Carbamazepine, phenobarbital, phenytoin, theophylline
What is the goal of urinary alkalinization?	To trap weak acids in their ionized form, once they are excreted into the renal tubules
Urinary alkalinization has been shown to be effective for which intoxications?	Aspirin and phenobarbital
What is the pH goal of the urine for urinary alkalinization?	A pH of 7–8

EFFECTS OF TOXINS

CARDIOVASCULAR EFFECTS

Name some toxins that cause tachycardia.	Cocaine, tricyclic antidepressants (TCAs), anticholinergics, amphetamines, and theophylline
Name some toxins that cause bradycardia.	β Blockers, calcium channel blockers, α agonists, clonidine, and digoxin
Name some toxins that cause hypotension.	β Blockers, calcium channel blockers, TCAs, clonidine, angiotensin-converting enzyme (ACE) inhibitors, and sedative–hypnotics
Name some toxins that cause hypertension.	Cocaine, amphetamines, anticholinergics, and sympathomimetics

NEUROLOGIC EFFECTS

Name some toxins that may cause central nervous system (CNS) depression.	Opioids, antidepressants, clonidine, carbon monoxide, organophosphates, and cyanide
Name some toxins that may cause CNS agitation.	Anticholinergics, salicylates, phencyclidine (PCP), cocaine, amphetamines, and xanthines

Name some toxins that may induce seizures.	Cocaine, ethanol (during withdrawal), amphetamines, lithium, TCAs, demerol, lidocaine, antihistamines, antidepressants, xanthines, and salicylates

RESPIRATORY EFFECTS

Name some toxins that cause tachypnea.	Salicylates, theophylline, and sympatho-mimetics
Name some toxins that cause bradypnea.	Opioids, sedative–hypnotics, and barbiturates

RENAL EFFECTS

Name some toxins that cause acute tubular necrosis (ATN).	Aminoglycosides, cyclosporine, intravenous contrast, and heavy metals
Name some toxins that cause interstitial nephritis.	Penicillins, nonsteroidal anti-inflammatory drugs (NSAIDs), and captopril

GASTROINTESTINAL EFFECTS

Name some toxins that cause hepatitis.	Acetaminophen, ethanol, toxic mushrooms, and heavy metals

ENDOCRINE AND METABOLIC EFFECTS

Name some toxins that may cause hypoglycemia.	Ethanol and salicylates
Name some toxins that cause hyperthermia.	Cocaine, anticholinergics, amphetamines, sedative–hypnotics, and thyroid hormones
Name some toxins that cause hypothermia.	Opioids, sedative–hypnotics, and ethanol
Name some toxins that predispose a patient to hyperthermia.	Cocaine, amphetamines, α agonists, anticholinergics, dopaminergic agonists (during withdrawal), salicylates, and ethanol
Name some toxins that predispose a patient to hypothermia.	Opioids, sedative–hypnotics, ethanol, and hypoglycemic agents

Name some toxins that can increase osmolar gap.	Methanol, ethylene glycol, isopropanol, ethanol, and propylene glycol

What is the differential of an anion gap metabolic acidosis?

MUDPILES
Methanol
Uremia
Diabetic ketoacidosis (DKA)
Paraldehyde
Iron (inhalation)
Lactate
Ethylene glycol
Salicylates

Name some other toxins that can also cause an acidosis.	Carbon monoxide and cyanide

SPECIFIC TYPES OF TOXINS

ANTICHOLINERGIC AGENTS

What are some commonly used anticholinergic agents?

Antihistamines, phenothiazines, antiparkinsonian drugs, TCAs, atropine, scopolamine, and jimsonweed

What is an anticholinergic syndrome?

A central and peripheral block of the muscarinic acetylcholine neuroreceptors, resulting from an overdose of, or abnormal reaction to, anticholinergic agents

What are the signs and symptoms of an anticholinergic syndrome?

Anhidrosis, or decreased sweating, and hyperthermia (hot as Hades)
Mydriasis, or dilated pupils (blind as a bat)
Urinary retention, decreased bronchial secretions, decreased gastrointestinal motility, decreased salivation, and decreased sweating (dry as a bone)
Flushed skin and hyperthermia (red as a beet)
Hallucinations, agitation, amnesia, anxiety, confusion, and disorientation (mad as a hatter)

What antidote is used to treat an anticholinergic syndrome?

Physostigmine

How does psysostigmine work?

Physostigmine is an anticholinesterase agent that causes acetylcholine to accumulate at the cholinergic receptor sites throughout the central and peripheral nervous system.

What are the indications for physostigmine?

Physostigmine is indicated in patients with refractory arrhythmias, refractory hypotension, intractable seizures, or uncontrolled agitation.

What are the complications associated with physostigmine?

Physostigmine can cause arrhythmias and seizures, and should be avoided in patients with TCA overdose or a wide QRS on their electrocardiogram (EKG).

What other treatment is available for an anticholinergic syndrome?

An anticholinergic syndrome can also be treated with supportive therapy and delayed gastric decontamination.

Why is delayed gastric decontamination beneficial in this intoxication?

Because the anticholinergic agents cause delayed gastric motility

CARDIOACTIVE AGENTS

What are some commonly used cardioactive agents?

Digitalis, β blockers, and calcium channel blockers

Digitalis

Name three plants from which digitalis can be obtained?

Foxglove, oleander, and lily of the valley

How does digitalis work?

Digitalis causes an inactivation of the ATPase-dependent sodium–potassium pump, resulting in a positive inotropic effect on the myocardium, as well as atrioventricular (AV) node blocking activity.

How does digitalis affect potassium and calcium distribution?

Digitalis increases potassium efflux from the cell and calcium influx into the cell.

What disorders can be treated with digitalis?

Digitalis can be used to treat congestive heart failure (CHF) and supraventricular tachydysrhythmias.

What is the therapeutic level of digitalis?	0.5–2.0 ng/ml
What is the most common digitalis-induced dys-rhythmia?	Digitalis frequently induces premature ventricular contractions (PVCs).
What are the symptoms of digitalis toxicity?	Nausea, anorexia, weakness and fatigue, headache, seizures, confusion, dizziness, chromatopsia (yellow and green), hallucinations, and delirium

What is the difference between chronic and acute toxicity of digitalis in terms of the following:

Incidence?	Chronic toxicity is more common in older patients than in younger ones.
Onset?	Chronic toxicity has an insidious onset, while acute toxicity has a rapid onset.
Cause?	Chronic toxicity is most often the result of abnormal renal function, which is more common in older patients. Acute toxicity usually results from the treatment of bradycardia or AV block.
The patient's potassium level?	In chronic toxicity, the patient usually has a lower potassium level, whereas in acute toxicity, the patient may have hyperkalemia.
Common dysrhythmias?	In chronic toxicity, the most common dysrhythmias are PVCs, ventricular tachyarrhythmias, and AV blocks. In acute toxicity, bradycardia and AV blocks, in addition to occasional atrial or ventricular dysrhythmias, are common.
How do you treat digitalis toxicity?	Digitalis toxicity can be treated with activated charcoal, electrolyte therapy (by replacing magnesium and treating hyperkalemia), phenytoin, and lidocaine (for tachyarrhythmias), and atropine and pacing (for bradyarrhythmias).

What antidote is used to treat digitalis toxicity?

Fab fragments of digoxin-specific antibody (Digibind)

What are the indications for Digibind?

Digibind is used to treat life-threatening ventricular dysrhythmias, hemodynamically significant bradydysrhythmias that are unresponsive to conventional therapy, hyperkalemia (potassium concentration > 5 mEq/L), and co-ingestion of other cardiotoxic drugs.

What should be avoided when treating a patient with digitalis toxicity?

Avoid using calcium to treat hyperkalemia.

Name three dysrhythmias that indicate digoxin toxicity.

1. Atrial tachycardia, with variable block
2. Accelerated junctional tachycardia
3. Fascicular tachycardia

Name some dysrhythmias occasionally caused by digoxin toxicity.

Atrial fibrillation, atrial flutter, ventricular tachycardia or fibrillation

How does digoxin affect the EKG?

Digoxin causes ST segment depression, with flattening or inversion of the T wave in leads with tall R waves.

β Blockers

How do β blockers work?

They inhibit the effects of catecholamines at the β receptor sites.

Describe the effects of β_1-receptor stimulation.

β_1-Receptor stimulation increases the force and rate of myocardial contractility and also AV node conduction velocity.

Describe the effects of β_2-receptor stimulation.

β_2-Receptor stimulation relaxes smooth muscle in blood vessels, bronchi, and the gastrointestinal or genitourinary tract. It also promotes glycogenolysis and gluconeogenesis.

What are some therapeutic uses of β blockers?

β Blockers are used to treat supraventricular dysrhythmias, hypertension, angina, thyrotoxicosis, migraines, and glaucoma.

What are the signs and symptoms of β blocker toxicity?

1. Bradycardia
2. AV block
3. Widening of the QRS complex
4. Hypotension
5. Altered mental status
6. Seizures
7. Coma
8. Respiratory arrest or insufficiency
9. Hypoglycemia (in diabetics and children)
10. Bronchospasm (rare)

How do you treat β blockers toxicity?

With supportive therapy and administration of glucagon

Calcium channel blockers

What are the effects of calcium channel blockers?

Calcium channel blockers promote coronary and peripheral vasodilation, reduce cardiac contractility and sinoatrial (SA) node activity, and slow AV node conduction.

What are some therapeutic uses of calcium channel blockers?

Calcium channel blockers are used to treat hypertension, angina, supraventricular dysrhythmias, and hypertrophic cardiomyopathy.

For a patient with calcium channel blocker toxicity, name the:

    Cardiac manifestations

Bradycardia, hypotension, AV conduction block or dissociation, asystole, junctional rhythm

    Systemic manifestations

Respiratory depression, apnea, vomiting, lethargy, confusion, coma, metabolic (lactic) acidosis with hypoperfusion

How is calcium channel blocker toxicity treated?

With aggressive supportive therapy

XANTHINES

Name two xanthines.

Theophylline and caffeine

What are the therapeutic uses of xanthines?

Xanthines are often used to treat asthma and apnea in preterm infants.

What are the signs and symptoms of xanthine toxicity?

The signs and symptoms are consistent with massive catecholamine release and include the following:
Agitation
Anxiety
Hyperventilation
Palpitations
Vomiting
Metabolic acidosis
Hypokalemia
Hyperglycemia
Seizures
Hypotension
Sinus tachycardia
Cardiac dysrhythmias (e.g., atrial fibrillation, multifocal atrial tachycardia, PVC, and ventricular tachycardia)
Tremor

What specific xanthine is more frequently associated with intoxication?

Theophylline

What is the main difference between acute and chronic theophylline toxicity?

Patients with chronic toxicity are much more prone to seizures than those with an acute overdose.

At what plasma concentrations would patients with the following types of toxicity develop seizures?

   Chronic theophylline toxicity

Patients develop seizure at concentrations as low as 40–60 μg/ml.

   Acute theophylline toxicity

Patients can tolerate higher concentrations—up to 90 μg/ml.

Why are patients with chronic theophylline toxicity unable to tolerate higher plasma concentrations?

Because they already have higher total body stores of the drug

How do you treat an overdosage of theophylline?

With supportive therapy and activated charcoal hemoperfusion

PSYCHOPHARMACOLOGIC AGENTS

What are some commonly prescribed psychopharmacologic agents?	Lithium, selective serotonin reuptake inhibitors (SSRIs), monoamine oxidase inhibitors (MAOIs), TCAs, and neuroleptic agents

Lithium

What is the therapeutic use of lithium?	The treatment of bipolar disorder
What are the therapeutic levels of lithium?	0.6–1.2 mEq/L
What levels of lithium are considered toxic?	Lithium levels greater than 2.0 mEq/L are considered toxic.
What are the signs and symptoms of lithium toxicity?	Vomiting Diarrhea Lethargy Confusion Tremor Ataxia Spasticity Stupor Seizures Coma Dysarthria Fasciculations Hyperreflexia Clonus
How do you treat lithium toxicity?	Consider whole-bowel irrigation and hemodialysis, and maintain the patient's urine output.
What are the indications for hemodialysis?	Hemodialysis is indicated if any of the following conditions are present: Clinical signs of severe poisoning (e.g., hyperreflexia, clonus) Deteriorating clinical condition (e.g., seizure, coma, ventricular arrhythmia) Decreased urine output or renal failure Lack of the expected 20% drop in serum lithium level after 6 hours of treatment Serum lithium level greater than 4.0

mEq/L with acute ingestion or greater
than 1.5 mEq/L with chronic ingestion

Selective serotonin reuptake inhibitors (SSRIs)

What are the therapeutic uses of SSRIs?

SSRIs are used to treat depression, panic disorder, and obsessive compulsive disorder.

What is a serotonin syndrome?

A serotonin syndrome is a syndrome of the CNS, in which cardiac and autonomic activity are increased as a result of increased stimulation of serotonin receptors.

What pharmacologic effect can increase the likelihood of subsequently developing serotonin syndrome?

An increase in serotonin neurotransmission, either as a result of decreased serotonin reuptake or increased serotonin release

Name some drugs that decrease serotonin reuptake.

Cocaine, amphetamines, TCAs, and meperidine

Name some drugs that increase serotonin release.

Cocaine, amphetamines, and dextromethorphan

What are the most common signs and symptoms of serotonin syndrome?

Agitation
Anxiety
Ataxia
Hyperthermia
Sinus tachycardia
Mild hypertension
Diaphoresis
Hyperreflexia
Myoclonus
Shivering
Tremors
Diarrhea
Muscular rigidity

How do you treat serotonin syndrome?

Serotonin syndrome can be treated with supportive therapy and the administration of cyproheptadine, if appropriate.

Monoamine oxidase inhibitors (MAOIs)

How do monoamine oxidase inhibitors (MAOIs) work?

Monoamine oxidase inhibition decreases inactivation of the biogenic amines (i.e., norepinephrine, dopamine, and serotonin).

What are MAOIs prescribed to treat?

Depression and Parkinson's disease

What substance should be avoided in patients being treated with MAOIs?

Tyramine, a substance found in cheese, beer, and chicken livers

Why should tyramines be avoided by patients taking MAOIs?

Tyramine, an exogenous biogenic amine, should be avoided because the mono-amine oxidase is not able to metabolize it.

What are the effects of the unmetabolized tyramine?

The unmetabolized tyramine has the ability to displace norepinephrine and serotonin into the neuronal synapse, causing a sympathomimetic storm.

What drugs should be avoided in patients being treated with MAOIs?

β Blockers, xanthines, codeine, anti-cholinergics, meperidine, dextromethorphan, ketamine, levodopa, SSRIs, TCAs, phenothiazines, amphetamines, bretylium, ephedrine, and dopamine

Name some of the symptoms associated with tyramine ingestion.

Headache
Diaphoresis
Mydriasis
Neck stiffness
Neuromuscular excitation
Hypertension

What is the most serious adverse effect of tyramine ingestion in patients on MAOIs?

Hypertensive crisis

What are the signs and symptoms of MAOI toxicity?

Initially (i.e., within 6–12 hours of ingestion), the patient will be in a hyper-adrenergic state, experiencing the following symptoms:
Headache
Agitation
Restlessness
Palpitations
Tremor
Sinus tachycardia
Mydriasis
Nystagmus
Muscle rigidity
Hypertension

Trismus
Diarrhea
Flushing
Confusion
Later, CNS depression and
cardiovascular collapse may occur.

**How do you treat MAOI
toxicity?**

MAOI toxicity can be treated with
supportive care, including cardiac
monitoring; activated charcoal; and
benzodiazepines. Hypotension can be
treated with norepinephrine or
epinephrine.

Tricyclic antidepressants (TCAs)

What are TCAs?

TCAs are aromatic compounds,
containing a 3-ring structure, that inhibit
uptake of biogenic amines (i.e., serotonin,
norepinephrine, and dopamine).

**What are TCAs prescribed
to treat?**

TCAs can be prescribed to treat
depression, peripheral neuropathies,
attention deficit disorder (ADD), chronic
pain syndromes, anxiety disorders, and
eating disorders.

**What is the toxic dose of
TCA?**

More than 2–4 mg/kg of TCA is
considered toxic.

**What are the four major
effects of TCA overdose?**

1. Anticholinergic symptoms
2. α-Adrenergic blockade
3. Norepinephrine reuptake inhibition
4. Sodium channel blockade

**What are the signs and
symptoms of TCA toxicity?**

Decreased level of consciousness
Anticholinergic symptoms
CNS depression
Seizures
Cardiac conduction delays
Hypotension
Arrhythmias
Respiratory depression

**What EKG changes are
seen with TCA overdose?**

TCA overdose has the potential to cause a
number of EKG changes, including sinus
tachycardia, widening of the QRS and QT
intervals, prolongation of the PR interval,

bradycardia, right axis deviation, and various conduction blocks.

How do you treat TCA intoxication?

With activated charcoal and bicarbonate.

What are the indications for bicarbonate?

Bicarbonate is indicated if the QRS prolongation is more than 100 msec. It is also appropriate in patients who develop hypotension refractory to fluid challenge, ventricular arrhythmias, or acidemia.

When is an asymptomatic patient considered at low risk for a lethal arrhythmia?

After 6 hours of observation, an asymptomatic patient would be considered at low risk for a lethal arrhythmia.

Neuroleptic agents

How do neuroleptic agents work?

Neuroleptic agents block dopaminergic, α-adrenergic, muscarinic, and histaminic neurotransmission receptors.

What are neuroleptic agents prescribed to treat?

Neuroleptic agents can be used to treat psychoses, particularly schizophrenia, and are also used as antiemetics.

What are some of the normal side effects of neuroleptics?

Dystonia
Akathisia
Parkinsonism
Tardive dyskinesia
Neuroleptic malignant syndrome (NMS)

What laboratory findings are associated with NMS?

Increased white blood cell (WBC) count and increased creatine phosphokinase (CPK) and liver enzyme levels
Metabolic acidosis
Hypoxia
Myoglobinuria

What are the general signs and symptoms of an acute overdose of a neuroleptic agent?

CNS depression
Hypo- or hyperthermia
Abnormal motor movements
Seizures
Anticholinergic symptoms
Hypotension, with reflex tachycardia

How do you treat neuroleptic toxicity?

With supportive care and gastric decontamination

SEDATIVE–HYPNOTIC AGENTS

Name three common sedative–hypnotic agents.	Benzodiazepines, barbiturates, and chloral hydrate

Benzodiazepines

How do benzodiazepines work?	Benzodiazepines potentiate the actions of γ-aminobutyric acid (GABA) in the CNS.
What are the signs and symptoms of benzodiazepine toxicity?	Lethargy Drowsiness Short-term memory loss Decreased level of consciousness Bradycardia Hypotension Respiratory depression
What antidote can be administered to reverse the effects of benzodiazepines?	Flumazenil
What is the risk factor associated with flumazenil administration?	Flumazenil can precipitate seizures in patients who are dependent on benzodiazepines.
How do you treat benzodiazepine toxicity?	With respiratory support

Barbiturates

How do barbiturates work?	Barbiturates inhibit GABA-mediated transmission in the CNS.
What are the signs and symptoms of barbiturate toxicity?	CNS depression and decreased deep tendon reflexes
What skin manifestations are found with barbiturate overdose?	Clear vesicles and bullae develop on an erythematous base, primarily over pressure points.
How do you treat barbiturate toxicity?	Barbiturate toxicity can be treated with airway support and hemodialysis, if persistent deterioration develops.

ANALGESICS

Name three common types of analgesics.	Acetaminophen, NSAIDs (including salicylates), and opioids

Acetaminophen

Why can acetaminophen be toxic?

Acetaminophen is a hepatotoxic metabolite that, after large doses, can deplete glutathione and cause hepatic necrosis.

What is the toxic dose of acetaminophen?

A dose of 140 mg/kg or more is toxic.

What is used to determine the likelihood of toxicity following an acute ingestion of acetaminophen

The Rumack-Matthew nomogram

Is the nomogram useful for subacute or chronic over-doses?

No.

Describe the signs, symptoms, and laboratory findings typically associated with acetaminophen toxicity at:

   1–24 hours post-ingestion

Nausea, vomiting, diaphoresis, and malaise

   24–48 hours post-ingestion

Abdominal pain in the right upper quadrant (RUQ) and increased liver enzyme levels

   72–96 hours post-ingestion

Peak in hepatic enzyme abnormalities, increased prothrombin time (PT), jaundice, and continued nausea and vomiting

   96 hours or more post-ingestion

Resolution of the hepatotoxicity or progressive hepatic failure

How do you treat acetaminophen toxicity?

With activated charcoal and N-acetylcysteine

How soon after the ingestion should N-acetylcysteine be administered?

Ideally, N-acetylcysteine should be administered within 8 hours of the ingestion; however, there can be benefits to administering it up to 24 hours after ingestion.

Nonsteroidal anti-inflammatory drugs (NSAIDs)

Name the three types of patients who are at risk for NSAID toxicity.

1. Elderly patients
2. Patients with renal or hepatic disease
3. Patients taking oral anticoagulation medications.

Salicylates

What are the toxic effects of salicylates?

With overdose, salicylates can cause gastritis, hyperventilation, respiratory depression, and oxidative phosphorylation impairment, such as acidosis and hypoglycemia.

How are salicylates eliminated from the body at:

   Therapeutic doses?

By hepatic metabolism

   Toxic doses?

By renal excretion

What is the toxic dose of aspirin?

200–300 mg/kg is generally considered toxic.

What are the signs and symptoms of aspirin toxicity?

Tinnitus
Respiratory alkalosis with metabolic acidosis
Vomiting
Dehydration
Diaphoresis
Agitation
Lethargy
Cerebral edema
Noncardiogenic pulmonary edema
Hyperthermia
Nephrotoxicity

How do you treat aspirin toxicity?

Aspirin toxicity can be treated with activated charcoal. It is also important to prevent dehydration, monitor serum glucose and urinary alkalinization, and consider hemodialysis in patients with serious conditions.

Opioids

How do opioids work?

Opioids bind to specific receptor sites, such as μ, κ, and δ, thus decreasing a patient's perception of pain.

What is the classic triad of opioid intoxication?

1. Miosis
2. Respiratory depression
3. Coma

What are the signs and symptoms of opioid over-dose in progressive order?

Excitation
Euphoria
Nausea and vomiting
Flushed skin
Pruritus
Slowing of gastric motility (i.e., constipation)
Stupor
Miosis
Respiratory depression
Noncardiogenic pulmonary edema
Orthostatic hypotension
Coma

How do you treat opioid intoxication?

With airway support and the administration of the antidote, naloxone.

What is the appropriate dosage of naloxone for adults and children, and what are the possible routes for administration?

Administer 2.0 mg/kg of naloxone to adults and .01 mg/kg to children. Naloxone can be administered by an intramuscular, intravenous, endotracheal, or subcutaneous route.

What is the half-life of naloxone?

The half-life is only 12–20 minutes, which is shorter than many other narcotics.

What symptoms are associated with opioid withdrawal?

Piloerection
Yawning
Lacrimation
Rhinorrhea
Diaphoresis
Insomnia
Myalgia
Vomiting
Abdominal cramping
Diarrhea
Irritability
Hyperactivity
Fever
Confusion

Drugs of abuse

Name the three most common drugs of abuse.

Cocaine, amphetamines, and hallucinogens

Cocaine

What is cocaine and how does it act on the CNS?

Cocaine is a CNS stimulant that blocks reuptake of norepinephrine, dopamine, and serotonin.

What are the signs and symptoms of cocaine intoxication?

Mydriasis
Euphoria
Tachycardia
Hypertension
Diaphoresis
Tachypnea
Hyperthermia

Name some of the cardiovascular complications associated with cocaine abuse.

Cocaine abuse can cause a number of cardiovascular complications, such as arrhythmias, myocardial ischemia or infarction, myocarditis, cardiomyopathy, and aortic rupture.

Name some of the CNS complications associated with cocaine abuse.

Cocaine abuse can also cause CNS complications, such as seizures, intracranial infarctions, and hemorrhages.

What is "crack eye"?

"Crack eye" is a term used to describe the corneal abrasions and ulcerations that occur from smoking crack.

What are some of the complications for the pregnant patient?

Cocaine can increase the patient's risk of spontaneous abortion, abruptio placentae, fetal prematurity, and intrauterine growth retardation.

How do you treat a patient with acute cocaine toxicity?

With supportive therapy and benzodiazepines

What drug should be avoided in patients with cocaine toxicity?

β Blockers

What treatment is indicated for body packers (body stuffers)?

Consider surgical consultation for the symptomatic patient.

Amphetamines

How do amphetamines work?

Amphetamines are structurally related to the endogenous catecholamines and, therefore, indirectly cause sympathomimetic, dopaminergic, and serotonergic actions.

What are the signs and symptoms of amphetamine toxicity?	Restlessness or sleep reduction Hyperactivity Repetitive behavior Anorexia Psychosis Arousal Mydriasis Peripheral vasoconstriction Tachycardia Bronchodilation Increased metabolism Diaphoresis Hypertension Flushing Nausea and vomiting Hyperpyrexia Rhabdomyolysis
How do you treat acute amphetamine intoxication?	With supportive therapy and activated charcoal
What drug should be avoided in patients with amphetamine toxicity?	β Blockers
What symptoms occur during amphetamine withdrawal?	During amphetamine withdrawal, the patient will experience depression, increased appetite, cramps, nausea, diarrhea, and headache.
When do the effects of these withdrawal symptoms peak?	The withdrawal symptoms will peak approximately 2–3 days after cessation of the drug.

Hallucinogens

What are some commonly abused hallucinogens?	PCP, lysergic acid diethylamide (LSD), marijuana, and psilocybin-containing mushrooms.

Phencyclidine (PCP)

What is PCP's effect on sensory perception?	It is a dissociative anesthetic.

What are the signs and symptoms of acute PCP intoxication?	Tachycardia Hypertension Nystagmus (vertical, rotary, horizontal) Violent, bizarre, agitated, or confused behavior Blank stare appearance Hyperthermia Rhabdomyolysis Seizures
Rhabdomyolysis is diagnosed using which laboratory studies?	Serum CPK and urine myoglobin levels
How do you treat PCP toxicity?	With sedation and gastric decontamination

Lysergic acid diethylamide (LSD)

What is LSD?	A hallucinogen primarily affecting the serotonergic and dopaminergic pathways at various levels in the CNS
What are the signs and symptoms of acute LSD intoxication?	Hallucinations Paranoia Anxiety Sympathomimetic symptoms
What is the treatment for hallucinogen abuse?	Provision of a calm environment and sedation with benzodiazepines

ALCOHOLS

What are the four common alcohols?	Ethanol, isopropanol, methanol, and ethylene glycol

Ethanol

Name the signs and symptoms of ethanol intoxication.	Slurred speech Disinhibited behavior Decreased motor coordination and control Hypotension Respiratory depression CNS depression Predisposition to hypothermia and hypoglycemia

What should be ruled out before treating a patient for ethanol intoxication?

It is important to rule out hypoglycemia, traumatic injury, and co-ingestion of other drugs as causes for the patient's decreased mental and respiratory status.

How do you treat ethanol intoxication?

With supportive therapy

What are the signs and symptoms of ethanol withdrawal?

Tremor
Anxiety
Agitation
Autonomic hyperactivity
Cardiac dysrhythmias
Hallucinations
Seizures

When do the most severe symptoms of ethanol withdrawal occur?

The most severe symptoms will occur within 48 hours of cessation of the drug.

What symptom may occur 72 hours after ethanol cessation?

Delirium tremens

Isopropanol

Where is isopropanol found?

Isopropanol is a component found in rubbing alcohol, antifreeze, paint thinner, jewelry cleaner, and detergents.

What are the signs and symptoms of isopropanol toxicity?

The signs and symptoms are clinically similar to those of ethanol intoxication, but with a longer duration and more profound CNS depression, respiratory depression, hypotension, and hemorrhagic gastritis.

What are three common laboratory findings?

1. Ketonemia or ketonuria, without elevated glucose or glucosuria
2. Increased osmolar gap
3. Possible hypoglycemia

How do you treat isopropanol intoxication?

Isopropanol intoxication can be treated with supportive therapy and, if necessary, hemodialysis for refractory hypotension.

Methanol

Where is methanol found?

Methanol is a component found in paint removers, varnishes, shellac, antifreeze, windshield washing solutions, and wood alcohol.

How does methanol cause toxicity?

Through its principal metabolites, formaldehyde and formic acid

How long after methanol ingestion do signs and symptoms present?

Signs and symptoms present 12–18 hours after ingestion.

What are the signs and symptoms of methanol toxicity?

Visual disturbances
CNS depression, with possible seizures
Abdominal pain
Vomiting
Optic papillitis
Retinal edema leading to blindness

What ophthalmologic conditions might you find when assessing a patient with methanol intoxication?

Patients with methanol intoxication often have nystagmus, fixed and dilated pupils with visual disturbances, optic atrophy, and hyperemia of the optic disc.

At what serum levels would the patient be symptomatic?

Levels greater than 20 mg/dl

At what serum levels would the patient have serious toxicity?

Levels greater than 50 mg/dl

What is the minimum lethal dose of methanol?

30 ml of a 40% solution

What is the common laboratory finding?

Metabolic acidosis with increased anion and osmolar gaps

How do you treat methanol toxicity?

With ethanol infusion and hemodialysis.

What serum concentration of methanol warrants ethanol infusion?

A serum concentration greater than 20 mg/dl.

Name some indications for hemodialysis for methanol toxicity.

Use hemodialysis if the patient develops signs of visual or CNS dysfunction, methanol levels greater than 25 mg/dl, or severe metabolic acidosis, regardless of the methanol level.

Ethylene glycol

Where is ethylene glycol found?	Ethylene glycol is a component found in coolant, preservative, glycerine substitute, lacquers, cosmetics, and polishes.
How does ethylene glycol cause toxicity?	Through its metabolites, glycolic acid, oxalic acid, and formic acid
What are the signs, symptoms, and laboratory findings of ethylene glycol toxicity?	Inebriation High anion gap metabolic acidosis, with increased osmolar gap Calcium oxalate crystalluria Leukocytosis Hypocalcemia
At what serum levels would the patient experience ethylene glycol toxicity?	Serum levels greater than 20 mg/dl are considered toxic.
What is a potentially lethal dose of ethylene glycol?	≥ 2 ml/kg
Describe the signs and symptoms during the initial phase of ethylene glycol toxicity (i.e., 1–12 hours after ingestion).	CNS depression, possible seizures, inebriation, slurred speech, ataxia
Describe the signs and symptoms during the cardiopulmonary phase of toxicity (i.e., 12–24 hours after ingestion).	Tachycardia, mild hypertension, tachypnea, CHF, acute respiratory distress, circulatory collapse
Describe the signs and symptoms during the nephrotoxic phase of toxicity (i.e., 24–72 hours after ingestion).	Flank pain and tenderness, oliguric renal failure, and ATN
At what serum level of ethylene glycol would the patient require treatment?	Treatment is necessary at levels greater than 20 mg/dl.
How do you treat ethylene glycol toxicity?	Ethylene glycol toxicity can be treated with pyridoxine, thiamine, ethanol, and

hemodialysis. Calcium gluconate can be used to treat severe hypocalcemia.

Why is ethanol used for treatment of ethylene glycol toxicity?

Because ethanol's affinity for alcohol dehydrogenase is 100 times that of ethylene glycol

Name the four indications for hemodialysis.

1. Elevation of the serum ethylene glycol level to more than 20–25 mg/dl
2. Concern of toxic ingestion
3. Signs of nephrotoxicity
4. Evidence of metabolic acidosis

What antidote inhibits the action of alcohol dehydrogenase?

4-Methylpyrazole

HYDROCARBONS

Which type of hydrocarbons have the lowest toxicity?

High viscosity hydrocarbons, such as lubricating oil, petroleum jelly, grease, and paraffin

What kinds of hydrocarbons have the most toxicity?

Those with high volatility (e.g., gasoline, natural gas) and those with low viscosity (e.g., kerosene)

What are the toxic effects of hydrocarbons or their metabolites?

Mitochondrial damage, as a result of lipid peroxidation

What type of patient is most likely to present with hydrocarbon toxicity?

Toddlers are most likely to present with hydrocarbon toxicity as a result of accidental ingestion.

What are the acute manifestations of hydrocarbon poisoning?

Neurologic dysfunction
Respiratory dysfunction
Cardiac dysrhythmias
Gastrointestinal upset
Malaise
Fever

What symptoms have a delayed presentation?

Hepatic dysfunction
Renal tubular dysfunction
Hemolysis

What pulmonary problem can develop with hydrocarbon ingestion?

Chemical pneumonitis can develop secondary to direct tracheal instillation.

When is gastric emptying indicated for patients with hydrocarbon ingestion?	Gastric emptying is indicated in patients who have ingested massive doses of the toxic agent or who have been in the presence of a toxic additive (e.g., chlorinated hydrocarbons).
Why is gastric emptying risky in a patient with hydrocarbon ingestion?	Gastric emptying can be risky because it increases the chance of pulmonary aspiration.
When can a patient with hydrocarbon poisoning be discharged from the hospital?	After 8 hours of observation, an asymptomatic patient with a normal chest radiograph may be discharged from the hospital.

HEAVY METALS

Name three heavy metal poisons that can cause gum discoloration.	Arsenic, lead, and mercury
What heavy metal intoxication can cause bullae and exfoliative dermatitis, such as that seen with barbiturate toxicity?	Arsenic
Name the six heavy metal poisons that can be treated with dimercaprol.	**LAGMAN** **L**ead **A**rsenic **G**old **M**ercury **A**ntimony **N**ickel
Name the five heavy metal poisons that cannot be treated with dimercaprol.	**CZITS** **C**admium **Z**inc **I**ron **T**ellurium **S**elenium
Name the five heavy metals for which calcium ethylenediamine tetraacetic acid (EDTA) is the antidote?	1. Cadmium 2. Cobalt 3. Copper 4. Lead 5. Nickel

Lead

What are some sources of lead poisoning?

Lead poisoning can result from the ingestion of flakes of lead-based paint often found in older homes. It can also result from the use of improperly glazed china and ceramics.

Name three antidotes that can be used to treat lead toxicity.

1. Calcium EDTA
2. Dimercaprol
3. Penicillamine

Arsenic

What are the signs and symptoms of arsenic ingestion?

Nausea
Vomiting, with a garlicky odor
Acute dysphagia
Acute abdominal pain
Watery diarrhea
Cyanosis

How do you treat arsenic poisoning?

Arsenic poisoning can be treated with dimercaprol or oral penicillamine, and hemodialysis if necessary.

Gold

Name the two diseases that can be treated with gold salts.

Rheumatoid arthritis and lupus erythematosus

What are signs and symptoms of gold toxicity?

Facial puffiness
Fever
Skin disorders
Intense pruritus
Nausea and vomiting
Abdominal pain
Diarrhea
Polyneuritis

What is the antidote for gold intoxication?

Dimercaprol

What is the prognosis for gold toxicity?

The prognosis for gold toxicity is generally good, unless agranulocytosis is present, in which case the mortality rate is increased to 30%.

Mercury

What are the symptoms of mercury poisoning?

Metallic taste
Whitish tongue

Choking sensation
Intense esophageal and gastric pain
Vomiting
Bloody diarrhea
Mental confusion
Anuria
Convulsions
Coma

What is the antidote for mercury poisoning?

Dimercaprol or penicillamine

Antimony

Where can antimony be found?

In weed killers, ant killers, snail baits, and the glaze used on cheap china and pottery

What are the signs and symptoms of antimony ingestion?

Nausea and vomiting
Dehydration
Extreme thirst
Choking and tightness in the throat
Cyanosis
Painful, profuse watery diarrhea

When do symptoms of antimony toxicity occur?

Symptoms usually develop about 0.5–2 hours after the ingestion.

What is the antidote used to treat antimony toxicity?

Dimercaprol

Nickel

What are the three symptoms of nickel toxicity?

Acute dermatitis, gingivitis, and stomatitis

Which complications with a delayed onset can develop secondary to nickel ingestion?

Headache, nausea, interstitial pneumonia, and hepatic complications

What agent is used to treat nickel toxicity?

Sodium diethyldithiocarbamate

Cadmium

What are the two ways a person can develop cadmium poisoning?

1. Inhalation of the fumes from solder
2. From food and drink containers or utensils with cadmium in the solder or glazing (uncommon)

What is unique about cadmium fumes?	Cadmium fumes are odorless.
What are the signs and symptoms of cadmium poisoning?	Pneumonitis and abdominal pain
When is renal involvement seen—with acute or chronic exposure?	Chronic exposure
When do symptoms begin to occur?	12 hours after exposure
How is cadmium poisoning treated?	There is no specific therapy.

Silver

What form of silver is nontoxic?	Halogen salts of silver are nontoxic.
What two forms of silver are acutely toxic if ingested?	Silver acetate and silver nitrate are acutely toxic if ingested.
How much silver can one ingest before symptoms start?	2 grams
What are the symptoms of silver poisoning?	Burning of the throat and epigastrium Black vomitus Violent abdominal pain Convulsions Coma
How do you treat a patient with silver poisoning?	Treatment consists of gastric emptying and gastric lavage with saline solution.
What is the prognosis for a patient who has ingested:	
2–10 grams of silver?	Poor (may be fatal)
More than 10 grams of silver?	Very poor (almost always fatal)

Iron

What is the minimum toxic dose of iron?	10 mg/kg

What is considered a potentially lethal dose of iron?	60 mg/kg
Serum iron levels are most useful how soon after an ingestion?	4–6 hours
What level of serum iron is associated with toxicity?	300–500 µg/dl
Which organ systems are affected by iron ingestion?	1. Gastrointestinal system 2. CNS 3. Cardiovascular system
How does iron affect liver function?	It disrupts aerobic metabolism in the hepatic mitochondria.

Describe the cause of the:

Gastrointestinal symptoms	The iron directly corrodes the mucosa of the gastrointestinal tract.
CNS symptoms	Diffuse systemic toxicity causes hypoperfusion, acidosis, and hepatic failure.
Cardiovascular symptoms	Cardiovascular symptoms result from direct toxicity to the heart, hypovolemia from bowel injury, and acidosis related to liver toxicity.
What are the initial symptoms of iron toxicity?	Nausea, vomiting, diarrhea, abdominal pain, hematemesis, melena, and lethargy
What are the symptoms of systemic toxicity?	Cyanosis, shock, coagulopathy, disorientation, and coma

What complications may occur after:

2 days?	Hepatic and renal failure
2 weeks?	Bowel or stomach obstruction
What can be given to bind serum iron?	Deferoxamine
Deferoxamine has what effect on urine in patients with iron toxicity?	It turns the urine reddish-orange.

Which patients are eligible for deferoxamine therapy?	1. Symptomatic patients 2. Asymptomatic patients who have ingested more than 60 mg/kg of iron 3. Asymptomatic patients with a serum iron level greater than 500 μg/dl

ORGANOPHOSPHATES AND CARBAMATES

Name four ways these chemicals can be absorbed into the body.	1. Inhalation 2. Across the gastrointestinal tract 3. Transdermally 4. Transconjunctivally
Which type of chemical penetrates the CNS, organophosphates or carbamates?	Organophosphates
Organophosphates and carbamates inhibit the function of which enzymes?	Acetylcholinesterase and plasma cholinesterase
What causes the symptoms of organophosphate or carbamate toxicity?	Excess acetylcholine stimulation
What is the difference in duration of effect between organophosphates and carbamates?	Carbamates spontaneously hydrolyze the enzyme within 48 hours; organophosphates do not.
What are the three classes of symptoms seen with organophosphate and carbamate poisoning?	1. CNS symptoms 2. Muscarinic symptoms 3. Nicotinic symptoms
What are the CNS symptoms?	Confusion, agitation, headache, ataxia, lethargy, coma, and seizure
What are the muscarinic symptoms?	**SLUDGE** **S**alivation **L**acrimation **U**rination **D**efecation **G**astrointestinal distress **E**mesis
What are the nicotinic symptoms?	Fasciculations, weakness, and cramping that may progress to paralysis and miosis

What tests may be ordered to verify the poisoning?
Red blood cell or plasma cholinesterase levels

What is the treatment for a patient with:

Mild symptoms?
Removal from exposure

Moderate or severe symptoms?
Atropine and pralidoxime chloride (2-PAM)

What is the endpoint for atropine administration?
Clearing of secretions and bronchospasm

What is the effect of 2-PAM?
It regenerates acetylcholinesterase and detoxifies the remaining organo-phosphate.

What symptoms of delayed neurotoxicity may occur following organophosphate toxicity?
Lower extremity weakness and paresthesias in a stocking–glove distribution that may progress to the upper extremities

CARBON MONOXIDE

What are the signs and symptoms of:

Mild carbon monoxide toxicity?
Headache, nausea, vomiting, and dizziness

Moderate carbon monoxide toxicity?
Chest pain, cognitive difficulties, tachycardia, tachypnea, blurred vision, myonecrosis, and ataxia

Severe carbon monoxide toxicity?
Myocardial ischemia, pulmonary edema, dysrhythmias, and seizures

What is the half-life of carboxyhemoglobin (COHb)?
2–7 hours

What is the half-life of COHb with 100% oxygen therapy at 1 atmosphere?
1 hour

What is the effect of hyperbaric oxygen therapy?
It decreases the half-life of COHb and increases the quantity of dissolved oxygen in the blood.

Which patients are candidates for hyperbaric oxygen therapy?

1. Patients with syncope, abnormal neurologic signs or symptoms, or cardiac symptoms
2. Pregnant patients with a COHb level > 15%
3. Patients with a COHb level > 25%
4. Patients with persistent symptoms after several hours of 100% oxygen therapy

What are possible delayed effects of carbon monoxide poisoning?

Memory problems, parkinsonism, blindness, peripheral neuropathy, dementia

CAUSTIC INGESTIONS

What test should be ordered for a patient with an alkali ingestion?

Radiographs to assess for perforation

What are the treatments for alkali ingestions?

1. Irrigation of exposed areas
2. Dilution of the ingestion with milk or tap water
3. Early airway control

What volume of fluid should be used for dilution?

250 ml in adults, 10–15 ml/kg in children

When should emesis be induced or gastric lavage performed?

Never!

What interventions are necessary after the patient has been treated in the ED?

Endoscopy and possibly the administration of antibiotics and steroids

How do acid ingestions differ from alkali ingestions?

Acid ingestions are often intentional; therefore, more acid is ingested.

How does the management of acid ingestions differ from that for alkali ingestions?

Nasogastric evacuation of large-volume acid ingestions should be done if there is no evidence of perforation.

What are the toxic effects of hydrofluoric acid?

Liquefaction necrosis, decalcification of bone, and the production of insoluble salts (i.e., calcium fluoride, magnesium fluoride)

What is the initial complaint of patients with hydrofluoric acid burns?

Pain out of proportion to physical findings

What systemic abnormality can occur with hydrofluoric acid ingestions?

Hypocalcemia

What are possible therapies for hydrofluoric acid burns?

1. Irrigation with cool water
2. Application of a calcium gluconate gel
3. Local injection of calcium gluconate or magnesium
4. Intra-arterial calcium injections

14

Environmental Emergencies

ELECTRICAL AND LIGHTNING INJURIES

State the range for high voltage.

600 V (as defined by National Electric Code) to 1000 V (as reported in medical literature)

Low-voltage sources cause what percent of deaths from electrical injuries?

60%–70%

What is the primary measure of the severity of an electric shock?

Current, in amperes (A)

What is Ohm's law and how is it important in determining extent of injury?

$I = V/R$ (current = voltage/resistance). Decreasing resistance will increase the injury current.

How can current (and the severity of injury) be increased from a given voltage exposure?

Decreased skin resistance from moisture, sweat, or a foreign substance (e.g., gel on defibrillator pads)

What three factors, other than amount of current, determine the severity of a shock?

Type, duration, and pathway of current

Which is more dangerous, alternating current (AC) or direct current (DC) at the same voltage?

AC

How do AC and DC differ in effects on skeletal muscle?

AC can produce tetanic contractions (may prevent voluntary release from the source); DC produces a single contraction (thrusting the victim from the source).

Which current pathway is more dangerous, hand-to-hand or hand-to-leg?

Hand-to-hand; current moving across the thorax may produce a life-threatening arrhythmia.

What are the two mechanisms for internal tissue damage from electrical current?

Direct conductive electrothermal injury, and nonconductive thermal injury

What kinds of tissues are most vulnerable to electrical damage?

Those tissues with the least resistance

Why?

The lower the resistance, the greater the current traveling through them.

List tissues in decreasing order of electrical resistance.

Bone, fat, tendon, skin, muscle, blood vessels, nerves

Which three tissues are most susceptible to electrical injury?

Nerves, blood vessels, muscle

List five mechanisms for cardiac arrest following electric shock.

1. Single direct tetanic cardiac contraction
2. Myocardial cell damage
3. Catecholamine release
4. "R-on-T" phenomenon
5. Coronary artery spasm

What is "R-on-T" phenomenon?

Cardiac depolarization occurring during repolarization may precipitate ventricular fibrillation.

How much current is needed to produce depolarization?

50–100 mA delivered during cardiac repolarization (the T wave)

What percentage of electric shock victims experience cardiac arrhythmias?

Up to 30%

How long after the shock can cardiac arrhythmias occur?

Arrhythmias have been reported up to 12 hours later.

Does an elevated creatine kinase-MB (CK-MB) level indicate cardiac damage?

Not necessarily, in electric shock patients

Name two events that may cause pulmonary arrest.

1. Diaphragmatic or thoracic muscle tetany
2. Central disruption of the medullary respiration center

List four common neurologic complications of electric shock.

1. Confusion
2. Short-term memory problems
3. Peripheral weakness
4. Spinal cord injury

Is delayed onset or persistence of neurologic symptoms common?

Yes.

What four vascular complications should be considered in electrical injury?

1. Direct damage
2. Spasm
3. Thrombosis
4. Compartment syndrome (sometimes)

Name three other complications that are common following electrical injury.

1. Renal failure [acute tubular necrosis (ATN)]
2. Gastrointestinal injury
3. Ophthalmologic injury (cataracts)

How do fluid requirements for patients who have experienced an electric shock compare with those of patients with a burn (assuming that the burn covers the same surface area on the skin)?

Patients who have experienced an electric shock have much greater fluid requirements.

What is the role of sodium bicarbonate in preventing renal failure?

Alkalinizing the urine increases myoglobin solubility and excretion.

Are there established criteria for disposition of the patient with electrical injury?

No, as long as there is no evidence of underlying trauma or need for cardiac monitoring.

Name six indications for admission for electrocardiographic monitoring.

1. Arrhythmia
2. Chest pain
3. Cardiac arrest

4. Cardiac disease
5. Abnormal electrocardiogram (EKG)
6. Concomitant injury

What types of injuries occur after electrocution?

Falls, injuries from muscle contraction, vertebral compression fractures, shoulder dislocation

How many lightning injuries involve two or more people?

30%

How does lightning injury differ from a high-voltage shock?

Lightning is extremely high voltage, but very short exposure. Cardiac arrest often develops with lightning exposure, but extensive tissue destruction, myoglobinuria, and renal failure are uncommon with lightning injury.

Why is there less tissue destruction with lightning injury than in high-voltage shock?

Lightning tends to "flashover" most victims, passing superficially over the skin.

How does the initial rhythm in cardiac arrest differ in lightning injury as compared with high-voltage shock?

Asystole is more common with lightning; ventricular fibrillation is more common with high-voltage shock.

What two additional complications may result from lightning injury?

1. Blunt trauma (from the shock wave)
2. Burns, with wet skin (from conversion of water to steam)

What is keraunoparalysis?

A flaccid paralysis that follows a lightning strike and usually resolves within 24 hours

How would an affected extremity appear?

The patient's extremities are mottled and cold owing to vascular spasm and instability.

What is keraunographic skin marking?

Fernlike erythematous markings where the electrical current passes over the skin (pathognomonic for lightning strike)

What are the most common long-term sequelae of lightning injury?

Neurologic sequelae, including coma, seizures, and cognitive disturbances

What otologic condition may result from lightning strike?	Tympanic membrane rupture (50% of of patients)
Name four ophthalmologic complications of lightning strike.	1. Uveitis 2. Hyphema 3. Retinal detachment 4. Cataracts
Are pupillary responses a reliable marker for intracranial injury after lightning injury?	No, because of ophthalmologic complications (decreased light perception)

RADIATION INJURIES

What are the two major types of radiation?	Ionizing (electromagnetic) and nonionizing (light, microwaves, radio)
What is a "rad"?	Radiation absorbed dose (absorbed energy)
What does "rem" stand for?	Roentgen equivalents man
Distinguish between rem and rad.	Rem indicates biologic impact of a dose, and is medically more useful than rad.
How much radiation does a person absorb from natural sources in the United States annually?	360 mrem
What is considered a large dose of radiation?	100 rem
What acute radiation dose will kill:	
50% of people exposed?	400 rem
100% (approximately) of people exposed?	600 rem
What radiation dose to fetuses has been associated with resultant mental retardation?	5 rem

**At how many weeks' gesta-
tion is the fetus most
vulnerable to radiation?**

8–15 weeks

**Name six acute signs of a
large radiation exposure.**

1. Erythema of the skin at the exposure
   site
2. Malaise
3. Nausea
4. Vomiting
5. Diarrhea
6. Seizures (in some patients)

**What are two consequences
of radiation exposure that
become apparent later?**

Internal bleeding (manifested by anemia)
and increased incidence of infection

**What is the latent period
and how long does it last?**

The period between the disappearance of
gastrointestinal symptoms and the
appearance of other symptoms, usually
lasting 1 week or longer

**What dose of radiation
should be suspected if
gastrointestinal symptoms
appear:**

Within 2 hours?

> 400 rem

After 2 hours?

≈ 200 rem

Not at all within 6 hours?

< 50 rem

**How can the white blood
cell (WBC) count be used
prognostically?**

After 48 hours:
$> 1200/mm^3$, good prognosis
$300–1200/mm^3$, fair prognosis
$< 300/mm^3$, poor prognosis

**Do people who have been
exposed to radiation be-
come radioactive?**

No. Although they may have radioactive
substances on or in them, people do not
become radioactive.

**What device is used to
check a person for radio-
active substances?**

A Geiger-Müller (GM) counter

**List three radiation decon-
tamination precautions for
staff in the emergency
department (ED).**

1. Lead shields
2. Special decontamination area
3. Rotation of caregivers to minimize
   exposure

How should treatment proceed?	Cover open wounds, remove the patient's clothing, and wash the patient's entire body with soap and water.
What medication will help protect the thyroid after radiation exposure?	Potassium iodide, given in the first several hours after exposure
What is decorporation?	Chelation of radiation with chelating agents in the gastrointestinal tract
When should decorporation be used?	After ingestion, inhalation, or wound contamination with a radioactive substance
What chelating agent is used?	Diethylenetriamine pentaacetic acid (DTPA)
Where is it available?	Radiation Emergency Assistance Center/Training Site (REAC/TS) in Oak Ridge, Tennessee

COLD-RELATED ILLNESS AND INJURIES

HYPOTHERMIA

What is the definition of hypothermia?	Core body temperature $< 35°C$ ($95°F$)
What part of the brain is responsible for temperature regulation?	The hypothalamus
What systemic conditions may cause hypothermia?	Hypothyroidism, hypoadrenalism, hypopituitarism, hypoglycemia, central nervous system (CNS) trauma, stroke, Wernicke's encephalopathy, drugs, sepsis, skin disease
What drugs are associated with hypothermia?	Ethyl alcohol, barbiturates, and sedative–hypnotic agents
What is the vasogenic effect of alcohol consumption?	Peripheral vasodilation, which leads to heat dissipation
What are two risk factors associated with hypo-thermia?	Exposure to cold weather; immersion in water

Name three signs of hypothermia.

1. Altered mental status
2. Decreased heart rate
3. Decreased respiratory rate

List four complications that are associated with hypothermia.

1. Coagulopathy
2. Acidosis
3. Ventricular arrhythmias
4. Asystole

What are the three levels of hypothermia?

Mild: Core body temperature of 32°C–34.9°C
Moderate: Core body temperature of 28°C–31.9°C
Severe: Core body temperature of < 28°C

What are the signs of:

Mild hypothermia?

Tachypnea, tachycardia, ataxia, dysarthria, shivering

Moderate hypothermia?

Loss of shivering, arrhythmias, Osborne (J) waves, decreased consciousness, combative behavior, muscle rigidity, dilated pupils

Severe hypothermia?

Coma, hypotension, acidemia, ventricular fibrillation, asystole, flaccidity, apnea

At what temperatures are hypothermic patients most susceptible to arrhythmias?

At core temperatures < 30°C

What EKG change is characteristic of hypothermia?

Osborne (J) waves

What are Osborne (J) waves?

Slow, positive deflections at the end of the QRS complex; most commonly seen in leads aVL and aVF, and in the left precordial leads

What other EKG changes are often observed?

T-wave inversions, PR/QRS/QT prolongation, arrhythmias

What is the typical series of arrhythmias observed in the hypothermic patient?

Sinus bradycardia, atrial fibrillation, slow ventricular response, ventricular fibrillation, asystole

How does hypothermia affect the defibrillation threshold?	Defibrillation is less effective in a hypothermic patient.
Do blood gas measurements reflect physiologic values?	No, the analyzed values reflect a slightly higher partial pressure of oxygen (PO_2) and partial pressure of carbon dioxide (PCO_2), and lower pH, than actual.
How does hypothermia affect the oxyhemoglobin dissociation curve?	The curve shifts to the left (oxygen is more tightly bound to hemoglobin).
How does hypothermia affect the kidney?	Increased urine output caused by exposure to cold ("cold diuresis") may cause volume loss.
Give three reasons why hypothermic patients are at increased risk for thrombus formation.	1. Dehydration 2. Fluid shift to the extravascular space 3. Cold-induced increase in blood viscosity
Why are hypothermic patients at risk for disseminated intravascular coagulation (DIC)?	The tissue release of thromboplastins, especially with rewarming, may induce DIC.
What warming techniques should be used for all hypothermic patients?	Administration of warmed oxygen and warm intravenous fluids
What are three general techniques for rewarming?	Passive rewarming, active external rewarming, and active core rewarming
What is passive rewarming?	External rewarming with blankets or by increasing room temperature
When is passive rewarming appropriate?	In the awake, cardiovascularly stable patient with mild hypothermia
What is active external rewarming?	Exposing the patient to heat lamps or another source of heat
What are the indications for active core rewarming?	Asystole Core temperature $< 28°C$ Failure of passive rewarming
What are three problems with active external rewarming?	Paradoxical decrease in core temperature Hypovolemia and hypotension "Rewarming acidosis"

Name five techniques for active core rewarming.	1. Gastrointestinal lavage 2. Bladder lavage 3. Peritoneal lavage 4. Pleural lavage 5. Extracorporeal rewarming
What are the dangers of overly aggressive treatment in severely hypothermic patients who have a pulse?	This has been thought to lead to refractory ventricular fibrillation. If the patient still has a pulse, treatment should include rewarming but not aggressive pharmacologic treatment unless absolutely necessary. A severely hypothermic patient without a pulse should undergo cardiopulmonary resuscitation (CPR) and other necessary treatments.
What is the best way to monitor body temperature?	With a core temperature reading by either an esophageal or rectal probe. Make sure it is a low-temperature probe.
What is the upper temperature limit for external rewarming devices?	A temperature > 45°C can damage the skin.
What is the treatment of choice for the patient with severe hypothermia and cardiac arrest?	Cardiopulmonary bypass
When is a hypothermic patient pronounced dead?	When the patient's body temperature is warmed to 32°C–35°C and the patient has no vital signs.

FROSTBITE

How is frostbite classified?	First through fourth degrees, or superficial and deep
What are the three zones of frostbite injury in an involved extremity?	Zone of coagulation, zone of hyperemia, zone of stasis
What is the "zone of coagulation"?	Irreversible injury
What is the "zone of hyperemia"?	Skin next to unaffected skin (most proximal); recovers without therapy in 10 days

What is the "zone of stasis"?	Potentially reversible injury (aim of therapy)
What is frostnip?	Pale skin with no tissue loss on rewarming
What is used to rewarm a frostbitten extremity?	Moving water, 40°C–42°C
Should dry heat (warm air, campfire) be used?	No. It could cause thermal injury.
What medication should be given prior to rewarming?	Analgesics (narcotics)
What are potential benefits of ibuprofen in the patient with frostbite?	Thromboxane inhibition and fibrinolysis production
How should the following types of blisters be treated?	
Clear blisters?	Consider aspiration or débridement (controversial).
Hemorrhagic blisters?	Consider aspiration (controversial).
What topical therapy may be used for both types of blisters?	Aloe vera
What type of antibiotics can be used for blistering?	Penicillin G 500,000 U, or topical antibiotics (controversial)
Is frostbite a tetanus-prone wound?	Yes.

HEAT-RELATED ILLNESS

What are the three major factors in determining body temperature?	1. Exogenous heat gain (temperature) 2. Endogenous heat production 3. Heat dissipation
What are the two major mechanisms of heat dissipation?	Sweating and peripheral vasodilation
What happens to cardiac output as peripheral vasodilation increases?	Cardiac output increases.

What are four examples of systemic conditions that may increase endogenous heat production?

1. Hyperthyroidism
2. Seizures
3. Drug withdrawal
4. Malignant hyperthermia

What drugs may increase endogenous heat production?

Salicylates, tricyclic antidepressants, cocaine, amphetamines, lysergic acid diethylamide (LSD), phencyclidine hydrochloride (PCP)

What factors may impair the body's ability to dissipate heat?

Age (old and young), obesity, improper clothing, cardiovascular disease, skin disease, drugs

What classes of drugs may decrease heat dissipation?

Anticholinergics, cardiac medications, diuretics, phenothiazines, sympathomimetics

Name three skin diseases that may predispose a patient to heat illness.

1. Scleroderma
2. Eczema
3. Psoriasis

What are three other names for "prickly heat"?

1. Heat rash
2. Lichen tropicus
3. Miliaria rubra

What causes heat rash?

Blocked sweat pores

How does heat rash present?

As a pruritic, erythematous, maculo-papular rash found on clothed areas of the body

What complication commonly results from prickly heat?

Secondary *Staphylococcus aureus* infection

What is "heat edema"?

Self-limited swelling of the hands and feet with heat exposure

What are three symptoms of heat exhaustion?

Weakness, fatigue, headache with normal mental status

What is the treatment for heat exhaustion?

Rest, fluids, electrolyte replacement

Distinguish heat exhaustion from heat stroke.

Heat exhaustion: Temperature < 40°C, normal mental status, sweating
Heat stroke: Hyperpyrexia (temperature usually > 40.5°C), CNS dysfunction, anhidrosis

Is anhidrosis a necessary diagnostic criteria for heat stroke?	No.
Is dehydration always present in a patient with heat stroke?	No.
Which part of the brain is particularly susceptible to heat?	The cerebellum; ataxia is a common finding.
What other CNS manifestations may be observed in heat stroke?	Confusion, drowsiness, disorientation, psychiatric symptoms
Laboratory studies reveal what abnormalities in heat stroke?	Hepatic injury, coagulation abnormalities, and renal failure
What cardiac complication may be seen in heat stroke?	Right-sided heart failure
What gastrointestinal complication may be seen in heat stroke?	Diarrhea
Which cooling method is most widely preferred in heat exhaustion and heat stroke, and how is it implemented?	Evaporative cooling
When should cooling efforts be stopped?	When the rectal temperature falls below 40°C
What complication may occur with continued cooling?	Overshoot hypothermia

VENOMOUS BITES AND STINGS

SNAKE BITES

What two families of poisonous snakes are found in North America?	Pit vipers (crotalids) and coral snakes

How does snake venom poison its victim?	The mix of enzymes may cause vascular damage, hemolysis, fibrinolysis, and neuromuscular dysfunction.
How often is venom not injected in a bite by a crotalid snake?	Approximately 25% of crotalid snake bites are "dry."
What are the local signs of a venomous snake bite?	Fang marks, pain, edema, ecchymoses, hemorrhagic blebs
What are the systemic signs and symptoms of a crotalid bite?	Sweating, nausea, vomiting, weakness, perioral numbness and tingling, tachycardia, hypotension, dizziness, mental status change, fasciculation
What are the neurologic signs and symptoms of a coral snake bite?	Diplopia, bulbar symptoms, drowsiness
What is the usual cause of death after a coral snake bite?	Respiratory paralysis
What measures should be taken "in the field" when administering first aid to the victim?	Immobilize the extremity, apply ice for comfort at the bite site, and identify the snake if possible
Why shouldn't incision and suction be performed?	No other measures should be taken "in the field" because they may increase tissue injury and cause the venom to spread.
What is the mainstay of treatment for snakebite in the ED?	Aggressive supportive therapy, which entails intravenous fluids, blood product replacement therapy, and advanced life support
What is the definitive treatment for a snake bite?	Antivenin (Crotalidae) polyvalent, also available for coral snake bites
Who should receive antivenin?	Crotalid bite victims who exhibit progression of symptoms, and all coral snake bite victims
What should be done prior to administration of antivenin?	Perform a skin test to determine the patient's sensitivity to the horse serum derivation.

Does a positive skin test rule out the use of anti-venin?	Not necessarily. Use of antivenin depends on the severity of symptoms.
Is compartment syndrome common after a snake bite?	No, not even with severe edema
Which patients with snake bites require hospital admission?	Any crotalid bite victim with symptoms after 8 hours of observation Any coral snake bite victim Anyone who received antivenin

INSECT AND ARACHNID BITES AND STINGS

Scorpion bites

What is the physiologic effect of scorpion venom?	Activation of sodium channels
What does this lead to?	Sympathetic, parasympathetic, and somatic nerve discharge
What symptoms may result?	Anxiety, roving eye movements, tachycardia, excessive secretions, opisthotonus, fasciculations, difficulty swallowing

Ant, bee, and wasp stings

What biologic order do stinging ants, bees, and wasps belong to?	Hymenoptera
What are the two types of reactions to Hymenoptera stings?	Toxic (nonantigenic) and systemic (antigenic)
Characterize a toxic re-action to a Hymenoptera sting.	Generally occurs with more than 10 stings Presents with gastrointestinal symptoms (nausea, vomiting, diarrhea)
Describe a systemic reaction.	An anaphylactic reaction, which may be mild to fatal
What are the symptoms of an anaphylactic reaction?	Itching eyes, urticaria, cough, and angioedema, which may proceed to bronchospasm

What medications are used to treat an anaphylactic reaction?	Subcutaneous epinephrine, antihistamines (H_1 and H_2 blockers), and steroids
How should hypotension be treated?	With crystalloid infusions and pressors
After a patient has experienced a systemic reaction, what preventive measures should be taken?	Patients should be advised to obtain a medical alert identification tag. In addition, they should be given a prescription for three insect sting kits (one for home, one for the car, and one for in the field).

Spider bites

What is the characteristic progression of a brown recluse spider (*Loxosceles reclusa*) bite?	Mild erythema, induration, blisters with bluish discoloration, necrosis
What systemic reactions may develop?	Fever, chills, nausea, myalgias, and hemolysis
Is there an antivenin for *Loxosceles reclusa*?	No.
What medication may help attenuate necrosis?	Dapsone
Black widow spider venom contains what type of toxin?	A neurotoxin
What is the progression of symptoms after a black widow spider bite?	Pain or numbness around bite, systemic symptoms, severe muscle cramps of large muscle groups, and hypertension
What are potential systemic symptoms?	Sweating, headache, hyperesthesia, paresthesia
Is there an antivenin for black widow spider bites?	Yes.
What other medical therapy can be given?	Analgesics, benzodiazepines (muscle relaxation), calcium gluconate (controversial)

Parasite bites

Where do body lice tend to bite?	The waist, shoulders, axillae, and neck

Describe body lice bites.	Red spots that become intensely pruritic wheals, leading to linear scratch marks
Where are scabies bites concentrated?	On the hands and feet, especially in the web spaces
How can chiggers, body lice, or scabies be treated?	With topical lindane or crotamiton (also permethrin for scabies)
Which of these agents should be used with caution in children?	Lindane is absorbed more readily by children's skin and can cause CNS toxicity.

MARINE ANIMAL STINGS

How do jellyfish (phylum Cnidaria) sting?	Nematocysts (hollow sharp tubes) puncture the skin and inject venom.
How can the nematocysts of a jellyfish be removed from a patient?	Acetic acid, rubbing alcohol, or baking soda applied for 30 minutes have all been shown to be effective.
How should sea urchin spine wounds be treated?	By removing the spines

HIGH-ALTITUDE ILLNESS

What percentage of travel-ers above 8500 feet (2590 meters) develop manifesta-tions of high-altitude illness?	25%
What are the three major forms of high-altitude sickness?	Acute mountain sickness (AMS), high-altitude pulmonary edema (HAPE), and high-altitude cerebral edema (HACE)
What are some conditions that may be aggravated by high altitude?	Chronic obstructive pulmonary disease (COPD), congestive heart failure (CHF), atherosclerotic heart disease, sickle cell disease
What are the effects of high altitude on pregnancy?	Pregnant women have an increased incidence of hypertension, low-birth-weight infants, and neonatal hyperbilirubinemia.
What is the primary factor in the pathophysiology of high-altitude sickness?	Decreasing arterial partial pressure of oxygen (PaO_2) at increasing altitude

What is the PaO_2 in a young, healthy person:

At sea level?	90–95 mm Hg
At 9200 feet (2800 meters)?	60 mm Hg
At 20,000 feet (6100 meters)?	35 mm Hg

At increasing altitude, what value of oxygen changes: the percentage or the partial pressure?

The partial pressure decreases.

What are the effects of decreasing PaO_2 on ventilation and acid-base status?

Respiratory alkalosis and tachypnea

ACUTE MOUNTAIN SICKNESS (AMS)

What is the clinical presentation of AMS?

Headache (frontal, bilateral), anorexia, nausea, overall weakness, sleep disruption

What is the fluid status in AMS?

Fluid retention occurs.

What are the physical findings in AMS?

Peripheral and facial edema from fluid retention

What is the definition of AMS?

Headache plus one of the following: gastrointestinal symptoms, dizziness or lightheadedness, difficulty sleeping

How should AMS be treated initially?

Stop ascent. Descend if symptoms persist.

What three pharmacologic treatment options are effective?

Low-flow oxygen, acetazolamide, steroids

When should steroids be used?

For moderate to severe cases of AMS

HIGH-ALTITUDE CEREBRAL EDEMA (HACE)

What symptoms indicate HACE?

HACE occurs when the cerebral edema of AMS progresses, resulting in altered mental status, ataxia, stupor, and eventually coma.

Are headache, nausea, and vomiting present in HACE?

Often, but not always

What focal neurologic signs may be present?

Third or sixth cranial nerve palsies may result from compression from the edema

How should symptoms of HACE be treated?

The patient should be removed to a lower altitude, oxygen and steroids should be administered, and measures should be taken to lower the intracranial pressure (ICP).

HIGH-ALTITUDE PULMONARY EDEMA (HAPE)

What are the pathophysiologic characteristics of HAPE?

Noncardiogenic edema (i.e., normal left ventricular function), increased pulmonary vascular resistance, and pulmonary hypertension

Which two symptoms suggest HAPE?

Decreased exercise performance and dry cough

Are rales audible?

Usually, but they may be absent in up to 30% of patients

What other symptoms occur?

Tachycardia, tachypnea, and fever; later, productive cough and cyanosis

What finding is characteristic on cardiac exam?

Tachycardia, a prominent pulmonic valve component (P_2) of the second heart sound, and right ventricular heave

What are the cornerstones of treatment?

Rapid diagnosis, descent from the high altitude, and administration of oxygen

What pharmacologic agent is helpful in HAPE?

Nifedipine (10–30 mg) reduces pulmonary artery pressure and increases oxygen saturation

MONGE'S DISEASE

What is Monge's disease?

Chronic mountain polycythemia (CMP), shown to affect long-term high-altitude residents around the world

What are the symptoms of CMP?	Headache, impaired concentration, difficulty sleeping, impaired peripheral circulation, chest congestion
What is the treatment of CMP?	Phlebotomy, relocation to a lower altitude, home oxygen use

DROWNING AND NEAR DROWNING

What age group is most at risk for drowning?	Bimodal: children younger than 4 years, and teenagers
What is "dry drowning"?	Respiratory block from laryngospasm
Which is more common, fresh or salt water drowning?	Fresh water drowning, even in coastal areas
What effect do fresh and salt water have on alveolar surfactant?	They both wash surfactant out of the alveoli.
How do fresh and salt water differ in their effect on alveolar surfactant?	Fresh water changes the surface tension of the surfactant.
How should water be removed from the patient's lungs and airways?	Only by suction (if available)
Should the Heimlich maneuver be used on patients who have inhaled water?	No.
Are cervical spine injuries commonly seen in near drowning victims?	Yes, after diving
Where are most spinal injuries located in divers?	The lower cervical spine
When should a patient be intubated following a near drowning?	If the patient fails to maintain an oxygen saturation over 90% despite the administration of 40%–50% high-flow oxygen
What type of ventilator manipulation may help a near-drowning patient after intubation?	Positive end-expiratory pressure (PEEP) or continuous positive airway pressure (CPAP) may help to recruit collapsed alveoli.

What complications can occur in near-drowning patients?

Blood volume shifts, electrolyte abnormalities, hemolysis, rhabdomyolysis, ATN, DIC

Which near-drowning patients may be discharged home from the ED?

Patients who are asymptomatic on arrival and after 4 hours of observation and evaluation

What other environmental condition is common with near-drowning victims?

Hypothermia

Which drowning allows for better cerebral recovery: cold-water drowning or ice-water drowning?

Ice-water drowning

15

Pediatric Emergencies

THE NEONATE IN THE EMERGENCY DEPARTMENT (ED)

List five nonsystemic causes of "fussing" in an infant.

1. Hair tourniquet
2. Testicular torsion
3. Corneal abrasion
4. Improper feeding
5. Fractures

SHOCK

What is the differential diagnosis for shock in a newborn?

1. Sepsis
2. Meningitis
3. Pneumonia
4. Heart disease
5. Metabolic disorder
6. Congenital adrenal hypoplasia
7. Dehydration
8. Posterior urethral valves

What are the causes of invasive bacterial disease (e.g., sepsis, meningitis, pneumonia, bacteremia) in the newborn?

Group B β-hemolytic streptococci, Gram-negative rods (e.g., *Escherichia coli, Klebsiella* species), and *Listeria monocytogenes*

Can viruses produce a septic-appearing infant?

Yes.

What is the most common viral cause for septic-appearing neonates or infants?

Herpes simplex virus (HSV) infection

What are the most common symptoms in septic newborns?

Respiratory symptoms

What approach should be taken when a newborn presents with a fever?	Thoroughly evaluate any child younger than 60 days who is brought to the ED with a fever: 1. History and physical examination 2. Complete blood count (CBC) 3. Blood cultures 4. Chest x-ray (if the symptoms are localized to the chest) 5. Urine culture 6. Lumbar puncture and cerebrospinal fluid (CSF) analysis 7. Initiation of empiric intravenous antibiotic therapy
What percentage of patients with congenital adrenal hypoplasia have the salt-wasting type?	75%
What are the most common enzyme deficits in congenital adrenal hypoplasia?	21-hydroxylase, 11-hydroxylase, or 3β-hydroxysteroid dehydrogenase
What are the physical signs of congenital adrenal hypoplasia in newborn girls?	Masculinization of the external female genitalia

JAUNDICE

What causes jaundice in the newborn?	Accumulation of (usually unconjugated) bilirubin
What causes unconjugated hyperbilirubinemia?	1. Infection 2. Hypothyroidism 3. Physiologic hyperbilirubinemia 4. ABO and Rh incompatibility
What causes conjugated hyperbilirubinemia?	1. Infection 2. Metabolic disorders 3. Hepatobiliary pathology (e.g., biliary atresia)
Why is jaundice a cause for concern in the neonate?	The complications of kernicterus (i.e., high levels of bilirubin in the blood) are severe, irreversible (e.g., deafness, cerebral palsy), and potentially fatal.

What is the treatment for:

**Unconjugated hyperbili-
rubinemia?**

Phototherapy

**Conjugated hyperbili-
rubinemia?**

Treatment of the underlying cause

CONJUNCTIVITIS

**When does gonococcal
conjunctivitis present?**

During the first 2–5 days of life

**When does chlamydial
conjunctivitis present?**

During the first 5–14 days of life

**Why are systemic anti-
biotics necessary for treating chlamydial conjunctivitis?**

To eradicate the carrier state and prevent
pneumonia

FLUID AND ELECTROLYTE REPLACEMENT IN THE PEDIATRIC PATIENT

**What are two ways in which
the fluid deficit can be estimated in a dehydrated child?**

1. Physical examination
2. Comparison of the child's current
   weight and his weight in the chart, if
   that weight was obtained recently

**What signs on physical
examination are consistent
with a fluid deficit of:**

Approximately 5%?

Increased urine concentration, decreased
urine output, decreased tear production,
tachycardia, dry mucous membranes

10%?

All of the above, plus decreased skin
turgor and sunken fontanelles

15%?

All of the above, plus acidosis and low
blood pressure

**What are the three types of
dehydration?**

Isotonic, hyponatremic, and
hypernatremic

**What are the three compo-
nents of fluid management?**

Replacement of the deficit, administration of maintenance fluids, and
replacement of ongoing losses

What intravenous fluid is used to resuscitate a child?	Isotonic solution (e.g., lactated Ringer's or normal saline)
What is the potential complication of rapid resuscitation with a hypotonic solution?	Cerebral edema
What is the typical initial fluid bolus used in resuscitation of a child?	20 ml/kg
What are the indications for a bolus of less than 20 ml/kg?	1. Underlying cardiac or renal disorder 2. Risk of cerebral or pulmonary edema
What is the endpoint for fluid resuscitation?	Adequate end-organ perfusion, often measured by urine output
After resuscitation, how is the fluid deficit replaced?	In the child with uncomplicated mild dehydration, repeat the fluid bolus. Otherwise, administer replacement fluids over a 24-hour period.
Describe 24-hour replacement fluid therapy.	1. Administer 50% of the deficit over the first 8 hours. 2. Administer the remaining 50% over the next 16 hours. 3. In addition to replacing the deficit, administer maintenance fluids to replace ongoing losses.
What are some examples of ongoing losses?	1. Losses as a result of emesis or diarrhea 2. Losses through drains placed postoperatively 3. Losses through breaks in the skin
How are fluid maintenance requirements calculated?	On the basis of the patient's weight
What is the fluid maintenance requirement for:	
The first 10 kg of weight?	Approximately 100 ml/kg/hr
The next 10 kg?	50 ml/kg/hr
Each subsequent 10 kg?	20 ml/kg/hr

What is the approximate maintenance intravenous fluid rate for a 22-kg child?	62 ml/kg/hr
For a child, what is the daily:	
Sodium requirement?	3–4 mEq/kg/day
Potassium requirement?	1–2 mEq/kg/day
What is the composition of a typical maintenance fluid?	One-fourth normal saline in 5% dextrose with 20 mEq potassium chloride (i.e., D5 1/4 NS with 20 mEq KCl)
When should hypertonic saline be considered for fluid replacement in the patient with hyponatremic dehydration?	When the patient is symptomatic, or has a serum sodium level of less than 125 mEq/L
What complication can occur as a result of rapid rehydration of the patient with hypernatremic dehydration?	Cerebral edema
Calculate an electrolyte deficit.	Deficit = (ideal electrolyte level − observed electrolyte level) × (fractional distribution of electrolyte) × (weight in kilograms)

CONGENITAL HEART DEFECTS

In what percentage of live births do congenital heart defects occur?	1%
When are the most serious cases of congenital heart defects diagnosed?	During the first year of life
What percentage of patients are diagnosed with serious congenital heart defects by:	
1 month of age?	35%

3–6 months of age?	40%
6–12 months of age?	25%
Congenital heart defects represent what percentage of heart disease in the pediatric population?	90%
What studies are helpful in evaluating a child with a suspected congenital heart defect?	Chest x-ray, CBC, electrocardiogram (EKG), arterial blood gases (ABGs), and echocardiography (if available)
Does the absence of a murmur exclude congenital heart defects?	No.
Is there a correlation between the severity of a congenital heart defect and the presence of:	
A murmur?	No.
Decreased pulses?	Occasionally; however, decreased pulses may also reflect shock owing to a noncardiac cause.
What are the common congenital heart defects that occur:	
On the left side?	Coarctation of the aorta, aortic stenosis, total anomalous pulmonary venous return (TAPVR), hypoplastic left heart syndrome
On the right side?	Transposition of the great vessels, tetralogy of Fallot, tricuspid atresia, truncus arteriosis, pulmonary atresia, pulmonary stenosis
What are common septal defects?	Ventricular septal defect (VSD), atrial septal defect (ASD), atrioventricular canal

LEFT-SIDED DEFECTS

What is coarctation of the aorta?	Narrowing of the aorta, usually at the ductus arteriosus

What is the prevalence of coarctation among children who have congenital heart defects?

8%

What are the common findings on physical examination and chest x-ray of the child with coarctation of the aorta?

1. Decreased femoral pulses
2. Rib notching secondary to intercostal vessel hypertrophy

How is coarctation diagnosed?

Using echocardiography

What is the prevalence of aortic stenosis among children who have congenital heart defects?

5%

What are common findings on physical examination of the child with aortic stenosis?

Harsh systolic ejection murmur, poor perfusion

What is a common EKG finding in the child with aortic stenosis?

Left ventricular hypertrophy

Describe TAPVR.

The pulmonary veins do not connect to the left atrium.

Describe the physiology of TAPVR.

Blood flow, as demonstrated by color Doppler echocardiography, may exhibit either nonobstructive or obstructive physiology.

What is nonobstructive physiology in TAPVR?

A left-to-right shunt similar to that seen with an ASD; patients may present with tachypnea

What is obstructive physiology in TAPVR?

Decreased filling of the left side of the heart; patients often present with cyanosis

What is hypoplastic left heart syndrome?

Congenital hypoplasia of the left ventricle and outflow tract

What percentage of children with congenital heart defects have hypoplastic left heart syndrome?

7%

How does it present?	Patients with hypoplastic left heart syndrome present with cyanosis and circulatory collapse. Poor perfusion develops as the patent ductus arteriosus (PDA) closes.
How is hypoplastic left heart syndrome treated?	With prostaglandin infusion until surgical intervention (e.g., the Norwood procedure or cardiac transplant) is feasible

RIGHT-SIDED DEFECTS

What is transposition of the great arteries?	The pulmonary artery originates from the left ventricle; the aorta originates from the right ventricle.
How does transposition of the great arteries present?	Cyanosis, circulatory collapse, and poor perfusion develop as the PDA closes.
How is transposition of the great arteries treated?	With prostaglandin infusion and balloon atrial septostomy until definitive surgical repair can take place
What complications are seen with prostaglandin infusion?	Apnea, hypotension, hyperthermia, irritability
What is tetralogy of Fallot?	Pulmonary stenosis, overriding aorta, VSD, and subsequent hypertrophy of the right ventricle
What is the physiology behind a "tet spell?"	A sudden increase in pulmonary outflow tract resistance increases the right-to-left shunt via the VSD
What is the main clinical feature of a tet spell?	Cyanosis that worsens with crying or exercise
How can a tet spell be treated?	Increase systemic pressure or otherwise relieve right-to-left shunting by placing the child in the knee-to-chest position.

RESPIRATORY TRACT INFECTIONS

SINUSITIS

When do the sinuses develop in childhood?	Small maxillary and ethmoid sinuses are present at birth. Frontal sinuses may not

develop at all (or may develop unilaterally) and, as with the sphenoid sinus, do not even begin to appear until around the age of 5 years.

Which is more common, viral rhinosinusitis or bacterial sinusitis?

Viral rhinosinusitis is 20–200 times more common than bacterial sinusitis.

What microorganisms cause bacterial sinusitis?

Streptococcus pneumoniae, nontypeable *Haemophilus influenzae, Moraxella catarrhalis*

What are the signs and symptoms of sinusitis?

Sinusitis is suggested by the presence of an unresolving upper respiratory tract infection (e.g., one with symptoms lasting longer than 10–14 days). Patients also complain of severe periorbital pain, swelling, a purulent nasal discharge, malaise, and a high fever.

What does a thick, opaque, discolored nasal discharge signal?

A viral upper respiratory tract infection

Is a nighttime cough specific for sinusitis?

No.

Can sinusitis be diagnosed by x-ray?

No.

What is the therapy for acute sinusitis?

Viral sinusitis usually resolves on its own. Bacterial sinusitis necessitates a 14-day course of an antibiotic (e.g., penicillin, amoxicillin–clavulanic acid, cefaclor). Decongestants and saline nasal irrigation can provide symptomatic therapy.

ACUTE OTITIS MEDIA

What is acute otitis media?

An acute infection of the middle ear

Who is most at risk for otitis media?

Male patients, young patients, children in daycare, patients with Down's syndrome or cystic fibrosis

What is the most common cause of otitis media?

Infection by bacteria from the nasopharynx commonly causes otitis media, which usually follows an upper respiratory tract infection.

Which bacteria cause otitis media?

Streptococcus pneumoniae, nontypeable *Haemophilus influenzae, Moraxella catarrhalis, Staphylococcus* species

Which bacteria most commonly cause otitis media in infants?

Staphylococcus aureus and *Escherichia coli*

How does one diagnose acute otitis media?

Pneumatic otoscopy is used to evaluate the color, mobility, translucency, and position of the tympanic membrane.

What are the symptoms of otitis media?

Fever, ear pain, and pulling on the ear are symptoms. However, many patients present only with fever and irritability.

What are the signs?

Injection of the tympanic membrane, purulent drainage, and an effusion behind the eardrum

What is the treatment for otitis media?

Administer antibiotics (e.g., amoxicillin) for 7–10 days. If the patient is allergic to penicillin, sulfamethoxazole–trimethoprim can be used. Broader spectrum agents can be used for recurrent infection.

Does acute otitis media resolve without antimicrobials?

It often resolves on its own.

Is a middle ear effusion expected after acute otitis media?

A middle ear effusion may persist for weeks after the acute otitis media resolves.

Does the presence of a middle ear effusion in an asymptomatic child immediately following the resolution of an episode of acute otitis media necessitate antimicrobial therapy?

No.

What are the complications of otitis media?

Labyrinthitis, tympanic membrane perforation, abscess, and chronic otitis media

PHARYNGITIS

Which is more common, viral pharyngitis or streptococcal pharyngitis?

Viral pharyngitis

What are the signs and symptoms of streptococcal pharyngitis?

Pharyngeal exudate, palatal petechiae, tender anterior cervical lymphadenopathy, headache, abdominal pain

What drug is used to treat a group A β-hemolytic streptococcal infection in a child?

Penicillin

LARYNGOTRACHEOBRONCHITIS (CROUP)

What causes croup?

Most cases are either caused by an influenzae virus, an adenovirus, or a parainfluenza virus

What are the signs and symptoms of croup?

A characteristic, "barking" cough; stridor; and a low-grade fever; most children are comfortable when being held by a parent and do not display signs of respiratory distress

What is the differential diagnosis for acute stridor?

1. Croup
2. Epiglottitis
3. Bacterial tracheitis
4. Retropharyngeal abscess
5. Diphtheria

What is the treatment for croup?

Supportive measures (e.g., vaporization) and the administration of racemic epinephrine or intramuscular corticosteroids

EPIGLOTTITIS

What are the clinical features of epiglottitis?

Acute onset of fever, "toxic-appearing" child, tripod position, drooling

How is the diagnosis of epiglottitis made?

Direct visualization of a swollen epiglottis (using direct or fiberoptic laryngoscopy), preferably in the operating room with a team of personnel skilled in airway management nearby

What is the therapy for epiglottitis?	Airway control (intubation) and antibiotics

BRONCHIOLITIS

What is bronchiolitis?	An acute viral infection of the lower respiratory tract that occurs in children younger than 2 years
What anatomy is involved?	The small airways
What is the pathophysiology of bronchiolitis?	The small bronchi and bronchioles are inflamed. There is necrosis, sloughing of the epithelium, mucus plugging, and destruction of ciliated cells.
How does bronchiolitis differ from:	
Bronchitis?	Bronchitis is characterized by large airway involvement.
Pneumonia?	Pneumonia affects the interstitium and the alveoli.
What causes bronchiolitis?	Viruses, such as respiratory syncytial virus (RSV), adenovirus, influenza virus, parainfluenza virus, or rhinovirus
Which children are at the greatest risk for death from RSV?	Children with congenital heart or lung disease or immunodeficiency disease
What are the signs and symptoms of bronchiolitis?	Fever, cough, rhinitis, dyspnea, and retractions
What signs merit hospitalization?	Hypoxia, cyanosis, lethargy, dehydration, and other signs of distress, especially in infants
Name some complications associated with bronchiolitis.	Apnea (particularly in the premature neonate), respiratory failure, atelectasis, and superinfection
What is the therapy for bronchiolitis?	Therapy is primarily supportive and includes the administration of oxygen; bronchodilator use is controversial

PNEUMONIA (SEE ALSO CHAPTER 4, "PULMONARY EMERGENCIES")

What type of pneumonia often presents with a low-grade fever and cough in a 6-week-old infant?	Pneumonia caused by *Chlamydia trachomatis*
What age group is most susceptible to pneumonia caused by *Mycoplasma pneumoniae?*	Children younger than 5 years
What is the most common cause of bacterial pneumonia in children?	*Streptococcus pneumoniae*

EXANTHEMS

What are the six common exanthems of childhood?	1. Measles (rubeola) 2. Scarlet fever 3. German measles (rubella) 4. Dukes' disease (fourth disease) 5. Erythema infectiosum (fifth disease) 6. Roseola infantum

MEASLES (RUBEOLA)

What are Koplik spots?	Koplik spots are elevations resembling salt grains that appear on the buccal mucosa, about 2 days before the measles exanthem appears.
Describe the measles exanthem.	It is an erythematous maculopapular eruption that appears first on the scalp and at the hairline.
What are several associated symptoms of measles?	Puffy red eyes, fever, and coryza
How is measles prevented?	By vaccine, given at 15–18 months of age
What may occur following vaccination?	An exanthem (5–15 days after vaccination)

SCARLET FEVER

What causes scarlet fever?	An erythrogenic toxin produced by group A β-hemolytic streptococci

What is the characteristic rash of scarlet fever?	An erythematous, fine punctate rash that feels like sandpaper
What are two late complications of group A β-hemolytic streptococcal infection?	Acute glomerulonephritis and rheumatic fever
Can rheumatic fever be prevented?	Yes. Rheumatic fever may be prevented by appropriate treatment of the streptococcal infection.

GERMAN MEASLES (RUBELLA)

What causes German measles?	The rubella virus
Describe the rash associated with rubella.	Light, reddish-pink discrete maculopapules, which usually start at the hairline

DUKES' DISEASE (FOURTH DISEASE)

What is Dukes' disease?	A mild, febrile disorder seen in children and characterized by a bright, rosy, generalized exanthematous rash
What causes Dukes' disease?	It has multiple causes.

ERYTHEMA INFECTIOSUM (FIFTH DISEASE)

What causes erythema infectiosum?	Infection with parvovirus B-19
What are the three stages of erythema infectiosum?	1. "Slapped cheeks" appearance 2. Erythematous maculopapular rash on the arms, trunk, and legs 3. Reticulated, lacy rash
What are three possible complications of parvovirus B-19 infection?	Reactive arthritis, arthralgia, and hemolytic anemia
What risk does parvovirus B-19 infection pose for pregnant women?	It may cause fetal hydrops during the first half of pregnancy.

ROSEOLA INFANTUM

What is roseola infantum?	A response, perhaps age-related, to any one of several viral infections

When does the rash of roseola infantum present?

Often at the end of a fever

What is the typical appearance of roseola infantum?

The child appears well until the appearance of the rash. The rash starts on the trunk and consists of discrete, rose-colored macules, 2–3 mm in size, which blanch with pressure.

OTHER EXANTHEMS

What is hand-foot-and-mouth disease?

A mild, self-limited disorder, often seen in preschool-age children and characterized by vesicular eruptions in the oral cavity and on the hands and feet

What causes hand-foot-and-mouth disease?

Coxsackie viruses

Describe the rash of chickenpox.

The rash begins as a maculopapular rash and develops into "teardrop" vesicles on an erythematous base.

What causes chickenpox?

Varicella-zoster virus

What percentage of patients with mononucleosis develop a rash?

About 10%–15% of patients

Describe the exanthem of mononucleosis.

A macular or maculopapular morbilliform eruption

How does pityriasis rosea present?

Pityriasis rosea typically presents on the thorax with a "herald patch," an oval area, 2–4 mm in size, of scaly dermatitis. The patch is pink-brown in the center and often has an elevated border.

What is the classic pattern of the exanthem of pityriasis rosea?

It is shaped like a Christmas tree.

What is a common variant pattern of pityriasis rosea in a young child?

It may appear as a papular, vesicular, urticarial, purpuric rash with lesions on the extremities rather than on the trunk.

KAWASAKI DISEASE (MUCOCUTANEOUS LYMPH NODE SYNDROME)

What is Kawasaki disease?

An acute, self-limited febrile disease of children (50% of patients are younger than 2 years; 80% are younger than 5 years)

What is its cause?

The cause of Kawasaki disease is unknown. The disorder may be caused by *Staphylococcus* or *Streptococcus* superantigen.

During which seasons is Kawasaki disease most common?

Winter and spring

What predisposes a patient to the development of Kawasaki disease?

A recent staphylococcal or streptococcal infection

What are the signs and symptoms of Kawasaki disease?

Patients appear ill, and have a history of a temperature greater than 102°F that has persisted for at least 5 days and is unresponsive to antibiotic therapy. In addition, four of the following five criteria must be present in order to diagnose Kawasaki disease:
1. Bilateral conjunctivitis (bright red eyes)
2. A nonpurulent morbiliform rash (any size, shape, or type, but it should be neither vesicular nor purulent)
3. Changes in the mucus membranes (e.g., dry, cracked, red lips; "strawberry tongue")
4. Limb edema progressing to desquamation
5. Unilateral cervical lymphadenopathy

What percentage of patients with Kawasaki disease have solitary cervical lymphadenopathy?

50%

Which conditions are in the differential diagnosis for Kawasaki disease?

1. Staphylococcal scalded skin syndrome (SSSS)
2. Toxic shock syndrome
3. Stevens-Johnson syndrome
4. Scarlet fever
5. Rocky Mountain spotted fever (RMSF)
6. Epstein-Barr virus (EBV) infection

(more than 80% of patients develop a
pruritic maculopapular rash following
misdiagnosis and treatment with
ampicillin)

What laboratory findings are commonly associated with Kawasaki disease?

Anemia, thrombocytosis (possibly more than 1 million platelets/mm^3), an increased ESR, and sterile pyuria

How is Kawasaki disease treated?

With large doses (i.e., 80–100 mg/kg) of acetylsalicylic acid

What are the emergent complications of Kawasaki disease?

1. Myocardial infarction
2. Aneurysm (especially of the axillary or coronary arteries)
3. Myocarditis (if the disease is untreated)
4. Hydrops of the gallbladder
5. Uveitis

What is the most common acquired pediatric heart disease in the United States?

Kawasaki disease

What percentage of patients, if left untreated, will develop coronary aneurysms?

20%

What therapy has been shown to decrease the risk of cardiac complications in patients with Kawasaki disease?

Intravenous immunoglobulin (IVIG), 2 g/kg

FEVER

What organisms are suspected in infants younger than 2 months with bacteremia?

Group B β-hemolytic streptococci, Gram-negative rods (e.g., *E. coli*, *Klebsiella* species), and *L. monocytogenes* (the same organisms responsible for bacteremia in a neonate)

What is the most common cause of bacteremia in children 3–36 months of age?

Streptococcus pneumoniae infection

What percentage of children with a fever higher than 39.5°C have invasive bacterial disease?	Approximately 5%
What percentage of children with a fever higher than 39.5°C and a white blood cell (WBC) count greater than 15,000 cells/ mm³ have invasive bacterial disease?	10%–15%
In what percentage of children younger than 1 year with a urinary tract infection (UTI) do radiographs reveal an abnormal urinary tract?	Approximately 50%
Can physical exam effectively exclude meningitis in a child younger than 3 years?	No.
Describe febrile seizures.	Generalized seizures lasting less than 15 minutes and lacking a postictal phase that occur in children between the ages of 3 months and 5 years and are associated with the onset of fever
What percentage of children will have a febrile seizure?	3%
What percentage will have recurrences?	More than 30%

GASTROINTESTINAL DISORDERS

GASTROENTERITIS

What are some common causes of viral gastro-enteritis?	Rotavirus, adenovirus, and calicivirus

Rotavirus infection

What is the peak age incidence for rotavirus
infection in children?

6–24 months

How is rotavirus
transmitted?

By the fecal–oral route (which is why
sporadic outbreaks in daycare settings are
common)

What are the signs and
symptoms of rotavirus
infection?

1. Explosive, watery, foul-smelling
   diarrhea that occasionally contains
   mucus, but no fecal leukocytes
2. Vomiting (early in the clinical course)
3. Fever (occasionally)
4. Malabsorption
5. Dehydration
6. Compensated metabolic acidosis

How is rotavirus diagnosed?

By means of an enzyme immunoassay

What is the treatment for
rotavirus infection?

Supportive measures

Adenovirus infection

Who is most susceptible to
adenovirus infection?

Children younger than 24 months

What are the signs and
symptoms of adenovirus
infection?

The signs and symptoms are similar to
those of rotavirus infection, but the
clinical course is generally less severe.

What is the quality of the
diarrhea?

It is watery, but contains no blood or
mucus.

PYLORIC STENOSIS

What is pyloric stenosis?

Gastric obstruction secondary to a
congenitally hypertrophied pyloric muscle

What is the clinical significance of pyloric stenosis?

It is the most common reason for
abdominal surgery in children younger
than 6 months.

How does pyloric stenosis
present?

Typically, with projectile, nonbilious
vomiting in the first 12 weeks of life

What other signs may be present?	Dehydration, weight loss, and peristaltic waves
Does pyloric stenosis have a sex predisposition?	Yes. It occurs more frequently in boys.
What is the "classic" physical finding in pyloric stenosis?	A palpable, olive-sized mass in the right upper quadrant (RUQ), near the midline
Can the physical exam exclude the diagnosis?	No.
How is the diagnosis made?	By ultrasound or radiographic evaluation of the upper gastrointestinal tract
What are some relatively common complications associated with pyloric stenosis?	Metabolic alkalosis, hypochloremia, hypokalemia, and hyponatremia
What is the treatment for pyloric stenosis?	Pyloromyotomy

ACUTE ABDOMEN

List causes of the acute abdomen in infants and toddlers.	1. Malrotation with volvulus 2. Appendicitis 3. Pneumonia 4. Henoch-Schönlein purpura 5. Hemolytic-uremic syndrome (HUS) 6. Diabetic ketoacidosis (DKA) 7. UTI 8. Intussusception 9. Testicular torsion

Malrotation

What is malrotation?	Failure of fetal gut rotation or fixation
What potentially devastating complication can occur as a result of malrotation?	Volvulus, or twisting of the gut onto itself, with subsequent obstruction and vascular compromise
What is the most common form of malrotation?	The cecum does not properly grow and fix to the right lower quadrant (RLQ), resulting in the formation of adhesions.

What is the name given to these adhesions?	Ladd's bands
How does a patient with malrotation present?	Typically, with bilious vomiting
How is malrotation diagnosed?	By radiographic evaluation of the upper gastrointestinal tract, or barium enema
How is malrotation treated?	Surgically (Ladd's procedure)

Meckel diverticulum and intussusception

What is Meckel diverticulum?	A small pouch from the antimesenteric side of the ileum resulting from persistence of part of the vitelline duct
What type of tissue is most commonly involved?	Ectopic gastric epithelium
What is the "rule of twos?"	The diverticulum is usually found within 2 feet of the ileocecal valve, typically occurs in children younger than 2 years, and is present in nearly 2% of the population.
How does a patient with Meckel diverticulum most commonly present?	With painless rectal bleeding or obstruction
What surgical emergency can a diverticulum mimic?	Appendicitis
How is a Meckel diverticulum diagnosed?	By means of a Meckel scan
What is the treatment for a Meckel diverticulum?	Surgical repair
A Meckel diverticulum can act as a lead point for what potential abdominal emergency?	Intussusception
What is an intussusception?	Telescoping of a portion of the bowel into a more distal component of the bowel
What is the classic triad of intussusception?	Colicky pain, a sausage-shaped mass, and "currant jelly" stools

When does intussusception most commonly present?	In infants between the ages of 3 and 12 months
How is it diagnosed?	By means of an air-contrast enema, which is often therapeutic
Should an air-contrast enema be performed in the ED?	Yes. A surgeon should be consulted in case of bowel perforation from the enema.

ORTHOPEDIC DISORDERS

ARTHRITIS

What are possible causes of arthritis in children?	1. Viral or bacterial infection (including infection with *Neisseria gonorrhoeae*) 2. Rheumatic fever 3. Juvenile rheumatoid arthritis (JRA) 4. Lyme disease 5. Systemic lupus erythematosus (SLE)
What is septic arthritis?	Bacterial infection of a joint space
What age group has a higher incidence of septic arthritis, young children or adolescents?	Young children (including infants)
How does the child with septic arthritis generally present?	The child appears ill, is febrile, and has a decreased appetite.
How does evaluation of septic arthritis in the hip differ from that of other joints?	In children, other joints may be aspirated, but a septic hip should be opened.
What is the gold standard for diagnosing septic arthritis?	Aspiration and culture of synovial fluid
What other studies may be used to help make the diagnosis of septic arthritis?	Magnetic resonance imaging (MRI), blood cultures, and the erythrocyte sedimentation rate (ESR) may support the diagnosis.
What causes most cases of osteomyelitis in children?	Hematogenous seeding of *Staphylococcus aureus*

SYNOVITIS

Which patients are most likely to present with transient synovitis?	Children between the ages of 3 and 10 years
How does the child with transient synovitis hold the lower extremity?	The child lies with the extremity in flexion, abduction, and external rotation.
Does the child with transient synovitis appear ill?	No.
What is the treatment for transient synovitis?	Bed rest

CONGENITAL HIP DISLOCATION

Describe the gait of a child with congenital hip dislocation.	The child walks with a painless limp secondary to unequal lower extremity length.

LEGG-CALVÉ-PERTHES DISEASE

What is Legg-Calvé-Perthes disease?	Avascular necrosis of the capital femoral epiphysis
When does Legg-Calvé-Perthes disease present?	Between the ages of 2 and 10 years
Does Legg-Calvé-Perthes disease have a sex predisposition?	Yes. Boys are more commonly affected.
How does Legg-Calvé-Perthes disease present?	The child typically presents with a limp and a joint that is tender to palpation. The disorder is bilateral in 15% of patients.
What do radiographs show?	1. Irregular epiphyses 2. Flat or wide femoral head 3. Shortening of the femoral neck
How long does Legg-Calvé-Perthes disease generally last?	18–24 months
How is Legg-Calvé-Perthes disease treated?	Maintain hip motion. The prognosis is good, but many patients later develop osteoarthritis in the affected hip.

SLIPPED CAPITAL FEMORAL EPIPHYSIS

What is the classic presentation of a slipped capital femoral epiphysis?	Wimpy blimp with a limp—an obese, tall, 10- to 15-year-old boy with a painful limp
What percentage of cases are bilateral?	One third
What should one do if the child is younger than 10 years old?	Consider an endocrine, metabolic, and renal work-up to rule out hypothyroidism and pseudohypoparathyroidism.

CHILD ABUSE AND NEGLECT

Distinguish between child abuse and child neglect.	Abuse is physical maltreatment of the child. Neglect is failure to provide the child with food, shelter, or care.
What are typical forms of:	
Neglect?	Emotional neglect Physical neglect (e.g., malnutrition)
Abuse?	Physical abuse (including Munchausen syndrome by proxy) Emotional abuse
Distinguish neglect from failure to thrive.	The child experiencing physical neglect may seem emotionally detached and difficult to console. He may have decreased muscle tone, be underweight for his height, and demonstrate delayed speech development and poor hygiene. An infant may have severe diaper dermatitis.
Is it easy to distinguish neglect from failure to thrive?	No.

PHYSICAL ABUSE

Who was Baron von Munchausen?	A German baron who would mimic the symptoms of gastrointestinal bleeding by running into taverns and spitting sheep's blood.
What is Munchausen syndrome by proxy?	A parent or caregiver fabricates an illness in a child and either demands unnece-

ssary medical treatments or harms the child through attempts to "treat" the imagined disorders at home

What mortality rate is associated with Munchausen syndrome by proxy?

10%

Who is the classic perpetrator of Munchausen syndrome by proxy?

Typically a woman caretaker who has had some medical training

Who is at risk for physical abuse?

Those unable to resist, with a poor attachment to the abuser

What is the age group most at risk for physical abuse?

Children younger than 4 years

Which adults are most likely to be the perpetrators in cases of physical abuse?

The child's parents

What factors can predispose a parent to be abusive?

1. Young parent
2. Substance abuse problem
3. History of being abused as a child
4. Previous loss of child
5. Violent personality with poor impulse control
6. Unrealistic expectations of the child

What are some typical characteristics of abusive families?

1. Poor emotional or financial support
2. Unwanted pregnancy

What factors predispose a child to abuse?

1. Physical or mental handicap
2. One or more same-age siblings (e.g., a twin or triplet)
3. Colic or a difficult temperament

What "red flag" should raise concern for abuse?

Abuse should be suspected when the mechanism of the injury described is not consistent with the injuries noted.

When are buttock burns most commonly noted?

During caregiver attempts at toilet training the child

Do burns from spills have distinct edges?

No. Distinct edges are consistent with immersion in scalding water.

What injuries are seen with shaken-baby syndrome?	Subdural hematomas and retinal hemorrhages
Are retinal hemorrhages easy to visualize?	No. An ophthalmologic exam may be needed.
What types of fractures are commonly associated with abuse?	1. Spiral fractures of the long bones 2. Rib fractures 3. Vertebral fractures 4. Epiphyseal-metaphyseal corner fractures 5. Multiple fractures of various ages
What laboratory and radiographic studies are indicated in cases of suspected abuse?	1. Skeletal survey 2. Platelet count, prothrombin time (PT) and partial thromboplastin time (PTT) 3. Computed tomography (CT) scan of the head (possibly)
Should all cases of suspected child abuse be reported to authorities?	Yes.
What is the disposition for the child if his safety at home cannot be guaranteed?	Admission to the hospital or placement in protective custody

SEXUAL ABUSE

What signs and symptoms may be seen in the child who is being sexually abused?	Enuresis, encopresis, sleep disturbances, abdominal pain, depression, behavior changes, dysuria, vaginal pain
Is sexual abuse more commonly reported in boys or girls?	In girls
What tests are indicated for victims of sexual abuse?	1. Throat, vaginal, and rectal cultures for *N. gonorrhoeae* and *Chlamydia trachomatis* 2. Syphilis serologies 3. Testing for HIV 4. Wet mount examination for *Trichomonas vaginalis* infection 5. Urinalysis

How long after a sexual assault can forensic evidence be collected?

It must be collected within 72 hours.

What will a Wood's lamp detect?

Semen

Should all cases of suspected sexual abuse of a child be reported to authorities?

Yes.

What is the disposition for the child whose safety at home cannot be guaranteed?

Admission to the hospital or protective custody

16

Dermatologic Emergencies

URTICARIA

What skin disorder is most commonly seen in the emergency department (ED)?

Urticaria

Describe the typical appearance of urticaria.

Palpable macules surrounded by an erythematous halo that can become pruritic

What are the classes of causes of urticaria?

1. Immunoglobulin E (IgE) dependent
2. Complement mediated
3. Non-immunologic
4. Idiopathic

What are the IgE-dependent causes of urticaria?

Antigen sensitivity (e.g., foods, drugs, mold, Hymenoptera venom)
Physical exposure (e.g., cold, light, exercise)

What are the complement-mediated causes of urticaria?

Angioedema (hereditary and acquired)
Blood-product reaction
Serum sickness

What are the non-immunologic causes of urticaria?

Histamine-releasing agents (e.g., opiates, antibiotics)
Drugs affecting arachidonic acid metabolism [e.g., aspirin, nonsteroidal anti-inflammatory drugs (NSAIDs)]

What foods can cause urticaria?

Nuts, shellfish, tomatoes, fresh fruits

What infections are associated with urticaria?

Viral infections, such as hepatitis and coxsackievirus (in children)
Fungal infections (e.g., candidiasis)

What is the treatment of urticaria?

Symptomatic therapy is with antihistamines and steroids. An attempt

392

should be made to define and treat the underlying cause.

What is urticaria called when it is associated with tachycardia and hypotension?	Anaphylaxis

HERPES ZOSTER

What causes herpes zoster?	Varicella-zoster virus
What are the signs and symptoms of herpes zoster?	Extreme pain in a dermatomal distribution; grouped vesicles with erythematous bases follow several days later
Which dermatomes are most commonly affected by herpes zoster?	The thoracic and trigeminal dermatomes
Patients with trigeminal involvement are prone to which type of complication?	Ocular complications
Who is at greatest risk for herpes zoster?	Elderly and immunocompromised patients
What is Ramsay Hunt syndrome?	Herpes zoster infection that involves the tympanic membranes and cornea
What medical therapy is available for herpes zoster?	Acyclovir may be helpful if started early in the course of the illness.

ERYTHEMA MULTIFORME

ERYTHEMA MULTIFORME MINOR

What is the typical dermal lesion of erythema multiforme?	Target lesions (i.e., "bull's eye" lesions consisting of an area of central erythema or a central papule surrounded by concentric rings of clearing and erythema, respectively)
What is the typical clinical presentation of erythema multiforme?	A prodrome, characterized by malaise, fever, arthralgia, myalgia, pruritus, and a generalized burning sensation, precedes

the appearance of the target lesions in a symmetric distribution on the palms of the hands, the soles of the feet, and the dorsum of the extremities.

Describe the clinical course of erythema multiforme.

Symptoms usually develop suddenly but can last 1–3 weeks.

What can cause erythema multiforme in adults?

1. Infection (e.g., herpes simplex, *Mycoplasma* infection, coxsackievirus virus infection)
2. Drugs (e.g., aspirin, antibiotics, anticonvulsants)
3. Vaccines [e.g., bacille Calmette-Guérin (BCG)]
4. Malignancy
5. Pregnancy
6. Rheumatoid disorders
7. Idiopathic

Is recurrence of erythema multiforme possible?

Yes, it can recur following re-exposure to the original trigger.

What is on the differential diagnosis list for erythema multiforme?

1. Herpes simplex
2. Vasculitis
3. Toxic epidermal necrolysis (TEN)
4. Blistering disorders (e.g., bullous pemphigoid, pemphigus vulgaris)

What is the treatment for erythema multiforme?

Administer topical steroids and arrange for follow-up with a dermatologist.

ERYTHEMA MULTIFORME MAJOR (STEVENS-JOHNSON SYNDROME)

What is Stevens-Johnson syndrome?

A severe form of erythema multiforme that is most often seen in children and young adults

How does the clinical presentation of Stevens-Johnson syndrome differ from that of erythema multiforme minor?

Erythema multiforme minor is associated with a diffuse papular eruption, whereas erythema multiforme major is associated with vesiculobullous lesions that involve the mucosa and multisystemic illness.

What etiologic factor is most commonly associated with the development of Stevens-Johnson syndrome in children?

Infection

What are possible complications of Stevens-Johnson syndrome?	1. Electrolyte imbalances 2. Fluid loss 3. Secondary infection leading to sepsis 4. Blindness 5. Multiorgan failure
What is the mortality rate associated with Stevens-Johnson syndrome?	Approximately 10%
What is the treatment for Stevens-Johnson syndrome?	The patient should be admitted to a burn unit or an intensive care unit (ICU). Symptomatic therapy should be provided, and an ophthalmologist should be consulted.

TOXIC EPIDERMAL NECROLYSIS (TEN)

What is TEN?	A severe form of erythema multiforme that involves the deposition of complement–immunoglobulin complexes in the cutaneous microvasculature
What is the mortality rate associated with TEN?	Approximately 30%
List five etiologic factors associated with the development of TEN.	1. Drugs (e.g., antibiotics, anticonvulsants, NSAIDs) 2. Malignancy 3. Radiation 4. Graft-versus-host disease (GVHD) 5. HIV infection 6. Vaccination
What are the signs and symptoms of TEN?	**Prodromal symptoms (7–14 days before the appearance of the rash):** Malaise, fever, upper respiratory tract infection, arthralgias **Skin lesions:** Warm erythema in the facial and genital areas that spreads to the entire body, may involve the mucous membranes, and develops into flaccid, ill-defined, tender bullae **Desquamation:** Sometimes includes the nails, hair, and lashes (75% of patients have ocular involvement)
What is the differential diagnosis for TEN?	1. Staphylococcal scalded skin syndrome (SSSS)

2. Erythema multiforme (TEN is thought to be the severe form of erythema multiforme)
3. Toxic shock syndrome (TSS)
4. Exfoliating drug reaction
5. Bullous diseases
6. Kawasaki syndrome

What is Nikolsky's sign?

Lateral pressure on normal skin adjacent to a bullous lesion dislodges the epidermis, produces a denuded dermis and, thus, extends the edge of the bulla

Where does the skin separate on skin biopsy in patients with TEN?

Between the dermis and epidermis

What are typical complications of TEN?

Like burn patients, patients with TEN are susceptible to infection (pneumonia and sepsis) and hypovolemia.

List three possible sequelae of TEN.

1. Scarring
2. Changes in skin pigmentation
3. Blindness

What is the treatment for TEN?

Patients should be admitted to the ICU. Therapy entails addressing the underlying cause and treating the skin damage in a way similar to that for burn injuries.

BACTERIAL SKIN INFECTIONS

TOXIC SHOCK SYNDROME (TSS)

Who is most susceptible to TSS?

In 85%–90% of cases, the patient is a menstruating woman between the ages of 15 and 34 years, although TSS is also seen in nonmenstruating women.

Is the mortality rate higher in menstrual-related or nonmenstrual-related TSS?

Nonmenstrual-related TSS—Because TSS is classically associated with the use of superabsorbent tampons, the diagnosis may be delayed if the patient is an older, nonmenstruating woman.

What is the cause of TSS?

Toxin-producing strains of *Staphylococcus aureus*

In TSS, what are the:

Major signs and symptoms?

Temperature greater than 102°F, sunburn-like rash that desquamates in 5–14 days, mucous membrane involvement, and hypotension

Minor signs and symptoms?

1. **Neurologic:** Change in mental status
2. **Cardiovascular:** Distributive shock, heart failure, arrhythmias and other electrocardiographic changes
3. **Pulmonary:** Acute respiratory distress syndrome
4. **Gastrointestinal:** Vomiting and diarrhea
6. **Musculoskeletal:** Myalgias and arthralgias

What might one find on laboratory studies?

1. Elevated blood urea nitrogen (BUN) and serum creatinine levels (as a result of rhabdomyolysis)
2. Hepatic enzyme levels greater than two times the upper limit of normal
3. Electrolyte imbalances, including hypocalcemia and hypophosphatemia
4. Negative cultures, except for *Staphylococcus* species
5. Negative serologies for leptospirosis, rickettsial infections, and rubeola

What are the criteria for diagnosis?

The sudden onset of all major signs and symptoms, accompanied by at least three minor signs and symptoms or suggestive laboratory findings

What is the differential diagnosis for TSS?

1. Scarlet fever
2. Rocky Mountain spotted fever (RMSF)
3. Leptospirosis
4. Rubeola
5. Meningococcemia
6. Streptococcal TSS
7. SSSS
8. Kawasaki syndrome
9. TEN
10. Stevens-Johnson syndrome
11. Gram-negative sepsis

What is streptococcal TSS?	Streptococcal TSS was discovered in 1983 and is similar to staphylococcal TSS. However, it is caused by an invasive species of Group A *Streptococcus* (*Streptococcus pyogenes*), is associated with soft tissue infection (75% of cases), and is **not** associated with tampon use. The treatment and differential diagnosis are the same as for staphylococcal TSS.
What is the treatment for TSS?	The patient should be admitted to the ICU for the administration of intravenous antibiotics.
Do antibiotics shorten the course of disease?	No, but they decrease the risk of TSS recurrence.

STAPHYLOCOCCAL SCALDED SKINS SYNDROME (SSSS)

What are two other names for SSSS?	Ritter's disease and staphylococcal epidermal necrolysis
Who is most susceptible to SSSS?	Children between the ages of 6 months and 6 years (62% of patients are younger than 2 years)
What is the cause of SSSS?	*S. aureus* phage group II, types 55, 71, 3B, and 3A
What is the exotoxin formed by these organisms?	Exfolatin
What are the signs and symptoms of SSSS?	1. Fever 2. Irritability 3. Skin tenderness 4. Diffuse erythroderma, without mucous membrane involvement, followed by exfoliation (positive Nikolsky's sign) and desquamation
What is the differential diagnosis for SSSS?	1. TSS 2. Drug reaction 3. Scarlet fever 4. Bullous diseases
Where does the skin separate on skin biopsy in patients with SSSS?	Within the epidermis (unlike TEN)

What is the treatment for SSSS?	Administration of fluids and antibiotics (do not administer steroids)
Can these patients be managed as outpatients?	Yes, if they appear well.

ECTHYMA GANGRENOSUM

What is ecthyma gangrenosum?	A necrotizing skin infection associated with septicemia caused by *Pseudomonas* species (classically)
Who is most susceptible to ecthyma gangrenosum?	Sick, neutropenic patients
What is the clinical presentation of ecthyma gangrenosum?	A red, swollen area becomes a hemorrhagic vesicle (the lesion looks like a "punched out" ulceration with a hemorrhagic border)
What is the treatment for ecthyma gangrenosum in the ED?	Systemic antibiotics

BULLOUS DISEASES

PEMPHIGUS VULGARIS

Who is most susceptible to pemphigus vulgaris?	Adults (often of Mediterranean or southern European descent) between the ages of 40 and 60 years
What is the clinical presentation of pemphigus vulgaris?	1. Large bullae on the head, neck, and trunk 2. Mucous membrane involvement (in 95% of patients); patient may stop eating because of mouth pain 3. Nikolsky's sign
Where do the bullae commonly appear first?	The nasopharynx or oropharynx
What is the clinical progression of the bullae?	Bullae are initially tense and clear. They eventually turn flaccid and then rupture, leading to a painful denuded area.
What is the differential diagnosis of pemphigus vulgaris?	1. TEN

2. Erythema multiforme
3. Burn
4. Contact dermatitis
5. Bullous diabeticorum

What is the treatment of pemphigus vulgaris?

Administer fluids and steroids and treat the denuded areas as you would treat a burn injury. Consultation with a dermatologist should be arranged.

What are the complications of pemphigus vulgaris?

Secondary infection; complications associated with high-dose steroids

What mortality rate is associated with pemphigus vulgaris when it is:

Untreated?   80%

Treated   10%

BULLOUS PYODERMA GANGRENOSUM

What is the clinical appearance of a patient with bullous pyoderma gangrenosum?

The patient does not appear ill, but exhibits large edematous, hemorrhagic, or necrotic bullae.

Bullous pyoderma gangrenosum is associated with what medical conditions?

Inflammatory bowel disease, rheumatoid arthritis, and myeloproliferative disorders

How is bullous pyoderma gangrenosum diagnosed?

Skin biopsy

What is the treatment for bullous pyoderma gangrenosum?

Administer steroids. Débridement exacerbates the condition.

NONTHROMBOCYTOPENIC PURPURA

PURPURA FULMINANS

What is purpura fulminans?

A nonspecific, hemorrhagic infection of the skin

Who is typically affected by purpura fulminans and when does it occur?

Children; following an infectious disease

What infections are associated with purpura fulminans?	Meningococcemia, group A streptococci, and pneumococcus

What is the appearance of purpura fulminans?	Massive ecchymoses with sharp, irregular borders appear and are often symmetric in the extremities. There may be surrounding erythema. Gangrene may occur.

What clinical manifestations usually occur with purpura fulminans?

1. Fever
2. Shock
3. Anemia
4. Extensive intravascular thromboses [disseminated intravascular coagulation (DIC)] and gangrene

What is the treatment of purpura fulminans?	Administration of antibiotics and treatment of DIC

HENOCH-SCHÖNLEIN PURPURA

Who is typically affected by Henoch-Schönlein purpura?	Children between the ages of 4 and 11 years

What are the signs and symptoms of Henoch-Schönlein purpura?

1. A rash, typically in dependent locations, characterized by swelling of the dorsum of the hands and feet, urticaria, and petechiae that coalesce into palpable purpura
2. Abdominal or testicular pain
3. Arthralgias
4. Renal involvement

What is the treatment of Henoch-Schönlein purpura?	Implementation of supportive therapy and monitoring for renal involvement

Section 2

Surgical Emergencies

17

Initial Evaluation of the Surgical Patient

The diagnosis and treatment of surgical diseases by the emergency medicine (EM) physician requires a thorough understanding of the pathophysiology and the expected course of many of these problems. Although many diagnostic adjuncts exist, a thorough history and physical examination help isolate the cause of many symptoms and allow prompt and directed treatment without expensive tests and procedures.

What types of patients require surgical evaluation?

Injured patients and those with abdominal or vascular complaints

What are the essential components of the surgical history?

1. Description of the pain (onset, character, ameliorating factors, enhancing factors)
2. Associated symptoms
3. Past medical history, including past surgical procedures
4. Medication history
5. Allergies
6. Social history

What are the essential components of the surgical physical examination?

1. Complete physical exam, including rectal and pelvic exams
2. Testing for signs of overt peritoneal irritation

What are the signs of significant peritoneal irritation?

Rebound tenderness, guarding, and diffuse rigidity or tenderness

How is the shake test performed, and what does it reveal?

Bump your hip against the side of the stretcher while distracting the patient. If the patient exhibits significant discomfort, this is a reliable sign of peritoneal irritation.

How is the heel-strike test performed, and what does it reveal?

Strike the patient's heel gently with your hand. If this elicits pain, peritoneal irritation is likely present.

In what sequence should you examine the abdomen?

Begin with the shake test or heel-strike test. Then try to begin the exam in an area away from the pain. If this area is tender, it suggests a more generalized peritoneal process. Slowly work your way toward the most tender area, while attempting to distract the patient with questions pertinent to the history. Finish with the rectal and/or pelvic exam.

When should laboratory tests be ordered?

It is not necessary to order all "belly labs" on every patient. If it is clear that the patient has simple gastroenteritis or another similar condition, a laboratory work-up may be avoided. However, whenever there is suspicion of a surgical process in the abdomen (symptoms include tachycardia, worsening pain, dehydration, hypotension, fever, extreme discomfort), laboratory tests should be obtained.

What laboratory tests should be ordered when a "surgical abdomen" is suspected?

1. Complete blood count (CBC) and differential
2. Serum electrolyte panel
3. Amylase and bilirubin levels
4. Liver function tests
5. Urinalysis

Which patients require an acute abdominal series of radiographs (i.e., flat and upright abdomen radiographs and an upright chest radiograph)

Patients with diffuse peritoneal irritation or signs of obstruction

What should be done before the patient leaves the emergency department (ED) for radiology?

Obtain the patient's history, perform a physical examination, and order appropriate laboratory studies.

When should surgical consultation be obtained?

Some surgeons want to be contacted as soon as you suspect a surgical problem, whereas others would rather the lab and x-ray results be in hand. The competent EM physician will recognize the patient with a likely surgical abdomen quickly and order appropriate tests. If there is any chance that the patient is unstable, surgery should be contacted immediately.

What is the least that should be done in the ED with a patient with a surgical abdomen?

1. Establish at least one large-bore intravenous (IV) line and initiate rehydration therapy.
2. Place a Foley catheter (in most patients).
3. Obtain "belly labs" and radiographs where appropriate.

18   Trauma

Major trauma care should be the domain of specialists. Trauma centers have significantly decreased morbidity and mortality rates in the areas where they have been developed. The role of the emergency medicine (EM) physician in trauma is to appropriately resuscitate and stabilize patients who have sustained major trauma before transferring them to trauma centers, and to work as part of the trauma team in a trauma center. The EM physician must be familiar with the mechanisms that cause severe injury, be aware of the subtle signs of occult injury, and avoid delays in the diagnosis and treatment of potentially life-threatening injuries. In many cases of severe trauma, the best action the EM physician can take in terms of providing safe, efficient care is to transfer the patient immediately to a trauma center.

What is a trauma center?

A trauma center is a full-service hospital that has been designated by a statewide or national agency as meeting the criteria to handle different degrees of service to injured patients.

What are the three levels of trauma centers?

Level I trauma centers are usually teaching hospitals that have 24-hour EM attending and senior surgical resident coverage. All specialties must be available. A trauma director must be appointed by the hospital and is responsible for outlining, coordinating, and auditing trauma care.

Level II trauma centers do not usually staff 24-hour surgical residents, but surgical consultants are immediately available. Level II hospitals are expected to care for most injured patients, but some groups of patients still require transfer to Level I or other specialty centers.

Level III trauma centers stabilize and transfer patients with major trauma. They are not expected to provide definitive care for multiple trauma, but are expected to provide coordinated, efficient stabilization and transport of trauma patients.

What is the role of the EM physician when confronted with a trauma patient?	The EM physician must be able to rapidly assess, resuscitate, and stabilize the patient for transfer or definitive therapy. Basically, EM physicians are members of the trauma team and are involved in the immediate resuscitation and stabilization of patients in the emergency department (ED).
What patients most likely will require surgical inter-vention?	Those with gunshot or stab wounds to the head, neck, torso, or extremities with vascular deficits; hypotensive patients; unconscious patients; patients with vascular or neurologic deficits
What are high-risk mech-anisms of injury?	Vehicular crashes involving ejection from the vehicle, speeds exceeding 50 mph, or the death of an occupant of the vehicle Motorcycle crashes Auto–pedestrian crashes Falls from heights of more than 12 feet
What is the significance of high-risk mechanisms of injury?	They should alert the physician to the possibility of injuries that require surgical intervention or critical care.

INITIAL TRAUMA EVALUATION

Where do I start?	Start with the ABCs: airway, breathing, and circulation. Do not go past airway unless the patient's airway is stable. Ask the patient to talk. Assess breath sounds, airway obstruction, chest rise, distal pulses, and perfusion.
Which patients need airway control?	The rule at our institution requires that we intubate anyone with severe facial trauma, hypotension, or the inability to respond to commands.
What should be done after the ABCs have been assessed?	1. Administer supplemental oxygen. 2. Establish electrocardiographic and pulse oximetry monitoring. 3. Undress the patient. 4. Ensure spinal stabilization. 5. Establish two large-bore intravenous lines. 6. Order trauma lab studies.

Which x-rays should be obtained immediately?

Chest and pelvis x-rays

Should a lateral C-spine x-ray be obtained?

There is no problem with obtaining a lateral C-spine film in stable patients; however, studies that could reveal immediately life-threatening injuries should be obtained first. The spine should be kept immobilized and the spine films obtained as soon as possible. Because most portable emergent lateral C-spine films are inadequate for visualizing the lateral view, obtaining this view often delays other needed interventions.

Now what?

When the ABCs have been stabilized and initial lab and x-ray studies obtained, a thorough physical exam and review of studies should be done. At this point, if severe injuries are found or suspected, trauma consultation should be initiated. If the patient is already being cared for by the trauma team, additional diagnostic studies and/or therapeutic interventions should be initiated.

AIRWAY

What is the preferred method of airway control for trauma patients?

Tracheal intubation. Aspiration is always a great risk in these patients and only a cuffed endotracheal tube can adequately protect the lungs. The tube can be inserted nasally in the patient with spontaneous respiration and the absence of facial injuries, or orotracheally in patients with in-line cervical stabilization.

Should drugs be used to intubate?

Yes, in most cases.

What dosage of drugs should be administered? Why?

The minimum amount of medication possible should be used for several reasons. First, in a patient with a decreased blood volume, many anesthetic agents and sedatives are sympatholytic and can precipitously decrease blood pressure. If paralytics are used, they should always be short acting because in the event the airway is lost and the intubation cannot be performed, the patient should regain spontaneous respirations as soon as possible. Often, etomidate or ketamine can be used initially and succinylcholine can be used if a paralytic is needed. Equipment for a surgical airway should always be nearby.

What is the first maneuver used to establish the airway?

Chin lift and/or jaw thrust. If successful, an oropharyngeal or nasopharyngeal airway can be used to temporarily maintain the airway.

What must be kept in mind when obtaining control of the airway in the trauma patient?

Do not turn a breathing patient with an airway into an apneic patient without one. If the airway appears difficult but the patient is respirating, get help, lights, exposure, and preparation before attempting any maneuvers. If the patient is not ventilating, prepare for endotracheal intubation, but avoid long-acting paralytics and always have the materials for the insertion of a surgical airway nearby. In addition, aspiration creates many long-term problems for the specialists that will be caring for these patients in the hospital, and it is better to control the airway definitively in a controlled manner then to allow an obtunded patient to aspirate.

BREATHING

How do you assess breathing?

Chest excursion, chest integrity, cyanosis, use of accessory muscles

What is a flail chest?

Two or more ribs broken in two or more places

How do you treat flail chest?

Search for associated injuries and hemo- or pneumothorax and treat appropriately. Admit the patient, administer pain control (via an epidural catheter if possible), and only intubate if necessary.

What is a sucking chest wound?

A wound (usually penetrating) where the diameter of the wound approaches the diameter of the trachea, thus causing air to move preferentially through the chest wound.

How do you treat a sucking chest wound?

Cover the wound with an occlusive dressing that is secured on three of four sides to allow trapped air to escape. Place the chest tube on the affected side, intubate if necessary. Remember, intubation and positive-pressure ventilation coupled with a thoracostomy tube takes care of the physiologic problems.

What is a tension pneumothorax?

A sufficient pneumothorax with persistent air leak from the lung that displaces the mediastinum away from the affected side

What are the physical signs of tension pneumothorax?

Hyperresonance on affected side, jugular venous distention, deviation of trachea to unaffected side

What is the mechanism of hypotension in tension pneumothorax?

Decreased venous return to the heart

What is a tension hemothorax?

Sufficient bleeding into the chest to displace the mediastinum

What is the treatment for tension hemothorax?

Chest tube placement, surgical consultation, blood transfusion, possible thoracotomy

When should tracheobronchial injury be suspected?

When bilateral pneumothoraces, pneumomediastinum, a large air leak, or the inability to expand the lung after chest tube placement is present

What are some relative indications for thoracotomy?

The removal of more than 1500 ml of blood following initial placement of the chest tube, or the removal of more than 200 ml blood/hour for 3 consecutive hours

CIRCULATION

What constitutes adequate access for a trauma patient?

Two large-bore intravenous lines (18-gauge or larger), preferably on both sides of the diaphragm if major abdominal trauma is suspected

Can you estimate the blood pressure from the status of the peripheral pulses?

Yes. The presence of pedal pulses equates to a systolic blood pressure of at least 80 mm Hg; the presence of femoral pulses equates with a systolic blood pressure of 60 mm Hg; and the presence of carotid pulses equates with a systolic blood pressure of 40 mm Hg.

What is cardiac tamponade?

Fluid within the pericardial sac that compresses the heart and prevents diastolic filling of the ventricles

How much fluid in the pericardial sac is required to cause hemodynamic compromise?

As little as 75 ml

What is Beck's triad?

Muffled heart sounds, hypotension, and jugular venous distention are present in pericardial tamponade.

How can you differentiate severe blood loss from tamponade in the patient with thoracic trauma?

The absence of jugular venous distention suggests blood loss, while the presence of jugular venous distention suggests cardiac tamponade.

Describe the initial fluid bolus used to treat hypotension in an adult.

Two liters of crystalloid solution

What is the initial fluid bolus for children?

20 ml/kg crystalloid $\times$ 3; if no response, 10 ml/kg packed red blood cells (RBCs)

What is likely occurring when a hypotensive patient who responds well to the initial bolus experiences recurrence of the hypotension?

Ongoing bleeding, cardiac contusion, cardiac tamponade

Define hypertonic saline.

Hypertonic is 7.5% NaCl saline. Normal saline is 0.9% NaCl.

What must be used in addition to large-bore intravenous catheters to ensure a high flow of fluids?

Large-bore intravenous tubing

Should a thoracotomy be performed in the ED on a patient with blunt trauma who arrives in full cardiac arrest?

No.

DISABILITY

What are some focal neurologic signs?

Unilateral dilated pupil, hemiplegia, unilateral posturing

What is decorticate posturing?

Flexion of the elbows and wrist toward the center of the body

What is decerebrate posturing?

Extension of the elbows and wrists

What does the absence of a bulbocavernosal reflex indicate in a patient with spinal trauma?

This is a spinal cord reflex. If it is not present in the patient with paraplegia, it indicates that the spinal cord is still in a "shock" state; thus, the level of sensation and motor loss may improve. If the reflex is intact and the patient has a dense paraplegia, the injury is considered complete.

Is hyperventilation indicated in patients with severe head injury without evidence of herniation?

No. Although controversial, the effects of hyperventilation decrease cerebral blood flow and are short lived. It should not be used prophylactically.

Is mannitol indicated for patients with head injury but no evidence of increased intracranial pressure (ICP)?

No. Mannitol should be used only if lumbar puncture, a computed tomography (CT) scan, or evidence of herniation suggest that the ICP is high. Mannitol should only be used in patients with adequate intravascular volume because hypotension may result.

FACIAL AND NECK INJURIES

FACIAL TRAUMA

What can you ask a patient in order to easily identify the existence of a mandible or midface fracture?

Ask her if her occlusion (teeth coming together) feels normal. If it does not, be very suspicious of facial fractures.

What is the x-ray of choice to evaluate mandibular fractures?

Panorex

In a patient with a mandibular fracture, what nerve can be injured, causing anesthesia of the lower lip and chin?

The infra-alveolar nerve

Describe the Le Fort system of categorizing midface fractures:

Le Fort I: Fracture through the maxilla

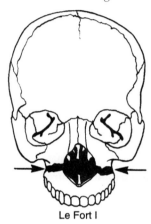

Le Fort I

Le Fort II: Pyramidal fracture separating the hard palate and maxilla from the midface

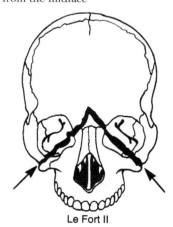

Le Fort II

Le Fort III: Craniofacial dissociation, facial skeleton separated from the neurocranium

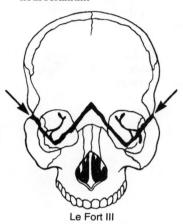

Le Fort III

What is a tripod fracture?

A fracture that separates the zygomatic process from the facial skeleton

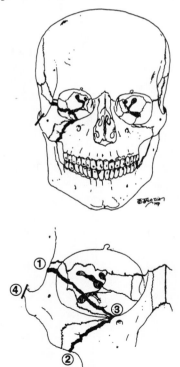

Tripod fracture

How can a tripod fracture be diagnosed clinically?	With the patient supine, stand at the head of the bed or examining table and look down the patient's face. The affected zygoma appears depressed. Also, palpate the suture at the infraorbital rim; a step-off and pain will be noted in this area.
What is the hallmark of orbital entrapment?	An inability to look upward

NECK TRAUMA

What are the zones of the neck with regard to penetrating trauma?	• **Zone I:** Sternal notch to cricoid cartilage • **Zone II:** Cricoid cartilage to angle of mandible • **Zone III:** Above the angle of mandible
What physical sign indicates a high risk of injury to critical structures in a patient with penetrating neck trauma?	Penetration of the platysma
What is the work-up for injuries in each zone?	**Zone I:** Angiography **Zone II:** Exploration or angiography/esophagography for stable patients **Zone III:** Angiography $+/-$ a head CT scan

CHEST INJURIES

What are the rapidly fatal intrathoracic injuries?	Tension pneumothorax, massive hemothorax, pericardial tamponade, ruptured thoracic aorta
Which patients with pneumothoraces require a thoracostomy tube?	Those with pneumothoraces that are visible on chest x-ray Those with an occult pneumothorax (i.e., one seen only on CT scan) who require positive-pressure ventilation
What hemothoraces should be treated?	All hemothoraces should be treated.
Why?	Although a few hemothoraces may resorb on their own, the risk of secondary

infection of the fluid collection leading to empyema, or late fibrothorax, can be devastating; thus, drainage is indicated for all hemothoraces identified on chest x-ray.

What risks are associated with rib fractures?

Pneumothorax, abdominal injuries, severe pain leading to pneumonia

Do most thoracic injuries require surgery?

No. Most patients with thoracic injuries only require a thoracostomy tube.

What is "the box" (in reference to penetrating injuries to the chest)?

"The box" is bordered by the nipples, the sternal notch, and the xiphoid process. Injuries to this area are likely to involve injury to the heart or great vessels.

What penetrating chest injuries require abdominal exploration?

Wounds below the nipples or the tips of the scapulae

What are some signs on chest x-ray that could indicate traumatic rupture of the aorta?

Mediastinum > 8 cm at the T3 vertebral body, loss of the aortopulmonary window, deviation of the nasogastric tube to the right, depression of the left main stem bronchus, pleural capping, left hemothorax

What are some signs of imminent traumatic rupture of the aorta?

Pseudocoarctation (different blood pressures in arms and feet), pulsatile left supraclavicular hematoma, left hemothorax larger than 500 ml

What are the most common mechanisms leading to traumatic rupture of the aorta?

Although any mechanism can lead to traumatic rupture of the aorta, head-on collision, falls greater than 12 feet, and T-bone collisions are the most common mechanisms of injury.

What percentage of patients with traumatic rupture of the aorta have a completely normal chest x-ray?

9%

What is the test of choice to identify traumatic rupture of the aorta?

Thoracic aortogram

What are two other tests and the problems with each?

Dynamic chest CT (high false-negative rate and requires experienced CT radiologist)

Transesophageal echocardiogram [cannot evaluate great vessels (5% of injuries) and requires experienced examiner]

What measures can be taken to prevent traumatic rupture of the aorta in a susceptible patient?

Administer a β blocker to maintain the systolic blood pressure below 120 mm Hg.

What chest x-ray maneuver can be done in an attempt to clearly visualize the mediastinum?

Place the patient in an upright position to obtain the x-ray. But remember, 9% of patients with traumatic rupture of the aorta have a normal chest x-ray.

ABDOMINAL INJURIES

What is the most common intra-abdominal organ injured in:

   Blunt trauma?

The spleen

   Penetrating trauma?

The liver

Do all patients with hemo-peritoneum have significant abdominal pain?

No. Fresh blood is not painful unless it is mixed with bile, succus, or urine. Old blood begins to hurt as it becomes more acidic.

What are some signs of intra-abdominal injury?

Lower rib fractures, hematuria, hemo-pneumothorax, pelvic fracture, thoracolumbar spine fractures

Other than laparotomy, what is the most sensitive test for abdominal injury?

Diagnostic peritoneal lavage

What is the most specific test for abdominal injury?

Abdominal and pelvic CT scans with oral and intravenous contrast

What patients need abdominal tests (e.g., CT, diagnostic peritoneal lavage) to rule out abdominal injuries?

Patients with hypotension, lower rib fractures, abdominal pain or tenderness, hematuria, pelvic fractures, mental obtundation with suspicious mechanism of injury, or spine fractures with deficits (i.e., an inability to detect pain)

What is the most common sign of hollow viscus injury?	Abdominal pain
What are the signs of diaphragmatic injury?	The presence of a thoracoabdominal penetrating wound (i.e., one below nipples and above the costal margins) Radiographic evidence of an elevated hemidiaphragm or curling of the nasogastric tube in the left thorax
What should be done immediately for the patient with suspected left diaphragm injury?	Place a nasogastric tube and place the patient on suction. Consider intubation to prevent respiratory compromise as a result of increasing movement of the abdominal contents into the chest.
What laboratory findings can indicate liver injury?	Elevated liver enzyme levels
What is Kehr's sign?	Pain in the left shoulder from diaphragmatic irritation, indicative of splenic injury
What is the best test for pancreatic injury?	Abdominal CT with oral and intravenous contrast
Are amylase levels sensitive for pancreatic injury?	Not really; 90% of patients with elevated amylase levels do not have significant pancreatic injury, and 30% of patients with pancreatic injury have normal amylase levels.
What are the types of pancreatic injury?	Laceration, contusion, transection
How does pancreatic transection most commonly occur?	The pancreas is crushed against the spine in blunt trauma.
Which abdominal injuries warrant surgical consultation?	All solid organ and hollow viscus injuries

GENITOURINARY INJURIES

Which injuries are most commonly associated with pelvic fracture?	Bladder and urethral injuries (15%)

What is the most common presenting sign of genito-urinary injuries?	Hematuria
What are the signs and symptoms of urethral injury?	Anterior pelvic ring injuries, blood at the meatus, inability to void, high-riding prostate, scrotal hematoma
How should a suspected urethral injury be diag-nosed?	Retrograde urethrography
Should you place a urinary catheter in a patient with suspected urethral injury?	Absolutely not. Placing a urinary catheter in a patient with suspected urethral injury may convert a partial urethral tear to a complete transection.
Where is the most common place for the bladder to rupture intraperitoneally?	The dome
What are the two types of bladder disruption?	Intraperitoneal and extraperitoneal
How are they diagnosed?	Cystogram
How do you evaluate the kidneys?	Abdominal CT with contrast or intra-venous pyelography (IVP)
Do a high percentage of patients with renal injuries require surgery?	No, the percentage of patients with renal injuries requiring surgery is very low (approximately 10%).
Which type of bladder rup-ture necessitates surgery most often?	Intraperitoneal
How do you differentiate intra- from extraperitoneal bladder rupture?	**Intraperitoneal bladder rupture:** Bowel loops outlined, dye outside of pelvis **Extraperitoneal bladder rupture:** Flame pattern, infiltrates perivesicle tissues (in pelvis exclusively)

NEUROTRAUMA

HEAD TRAUMA

What is the annual inci-dence of head trauma in the United States?	70,000 fatal head injuries occur annually in the United States.

What is the Glasgow Coma Scale (GCS) and how is it used?

The GCS is a measure of brain dysfunction and is used as a predictor of prognosis in head injury patients. Responses are graded by verbal, motor, and ocular ability. A score of 3–8 suggests severe head injury (coma); 9–12, moderate head injury; and 13–14, mild head injury.

Outline the GCS.

Eyes (4 possibilities—think "4 eyes")
Open spontaneously
Open to voice
Open to pain
Do not open

Motor (6 possibilities—think "6 cylinder motor")
Obeys commands
Localizes painful stimuli
Withdraws from pain
Decorticate posturing
Decerebrate posturing
No movement

Verbal (5 possibilities)
Oriented
Confused
Inappropriate words
Incomprehensible sounds
No sounds

What do unilateral, dilated, nonreactive pupils suggest?

A focal mass lesion (e.g., epidural or subdural hematoma)

What do bilateral fixed and dilated pupils suggest?

A diffusely high ICP

What are four signs of basilar skull fracture?

Raccoon eyes, Battle's sign (retroauricular ecchymoses), hemotympanum, oto- or rhinorrhea (i.e., leaking of the CSF)

What is the best test for intracerebral injury?

Noncontrast head CT scan

What is Cushing's triad?

A response to a high ICP characterized by an increasing blood pressure, a decreasing pulse rate, and irregular respirations

List nonoperative techniques to lower ICP.

Elevation of the head of the bed, administration of mannitol, hyperventilation, sedation

What is an epidural hematoma?	Blood between the calvaria and dura
What does it look like on head CT?	Convex shape, temporal region, does not outline sulci
What artery is usually involved?	The middle meningeal artery
What is a subdural hematoma?	Blood between the brain and the dura
What causes it?	Tearing of the bridging veins that pass through the space between the cortical surface and the dural venous sinuses, or injury to the brain itself with bleeding from cortical vessels
Do these diagnoses require neurosurgical consultation in all cases?	Absolutely, unless a small chronic subdural hematoma has been confirmed to be stable from a previous head CT and there has been no change in the patient's neurologic status.
What are the most important emergency treatments for severe head injury?	Ensure oxygen delivery to the brain through intubation, prevent hypercarbia, and maintain blood pressure. Exclude intracranial mass lesions. Transport the patient to neurosurgical care rapidly.

SPINAL TRAUMA

What are the two general types of spinal cord injury?	**Complete:** No motor or sensory function below the level of injury **Incomplete:** Residual function below the level of injury
What is an anterior cord syndrome?	Anterior cord syndrome is paraplegia with loss of pain and temperature sensation. The corticospinal and lateral spinothalamic tracts are affected.
What is the cause of an anterior cord syndrome?	Occlusion of the anterior spinal artery
What is central cord syndrome?	Preservation of some lower extremity motor and sensory function

What is Brown-Séquard syndrome?	Hemisection of the spinal cord with ipsilateral motor weakness and contra-lateral pain and temperature loss
Cauda equina syndrome can occur with spinal canal injury below which vertebral body?	Vertebra T10
What are the symptoms of cauda equina syndrome?	Incontinence, anterior thigh pain, quadriceps weakness, abnormal sacral sensation, variable reflexes

What spinal cord level is responsible for the follow-ing reflexes:

Biceps?	C5–C6
Triceps?	C7–C8
Cremaster?	L2–L3
Quadriceps?	L3–L4
Achilles?	S1–S2
Anal wink and bulbo-cavernosis?	S2–S3 and S3–S4

What spinal cord sensory level corresponds with the following locations:

Index finger?	C6
Nipple?	T4
Umbilicus?	T10
Great toe?	L5

What skeletal muscle function is mediated by each of the following levels of spinal innervation:

C5–C6?	Biceps function

C6–C7?   Wrist extension

C7–C8?   Triceps function

C8–T1?   Grasp

L3–L4?   Quadriceps

L4–L5?   Ankle dorsiflexion

L5–S1?   Great toe extension

S1–S2?   Ankle plantar flexion

S2–S3 and S3–S4?   Voluntary anal contraction

What is a normal Babinski sign?

Plantar flexion of the great toe with stimulation of the foot

List six important initial interventions in patients with a spinal cord injury.

1. Evaluate the ABCs.
2. Maintain the blood pressure above 100 mm Hg.
3. Place a nasogastric tube to prevent aspiration.
4. Place a Foley catheter.
5. Administer high-dose steroids within 6 hours.
6. Perform a complete radiologic spinal evaluation.

Describe the following types of vertebral fractures:

Jefferson's fracture

A fracture through the arches of vertebra C1 that results from axial loading; usually unstable

Hangman's fracture

A fracture through the pedicles of vertebra C2, usually stable [Hint—think "Hangman is below Jefferson" (C2 is below C1)]

Chance fracture

A fracture that is transverse through the vertebra; often occurs secondary to seatbelt restraint in a motor vehicle collision (MVC); can be associated with bowel injuries

Compression fracture	Anterior wedging of a vertebra secondary to axial loading
Burst fracture	Compression of a vertebra both anteriorly and posteriorly with high force, often with retropulsion of fragments into the spinal canal
Odontoid fracture	A fracture through the odontoid process of vertebra C2
Which patients require spinal x-rays?	Patients with deficits or pain over the spine Patients who were ejected from a vehicle or involved in motorcycle or bicycle crashes with significant force Unconscious patients
Do you need to keep the patients on the backboard until the spine is cleared?	No. The board can be removed and the patient carefully log-rolled when the initial evaluation is completed.
Who needs flexion–extension films?	Patients with neck pain and normal plain films. Never flex–extend a patient with known fractures unless a spine specialist instructs you.
Does a patient with a spinal fracture require an evaluation of the entire spine?	Yes.
Which patients require evaluation by a specialist?	Any patient with a spinal fracture should be evaluated by a specialist. Patients with negative plain films but significant pain can be considered for specialist follow-up. These patients should be sent home in a cervical collar for comfort and given appropriate follow-up.

ORTHOPEDIC TRAUMA

What factors determine the extent of injury?	Age, direction of forces, magnitude of forces
How are fractures generally described?	Open versus closed Bone (by thirds: proximal/middle/distal) Pattern of fracture (e.g., comminuted) Degree of angulation

| **How do you define the degree of angulation, displacement, or both?** | Define lateral/medial/anterior/posterior displacement and angulation of the distal fragments in relation to the proximal bone. |

Define the following terms.

Diaphysis	Main shaft of bone
Metaphysis	Flared end of long bone
Physis	Growth plate, only found in immature bone
Epiphysis	End of long bone

Define the following types of fractures.

Closed fracture	Intact skin over fracture/hematoma
Open fracture	Wound overlying fracture through which fracture fragments are in continuity with the environment
Simple fracture	One fracture line, two fragments
Comminuted fracture	Results in more than two fragments

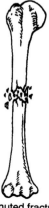

Comminuted fracture

Transverse fracture   Fracture line is perpendicular to long axis
                               of bone

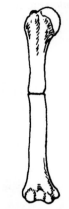

Transverse fracture

Oblique fracture   Fracture line creates oblique angle with
                               long axis of bone

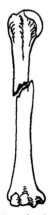

Oblique fracture

Spiral fracture

Severe oblique fracture in which fracture plane rotates along the long axis of bone; caused by a twisting injury

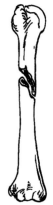

Spiral fracture

Pathologic fracture

Fracture through abnormal bone

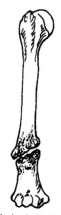

Pathologic fracture

Greenstick fracture

Incomplete fracture in which cortex is disrupted on only one side; usually seen in children

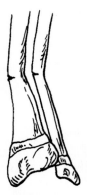

Greenstick fracture

Torus fracture (buckle fracture)

Impaction injury in children where cortex is buckled but not disrupted

Displaced fracture

Occurs when the cortices of the fractured bone are knocked out of alignment without angulation

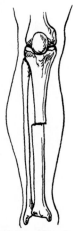

Displaced fracture

Angulated fracture

Occurs when an angle is created between the long axes of the two bone fragments; the angulation should be measured and noted

Avulsion fracture

Fracture in which the tendon is pulled from bone, carrying with it a bone chip

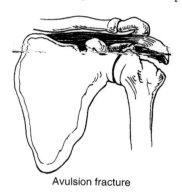

Avulsion fracture

Intra-articular fracture

Fracture through the articular surface of the bone

Colles' fracture

Fracture of the distal end of the radius, usually from falling on an outstretched hand

Jones fracture

Fracture at the base of fifth metatarsal diaphysis

Bennett's fracture

Fracture of the base of the first metacarpal with involvement of the carpometacarpal joint

Smith's fracture

Opposite of Colles' fracture; fracture of distal radius, but from falling on the dorsum of the hand

Boxer's fracture

Fracture of the neck of the metacarpal, typically the fifth digit

Clay shoveler's fracture

Fracture of the spinous process of C7

Hangman's fracture

Fracture of the pedicles of C2

Transcervical fracture

Fracture through the neck of the femur

Monteggia's fracture	Fracture of the proximal one-third of the ulna with dislocation of the radial head
Galeazzi's fracture	Fracture of the radius at the junction of the middle and distal thirds, accompanied by disruption of the distal radioulnar joint
Pott's fracture	Fracture of the distal fibula

Define the following terms relating to fracture treatment.

Reduction	Maneuver to restore proper alignment of a fracture or joint
Closed reduction	Reduction done without surgery
Open reduction	Surgical reduction
Fixation	Stabilization of a fracture by the placement of surgical hardware (internal or external)
Unstable fracture	Fracture or dislocation in which further deformation will occur if reduction is not performed
Varus deformity	Extremity abnormality with apex of defect pointed away from midline

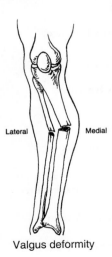

Valgus deformity

Valgus deformity	Extremity abnormality with apex of defect pointed toward midline
Dislocation	Total loss of congruity between articular surfaces of a joint
Subluxation	Anything less than total loss of congruity between articular surfaces

ORTHOPEDIC EMERGENCIES

What are the major orthopedic emergencies?
Open fractures and hip dislocations

What is the main risk associated with an open fracture
Infection

What are the classifications of open fractures?
Grade I: < 1 cm soft tissue laceration
Grade II: > 1 cm soft tissue laceration
Grade IIIA: Usually > 10 cm severe tissue injury with high contamination
Grade IIIB: Grade IIIA fracture requiring a skin graft for soft tissue coverage
Grade IIIC: Grade IIIA or IIIB fracture plus vascular injury requiring repair

What is the initial treatment of open fractures?
Administration of an antibiotic (e.g., cefazolin, gentamicin), surgical débridement, tetanus inoculation, wound lavage within 6 hours of injury, open reduction and stabilization of fracture

What are the major complications of orthopedic injuries?
Osteomyelitis and other types of infections, vascular or neural compromise, compartment syndromes

What is an acute compartment syndrome?
Increased pressure in the osseofascial compartment that leads to compromised circulation and function

What can cause acute compartment syndrome?
Fractures, vascular injury, and reperfusion injury

What fractures are associated with compartment syndrome?
Supracondylar humerus fracture, midshaft or proximal tibia fracture

What signs and symptoms are associated with compartment syndrome?	Pain on passive movement in the compartment, paresthesias distal to the compartment, vascular compromise
How is the diagnosis made?	Clinical suspicion, compartment pressures greater than 30–40 mm Hg, pain, pallor, paresthesias, paralysis, pulselessness (or diminished pulses)
Can a patient with compartment syndrome have a palpable pulse or a pulse that is evident on Doppler echocardiography?	Yes.
What is the treatment for compartment syndrome?	Fasciotomy (as soon as possible)
What is likely if there is a fracture and no pulse, but no compartment syndrome?	Vascular injury; consider arteriogram or exploration

SHOULDER INJURIES

Dislocation

What is the most common type of shoulder dislocation?	Anterior (95%)
Which structures are at risk with shoulder dislocation?	Axillary nerve and artery
How is shoulder dislocation diagnosed?	Indentation of soft tissues beneath acromion
How are shoulder dislocations treated?	Reduction, immobilization for 3 weeks in internal rotation, range-of-motion exercises

Rotator cuff injury

Which muscles form the rotator cuff?	The supraspinatus, infraspinatus, teres minor, and subscapularis muscles
What is the most common history?	Intermittent shoulder pain, followed by an episode of acute pain, weakness of abduction

What is the treatment for rotator cuff injury?	Most patients require only symptomatic pain relief. If poor function persists, surgical repair may be indicated.

ELBOW INJURIES

What is the most common type of elbow dislocation?	Posterior
Which structure is at risk?	The brachial artery
What is the treatment?	Reduce and splint for 7–10 days

HIP INJURIES

What is the most common type of hip dislocation?	Posterior (i.e., dashboard dislocation)
What is the most common mechanism of injury?	High-velocity injuries (e.g., those caused by MVCs)
Which structures are at risk?	The sciatic nerve and the arteries that supply the femoral head
How are hip dislocations treated?	With closed or open reduction (to prevent avascular necrosis of the hip joint, reduce on an x-ray table)

KNEE INJURIES

What is the most common type of knee dislocation?	Anterior or posterior
Which structures are at risk?	The popliteal artery and nerve (an arteriogram is usually recommended for patients with posterior dislocation)
What is the treatment?	Dislocation usually requires ligament repair but can be treated initially with knee immobilization.
How do you reduce a patellar dislocation?	With the patient's knee extended, move the patella back into anatomic position.
How is an abduction and adduction test of the knee performed?	Apply lateral pressure to the knee while the patient holds it in 30° of flexion. Compare the laxity of the injured knee to that of the uninjured knee.

How is Lachman's test performed and what does it evaluate?	Stabilize the patient's femur using your left hand and grasp the posterior knee with your right hand. With the patient's knee held in 20° of flexion, apply anterior force with your right hand. A displacement of more than 5 mm is considered evidence of an anterior cruciate ligament tear.
How is a drawer test performed and what does it evaluate?	Place the patient's knee in 90° flexion and pull forward (like opening a drawer). If the tibia is pulled forward, the test is positive (i.e., the patient has an anterior cruciate ligament tear).
What is the "unhappy triad?"	A lateral knee injury resulting in an anterior cruciate ligament tear, a medial collateral ligament tear, and a medial meniscus injury
What is a knee sprain?	A minimal ligament injury without instability
How are knee sprains treated?	With ice packs, elevation, splinting, and ambulation as tolerated

LONG BONE INJURIES

What is the Salter classification used for?	To classify fractures involving the physis in children (these injuries place the patient at risk for growth arrest)
Describe the Salter classification scheme.	**Salter I:** Through the physeal plate only **Salter II:** Through the physis and metaphysis **Salter III:** Involves the physis and metaphysis **Salter IV:** Extends from the metaphysis through the physis, into the epiphysis **Salter V:** Crushing of the physeal plate as a result of axial force
Which structure is at risk in humeral shaft fractures?	The radial nerve (look for wrist drop)
What must be done when both forearm bones are broken?	Open reduction and fixation

How are femoral fractures repaired?	With intramedullary rod placement (traction for 4–6 weeks is the traditional treatment)
What are the advantages of intramedullary rod placement in patients with femoral fractures?	Nearly immediate mobility with reduced morbidity and mortality

WRIST AND HAND INJURIES

What causes pain in the anatomic snuff box?	Fracture of the scaphoid bone (i.e., navicular fracture)
What is a paronychia?	Paronychia (an abscess around the nail root) is the most common hand infection. Patients present with erythema, pain, and tenderness at the base of the nail.
How is paronychia treated?	With drainage
What is a felon?	Painful infection of the pulp of the tip of a digit, usually caused by *Staphylococcus* species
How is felon diagnosed?	Clinically (think "rubor, calor, dolor, and tumor" of the fingertip, accompanied by throbbing pain)
When is it appropriate to obtain an x-ray of the affected digit?	When the infection is long-standing; the patient is immunosuppressed; or foreign body, fracture, or osteomyelitis is suspected
How is felon treated?	Drained by lateral incision to avoid injury to the digital nerves
Are antibiotics routinely administered?	Yes.
What are common complications of untreated felon?	Necrosis, abscess, osteomyelitis, and tenosynovitis
What is a mallet finger?	Detachment of the extensor tendon from the distal phalanx
What are the symptoms?	Pain at the distal interphalangeal joint and inability to fully extend finger.

How is mallet finger treated?   With a dorsal splint for 6 weeks if there is no associated fracture

What is a boutonnière deformity?   Disruption of the extensor hood apparatus near the proximal interphalangeal joint

How is boutonnière deformity treated?   Dorsal splinting with the proximal interphalangeal joint in extension; requires close follow-up

ANKLE AND FOOT INJURIES

What are the symptoms and signs of Achilles tendon rupture?   Patients present with severe calf pain and swelling and bruising of the calf. The two ends of the ruptured tendon may be palpable, and the patient will have weak plantar flexion owing to the great toe flexors, which should be intact.

What test can be used to assess for an intact Achilles tendon?   Thompson's test (squeezing the gastrocnemius muscle results in plantar flexion of the foot)

19

Emergency Medical Services

Which act of Congress was responsible for formalizing the approach taken to providing prehospital care in the United States?	The Highway Safety Act of 1966
What did the Highway Safety Act of 1966 call for?	The creation of a Department of Transportation and the development of highway traffic safety programs in each state, federal funding for improvement of the existing emergency medical services (EMS) system, and the development of a 70-hour curriculum for emergency medical technicians (EMTs)

EMERGENCY MEDICAL SYSTEMS (EMS) TRAINING

How has EMS training changed since the Highway Safety Act of 1966?	Developments in the field of medicine (e.g., new equipment, new medications) have necessitated the development of new curricula for the training of EMTs. Four levels of training are currently offered: first responder, EMT–basic (EMT-B), EMT–intermediate (EMT-I), and EMT–paramedic (EMT-P).
What training does a first responder receive?	A first responder receives 40 hours of training in basic first aid and cardio-pulmonary resuscitation (CPR).
What is the role of a first responder?	To stabilize the patient at the scene before other EMS personnel arrive
What type of personnel are generally trained as first responders?	Police officers, sports trainers, and firefighters

What is the role of an EMT-B?

EMT-Bs are trained to provide basic, noninvasive life support to a patient.

What training does an EMT-B receive?

The EMT-B receives approximately 110 hours of training, covering oxygen therapy, the operation of automated external defibrillators, splinting, immobilization, and assisting patients with self-administration of medications (in addition to advanced first aid techniques and CPR).

What is the role of the EMT-I?

People who complete EMT-I training are capable of performing some, but not all, advanced life support procedures.

What training does an EMT-I receive?

The EMT-I curriculum requires 150 hours of training, and completion of the EMT-B curriculum is a prerequisite. EMT-Is are trained in the provision of intravenous therapy, the administration of certain medications [e.g., those used in advanced cardiac life support], defibrillation, cardioversion, and advanced airway techniques.

What is the role of an EMT-P?

The EMT-P can perform a full range of advanced life support procedures.

What training does an EMT-P receive?

The EMT-P is the highest level of certification, requiring more than 1000 hours of training in advanced airway skills (e.g., surgical cricothyrotomy), pediatric advanced life support, and basic trauma life support. EMT-Ps also receive certification in ACLS.

Name two types of EMS systems.

Single-tiered and multi-tiered

What is a single-tiered EMS system?

All ambulances and EMT personnel are capable of providing advanced life support and respond to all calls, regardless of the complaint

What is a multi-tiered system?

Some ambulances and staff are equipped to provide only basic life support, while others are prepared to provide advanced life support. Decisions regarding the response to the call depend on the complaint and the availability of resources.

INTERACTION BETWEEN PHYSICIANS AND EMERGENCY MEDICAL SERVICES (EMS) PERSONNEL

What is medical direction?

Medical direction in the legal sense involves a physician extending her license to practice medicine to field providers. However, there are many responsibilities involved, including administration tasks (e.g., training, development of protocols) and involvement in patient care through direct observation or direct communication with the field provider via the radio (i.e., on-line medical direction). Finally, medical directors are also responsible for risk management, quality control, and retrospective call review.

What are the two types of medical direction?

Direct (on-line) and indirect (off-line)

What is direct medical direction?

The emergency physician directly observes or communicates with the non-physician provider in the field, offering advice or orders.

What is indirect medical direction?

Indirect medical direction is both proactive (i.e., an emergency physician provides written protocols for the training of EMS personnel) and reactive (i.e., an emergency physician evaluates the system and the providers to ensure ongoing quality of the care provided).

What information should the prehospital provider report before leaving the emergency department (ED)?

1. Pertinent details regarding the scene (e.g., a partially empty pill bottle near the patient, notable odors)
2. The mechanism of injury
3. Reports from bystanders

AEROMEDICAL TRANSPORT

When was aeromedical transport first used?

During World War I

When were helicopters first used for aeromedical transport?	During the Korean War
When did aeromedical transport become an integral part of civilian EMS in the United States?	The first civilian hospital-based aeromedical program began in 1972.
When is aeromedical transport indicated over ground transport?	Aeromedical transport is indicated when time is critical (traffic delays can be avoided) or when a higher level of care is necessary (flight paramedics and nurses receive a higher level of training).
What types of aeromedical transport are available?	Fixed-wing aircraft (i.e., airplanes) and rotor-wing aircraft (i.e., helicopters)
What are the advantages of fixed-wing aircraft over rotor-wing aircraft?	Fixed-wing aircraft are faster, have a greater geographic range, can transport more patients, and are subject to fewer weather limitations.
What are the disadvantages of fixed-wing aircraft?	A runway (i.e., an airport) is necessary in order to land.
What are the advantages of rotor-wing aircraft over fixed-wing aircraft?	Rotor-wing aircraft enable a rapid response and have "on-scene" capability. Furthermore, an airport is not necessary in order to land.
What are the disadvantages of rotor-wing aircraft?	They are expensive to operate, they may not be operable under certain weather conditions, and they come with weight restrictions.
What is the crew complement of an aeromedical team?	The crew can vary, but may include a nurse; an EMT-P with additional training in pediatrics, trauma, burn care, and ventilator management; a physician; a respiratory therapist; or any combination of these.
What is the most common crew configuration?	Most crews consist of a paramedic and a nurse.
What training must aeromedical crew members undergo?	These professionals receive training in critical care medicine, emergency medicine, pediatrics, flight and altitude

physiology, and special medical procedures (e.g., rapid sequence intubation, central line placement, cricothyroidotomy, pericardiocentesis, tube thoracostomy).

What is altitude physiology?

The study of the effect of altitude on gas volume, temperature, partial pressure, and solubility

What is Boyle's law?

As the altitude increases, the atmospheric pressure decreases and the gas volume increases ($P_1/V_1 = P_2/V_2$)

Why is Boyle's law clinically significant to a member of an aeromedical transport team?

At high altitude, a patient's pneumothorax or ileus will expand. In addition, balloons on endotracheal tubes or Foley catheters, bubbles in intravenous tubing, and patients in military antishock trousers (MAST) trousers require careful monitoring.

What is Charles' law?

The ambient temperature decreases as the altitude increases

How much does the temperature change?

About 2°C per 1000 feet of altitude

What clinical significance does Charles' law have in aeromedical transport?

Patients may develop hypothermia.

What is Dalton's law?

The pressure of a gaseous mixture is equal to the sum of the partial pressure of the gases in the mixture.

Why is Dalton's law an important consideration for people involved in aeromedical transport?

Most patients require supplemental oxygen.

What is Henry's law?

Less gas can be dissolved in a solution at high altitudes

Why is Henry's law important in aeromedical transport?

Patients with decompression sickness must be transported with high-flow oxygen and at a low altitude.

TRIAGE

What is a mass casualty incident (MCI)?

Any event that results in more than one significantly injured victim

How many people must be injured in order for an event to qualify as an MCI?

There is no set number; generally if the local EMS and hospital systems are able to respond effectively and are not overwhelmed, the event is categorized as an MCI.

What is a disaster?

An event that overwhelms the usual health care resources of a community or hospital

What is the goal of triage in the ED?

To prioritize the care of all patients

What is the goal of triage in the field, following an MCI or a disaster?

To do the most good for the most people

In an MCI or a disaster, which four triage categories are used to classify patients?

1. First priority (patient has severe injuries but is potentially salvageable)
2. Second priority (patient has moderate injuries but is temporarily stable)
3. Third priority (patient has minor injuries and is ambulatory)
4. No treatment (the patient is dead or expected to die)

Should CPR be performed at the scene of an MCI or disaster?

Typically, no.

What are the highest priority medical treatments at the scene of an MCI or disaster?

Airway control, control of bleeding, backboarding, and oxygen administration

20

Emergency Procedures and Wound Care

DRAINS AND TUBES

How can a tube diameter in mm be determined from a French measurement?	Divide the French size by π or 3.14 (e.g., a 15 French tube has a diameter of 5 mm).
How can the needle-gauge size be determined?	A 14-gauge needle is 1/14 of an inch; thus, a 14-gauge needle is larger than a 21-gauge needle.

CHEST TUBES

How is a chest drain inserted?	1. Administer local anesthetic.
	2. Incise the skin in the fourth intercostal space between the mid- and anterior-axillary lines.
	3. Perform a blunt Kelly-clamp dissection over the rib into the intrapleural space.
	4. Perform a finger exploration to confirm intrapleural placement.
	5. Place the tube posteriorly and superiorly.

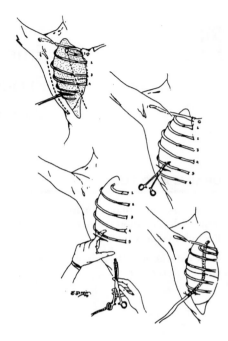

What are the goals of chest tube insertion?

Drainage
Appose parietal and visceral pleura to seal any visceral pleural holes

In most cases, where should the chest tube be positioned?

Posteriorly into the apex

How can you tell on a chest x-ray if the last hole on the chest tube is in the pleural cavity?

The last hole is cut through the radiopaque line in the chest tube. This can be seen on a chest x-ray as a break in this line, which should be within the pleural cavity.

To what is the chest tube connected?

A Pleurovac (a three-chambered box that replaces the old three-bottle systems)

What are the three chambers of the Pleurovac box?

1. Collection chamber
2. Water seal chamber
3. Suction-control chamber

Describe the old three-bottle system:

    Collection chamber

Collects fluid, pus, blood, or chyle and measures the amount

Connects to the water seal chamber and
to the chest tube

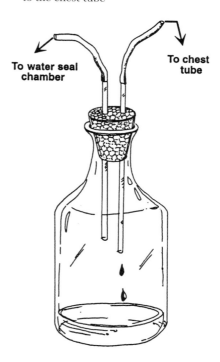

**To water seal
chamber**

**To chest
tube**

Water seal chamber

One-way valve allows air to be removed
from the pleural space but does not
allow air to enter pleural cavity
Connects to the suction-control bottle
and to the collection chamber

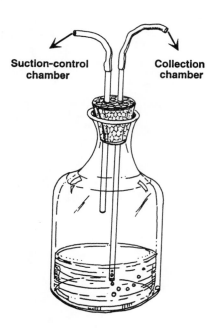

Suction-control chamber   Controls the amount of suction by the
height of the water column

Excessive suction is released by sucking
in room air

Connects to wall suction and to the water
seal chamber

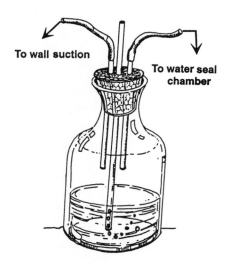

How is a chest tube placed on a water seal?

By removing the suction; a tension pneumothorax cannot form because the one-way valve allows the release of air build-up.

Should a test tube ever be clamped off?

No, except momentarily to run the system

What does it mean to "run the system" of a chest tube? How is this done?

Running the system checks if the air leak is from a leak in the pleural cavity (i.e., a visceral hole) or from a leak in the tubing. To "run the system," momentarily occlude the chest tube, and if the air leak is still present, the leak originates in the tubing or tubing connection, not from the chest.

How can you check for an air leak?

Look at the water seal chamber on suction; if bubbles pass through the water seal fluid, a large leak (i.e., air leaking into the chest tube) is present. If no air leak is evident on suction, remove the suction and ask the patient to cough. If air bubbles through the water seal, a small air leak is present.

What is the usual course for removing a chest tube placed for a pneumothorax?

1. Suction until the pneumothorax resolves and the air leak is gone.
2. Place the chest tube to the water seal for 20 hours.
3. Remove the chest tube if no pneumothorax or air leak is present after 24 hours of water seal.

How fast is a small, stable pneumothorax absorbed?

Approximately 1% daily; therefore, a 10% pneumothorax by volume will absorb in 10 days.

How should a chest tube be removed?

1. Cut the stitch.
2. Ask the patient to exhale.
3. Rapidly remove the tube as the patient forcefully exhales; at the same time, place a petroleum jelly gauze covered by a 4×4 gauze pad, and tape the pad and gauze to the chest.
4. Obtain a chest x-ray.

NASOGASTRIC TUBES

How should a nasogastric tube be placed?	1. Use lubrication and have suction hooked up and functioning. 2. Slightly numb the nose. 3. Place the head in flexion. 4. Ask the patient to drink a small amount of water when the tube is in the back of the throat and to swallow the tube; if the patient can talk without difficulty and gastric contents appear in the tube, the tube should be in the stomach (obtain an x-ray if there is any question of tube placement).
What test should be performed before feeding via any tube?	Low chest x-ray to confirm the tube placement in the gastrointestinal tract
How does a nasogastric tube work?	The nasogastric tube is a dual-lumen tube, consisting of a large clear tube and a small blue tube. The large clear tube is hooked to suction, forming an air sump with the small blue tube (i.e., a circuit sump pump). Air is contained in the blue tube and air and succus are sucked out through the large clear tube.
Should a nasogastric tube be placed on continuous or intermittent suction?	Continuous low suction; side holes disengage if they are against mucosa because of the sump mechanism and multiple holes.
What happens if the nsogastric tube is clogged?	The tube will not decompress the stomach and keeps the low esophageal sphincter open (i.e., a setup for aspiration).
How should a nasogastric tube be unclogged?	The clear port should be flushed with saline. Reconnect the tube to suction. Flush air down the blue sump port.
What is a common cause of excessive nasogastric tube drainage?	When the tip of the nasogastric tube is inadvertently placed in the duodenum, it drains the pancreatic fluid and bile; an x-ray should be taken and the tube repositioned in the stomach.

CATHETERS

What is a Foley catheter?	A catheter placed in the bladder that allows accurate urine output determination
What is a catheter coudé?	A Foley catheter with a small, curved tip to help maneuver around a small prostate
If a Foley catheter cannot be inserted, what are the next steps?	1. Anesthetize the urethra with a sterile local anesthetic (e.g., lidocaine jelly). 2. Try a larger Foley catheter.
What is a Tenckhoff catheter?	A Tenckhoff catheter is placed into the peritoneal cavity for peritoneal dialysis.

CENTRAL LINES

What are central lines?	Catheters placed into the major veins (central veins) via femoral-, jugular-, subclavian-, or internal-vein approaches
What major complications result from central-line placement?	Pneumothorax (always obtain a postplacement chest x-ray), bleeding, malposition (e.g., into the neck from the subclavian approach)
In long-term central lines, what does the "cuff" do?	The "cuff" allows the ingrowth of fibrous tissue, which holds the line in place and forms a barrier to bacterial growth.
What is a Hickman or Hickman-type catheter?	An external central line tunneled under the skin with a "cuff"
What is a Portacath?	A central line that has a port buried under the skin that must be accessed through the skin (percutaneously)

Femoral access

What are the advantages of femoral access?	No risk of pneumothorax, keeps procedures away from the head during a trauma resuscitation
What are the disadvantages of femoral access?	Not truly "central;" can cause retroperitoneal bleeding if the vessel is stuck above the inguinal ligament; higher infection risk

What are the landmarks and the procedure for femoral access?

Landmarks: A midpoint between the **anterior superior iliac spine** and the **pubic tubercle**

Procedure: Identify the femoral artery pulse and stick 1–2 cm medial to this point. Be sure to enter the vessel below the inguinal ligament.

Jugular access

What are the relative advantages of jugular access?

There is a slightly lower chance of pneumothorax with jugular access (as compared with subclavian access), and landmarks (i.e., the sternal and clavicular heads of the sternocleidomastoid muscle and the carotid pulse) may be easier to identify.

What are the disadvantages of jugular access?

Can be positional (i.e., the intravenous line could stop running when the patient turns her head); risk of carotid artery laceration; more tortuous course to the heart

Subclavian access

What are the advantages of subclavian access?

Stable site; more comfortable for the patient; straight course to the heart

What are the disadvantages of subclavian access?

Less clear landmarks; risk of arterial injury; more painful insertion for the patient; harder to find the landmarks and place the catheter in obese or muscular patients (also plays a role for internal jugular)

WOUND CLOSURE

What are the three types of wound closure?

1. Primary intention
2. Secondary intention
3. Tertiary intention (delayed primary intention)

What is primary intention?

When the edges of a relatively clean wound are closed in some manner (e.g., suture, Steri-Strips, staples)

What is secondary intention?

When a wound is allowed to remain open and heal by granulation

What is tertiary intention?	When a wound is allowed to remain open for a time and is closed later, allowing for débridement and other wound care to reduce bacterial counts before closure (i.e., delayed primary closure)
What rule is constantly told to medical students about wound closure?	"Approximate, don't strangulate!"
What does this rule mean?	If a suture is tied too tightly, the wound edges may become ischemic and either fail to heal or even become necrotic.

SUTURES

What is a suture?	Any strand of material used to ligate blood vessels or to approximate tissues
What is the purpose of a suture?	To approximate divided tissues in order to enhance wound healing
How are sutures sized?	By diameter; stated as a number of Os: the higher the number of Os, the smaller the diameter (e.g., a 2-O suture has a larger diameter than a 5-O suture)
Which is thicker, a 1-O suture or a 3-O suture?	A 1-O suture (pronounced "one oh")
What are the two most basic suture types?	Absorbable and nonabsorbable
What do these terms mean?	Absorbable sutures are broken down and eventually absorbed by the body. Nonabsorbable sutures are not broken down and need to be removed.

Suture materials

Absorbable materials

What materials are used to make "catgut" sutures?	Purified collagen fibers from the intestines of healthy cows or sheep (not cats)
What are the two types of gut sutures?	Regular and chromic

What are the differences between regular and chromic gut sutures?	Chromic gut is soaked in chromium salts, which cause it to resist breakdown and to be less irritating to tissues than regular gut.
What materials are used to make vicryl sutures?	Absorbable, braided, multifilamentous copolymer
How long do vicryl sutures retain their strength?	60% at 2 weeks, 8% at 4 weeks
What materials are used to make polydioxanone sutures (PDS)?	Absorbable, monofilament polymer of polydioxanone (absorbable fishing line)
How long do PDS maintain their tensile strength?	70%–74% at 2 weeks, 50%–58% at 4 weeks, 25%–41% at 6 weeks
How long does it take to complete absorption with PDS?	180 days (6 months)

Nonabsorbable materials

What is silk?	Braided protein filaments spun by the silkworm larva; known as a nonabsorbable suture
What is prolene?	A nonabsorbable suture used for vascular anastomoses
What is nylon?	Nonabsorbable "fishing line"

Suture techniques

What is a taper point needle?	A needle with a round body that leaves a round hole in the tissue

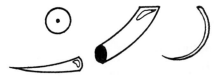

For what is a taper point needle used?	Suturing of soft tissues other than skin (e.g., gastrointestinal tract, muscle, nerve, peritoneum, fascia)
What is a conventional cutting needle?	A needle with a triangular body with the sharp edge toward the inner

circumference; leaves a triangular hole in the tissue

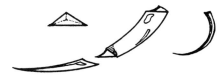

For what is the conventional cutting needle used?

The suturing of skin

What is a simple interrupted stitch?

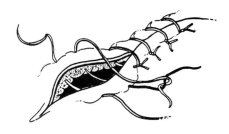

What is a vertical mattress stitch?

A simple stitch is made, the needle is reversed, and a small bite taken from each wound edge; the knot ends up on one side of the wound.

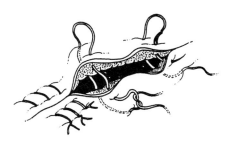

What is another name for the vertical mattress stitch?

Far-far, near-near stitch

For what is this stitch used?

Difficult-to-approximate skin edges; everts tissue well

What is a horizontal mattress stitch?

A simple stitch is made, the needle is reversed, and the same size bite is taken again.

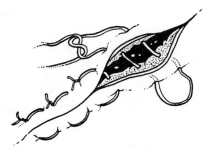

What is a simple running (continuous) stitch?

Stitches made in succession without knotting each stitch

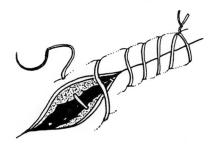

What is a subcuticular stitch?

A stitch, usually running, placed just underneath the epidermis; allows suture to remain in longer without leaving scars; can be either absorbable or nonabsorbable

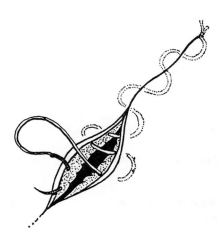

What is a "Z-plasty?"

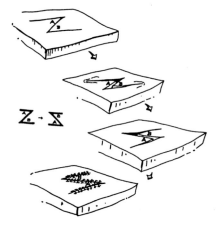

KNOT TYING

What is the first knot that should be mastered?

The instrument knot

How is an instrument knot tied?

Always start with a double wrap, known as a "surgeon's knot," and then use a single wrap, pulling the suture in the opposite direction after every "throw."

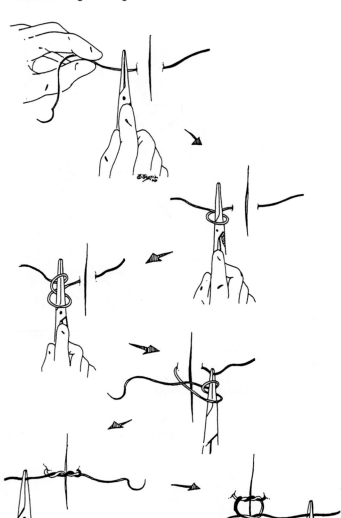

Does a student need to know a one-hand tie?

No! Master the two-hand tie and the instrument tie.

What is the basic position for the two-hand tie?

The "C" position, formed by the thumb and index finger; the suture will alternate over the thumb and then the index finger for each throw.

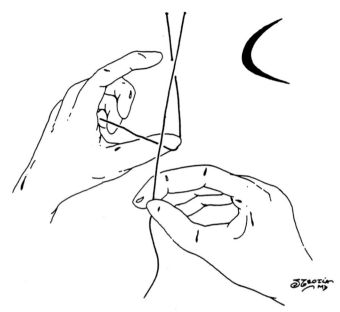

How is the two-hand knot tied?

First, use the index finger to lead. Then, use the thumb to lead. Ask a resident to help you after you have tried for a while.

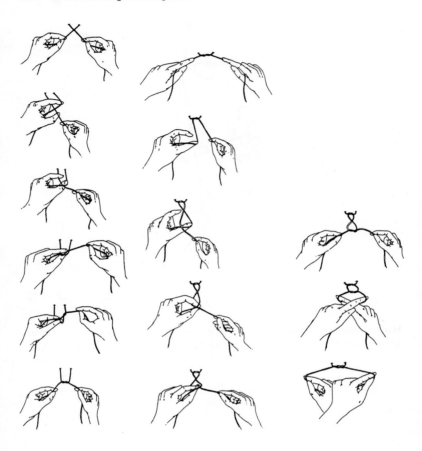

COSMETIC REPAIRS AFTER TRAUMA

What are the essentials of facial laceration repair?

Fine suture
Accurate approximation of the tissue
Avoidance of tissue strangulation
Early suture removal
Adequate but not aggressive débridement

Which lacerations require a specialty consultation?

Ear lacerations through or including the cartilage
Nasal lacerations involving cartilage or associated with nasal fracture
Eyelid lacerations or lacerations that involve the lacrimal complex
Lacerations associated with skull fractures
Any sufficiently complex lacerations

where there is a significant loss of tissue or underlying structure

Lacerations involving the parotid duct or gland

Lacerations associated with the fracture of facial bones

In lacerations involving the eyebrow, what should not be done?

The eyebrow should not be shaved because this can eliminate landmarks and lead to incorrect approximation.

What is essential in lacerations of the lip?

Very accurate approximation of the vermillion border

What are the essential aspects of closure in through-and-through cheek lacerations?

Approximation of mucosa (with absorbable suture, usually catgut)

Approximation of muscles (using vicryl sutures)

Approximation of skin and subcutaneous tissues using a fine, permanent suture that is removed in 3–5 days

Why must aggressive débridement be avoided in facial lacerations?

The face is extremely well vascularized and often ischemic-appearing tissue heals without incident. Loss of tissue through débridement, which leaves tension on a closure, can lead to a worse cosmetic result.

What type and style of suture is best for facial lacerations?

Interrupted suturing is best. A running suture can be used as long as you are certain that you are not strangling tissue in between bites. A simple suture will usually suffice. Take fine bites near the skin edge. Avoid an absorbable suture.

What new technologies are currently being developed?

Different types of skin cement are being developed. Effective use of these cements include careful approximation of the skin edges, keeping the wound free of cement, and achieving adequate hemostasis.

What anesthesia should be avoided in patients with facial trauma?

Lidocaine with epinephrine in the nasal area (leads to necrosis)

What should make you suspect parotid duct injury?

A laceration that crosses inferior to the line connecting the tragus and the corner of the mouth

21

General Surgical Emergencies

ESOPHAGEAL DISORDERS

What is Boerhaave's syndrome?

Rupture of all three layers of the esophagus that occurs at the postero-lateral aspect of the esophagus on the left, 3–5 centimeters above the gastro-esophageal junction

Describe two causes of Boerhaave's syndrome.

1. A sudden, violent, and often repeated increase in the intra-abdominal pressure (i.e., a Valsalva maneuver), such as that caused by violent emesis, retching, hiccuping, weight lifting, defecation, and seizures
2. A weakened esophageal wall (rare)

What are the symptoms of Boerhaave's syndrome?

Severe chest and abdominal pain that radiates to the back and neck, often occurring following an episode of vomiting

What are the signs of Boerhaave's syndrome?

Hamman's sign (i.e., "mediastinal crunch," or the sound of the heart beating against air-filled tissues in the thorax), left pleural effusion, subcutaneous emphysema, neck crepitus, dysphagia, fever, tachycardia, and tachypnea; after 48 hours, patients can develop shock and septicemia

What is the treatment for Boerhaave's syndrome?

Resuscitation, antibiotics, and surgical consultation

PEPTIC ULCER DISEASE

What is peptic ulcer disease?

A disease characterized by discrete erosions of the upper gastrointestinal tract mucosa

What are the two most common sites of peptic ulcer disease?	1. Duodenum, within 2 centimeters of the pylorus 2. Stomach (95% along lesser curvature; 60% within 6 centimeters of the pylorus)
Which site is more common?	The duodenum is 10 times more likely than the stomach to be affected.
What percentage of the population of the United States has peptic ulcer disease?	10%
What is one cause of peptic ulcer disease?	*Helicobacter pylori* infection
What are risk factors for developing peptic ulcer disease?	1. Male gender (male:female ratio is 2:1 in patients under 40 years of age) 2. Alcohol use or smoking 3. Therapy with nonsteroidal anti-inflammatory drugs (NSAIDs) or steroids
What medical conditions can be associated with peptic ulcer disease?	1. Trauma, burns, or severe stress or shock 2. Central nervous system (CNS) tumors (treated with high doses of steroids) 3. Zollinger-Ellison syndrome
What are the common symptoms of peptic ulcer disease?	Abdominal pain, vomiting, anorexia, weight loss
Characterize the abdominal pain associated with peptic ulcer disease.	1. Burning, gnawing, or sharp 2. Located in the epigastrium, left upper quadrant, or right upper quadrant; may radiate to the back 3. Transiently relieved by food or antacids but recurs 30 minutes to 3 hours after eating 4. Worsens at night (attributable to the circadian-increased release of acid at night) 5. Present daily, with intermittent asymptomatic periods

What is the differential diagnosis for peptic ulcer disease?	1. Other gastrointestinal conditions (e.g., esophagitis, pancreatitis, cholecystitis, gastritis, Zollinger-Ellison syndrome) 2. Cardiovascular conditions (e.g., myocardial infarction, abdominal aortic aneurysm) 3. Pulmonary problems

UNCOMPLICATED PEPTIC ULCER DISEASE

What is the initial treatment for uncomplicated peptic ulcer disease in a stable patient?	Therapy with a liquid antacid (e.g., Maalox) and a H_2 blocker (e.g., cimetidine) is usually sufficient; the need for analgesia suggests another, more serious illness. If *H. pylori* is implicated as the cause of the peptic ulcer disease, antibiotic therapy should be initiated. The patient should be advised to avoid activities and substances that can aggravate the condition (e.g., smoking, alcohol, NSAIDS, caffeine).
What other medical therapies are available for the treatment of uncomplicated peptic ulcer disease?	Sucralfate (a coating agent) and omeprazole (a proton pump inhibitor)
Which patients require more intensive work-up and follow-up?	Elderly patients with weight loss of more than 20 pounds in a short period of time; patients with symptoms that persist after 6 weeks of adequate medical therapy

COMPLICATED PEPTIC ULCER DISEASE

Name three possible complications of peptic ulcer disease.	Hemorrhage, perforation, and pyloric stenosis (obstruction)
What percentage of patients with peptic ulcer disease present with a serious complication?	15%
Peptic ulcer disease accounts for what percentage of upper gastrointestinal tract bleeding?	50% of cases

Which artery is most commonly involved in bleeding from a duodenal ulcer?

The gastroduodenal artery

What laboratory and imaging studies may be appropriate when the diagnosis is uncertain or the patient is hemodynamically unstable?

1. Complete blood count (CBC) with differential
2. Prothrombin time (PT) and partial thromboplastin time (PTT)
3. Serum electrolyte levels
4. Liver function tests (LFTs)
5. Amylase and lipase levels
6. Blood urea nitrogen (BUN) and creatinine levels
7. Blood type and cross match
8. Upper gastrointestinal studies (endoscopy or fluorography)
9. Electrocardiography
10. Abdominal radiographs

What is the treatment for acute hemorrhage?

Fluid resuscitation, lavage, and, if the patient is stable, endoscopy. If the patient is unstable, surgery is necessary.

What are the signs and symptoms of perforation?

1. Pain that is usually located in the upper quadrants, but may radiate to the lower quadrants or back
2. Decreased or tympanitic bowel sounds
3. Rigid, guarded, "board-like" (peritonitic) abdomen
4. Shock

Which is more common—anterior or posterior perforations?

Anterior perforations

What are the possible complications of a posterior perforation?

Bleeding (if the gastroduodenal artery is involved) or pancreatitis

What studies are useful for the assessment of a patient with suspected perforation?

1. Chest radiograph (the finding of free air on a plain film is most sensitive, with a sensitivity of approximately 80%)
2. Computed tomography (CT) scan
3. Lavage in an obtunded patient (be sure the airway is secured)

How is perforation treated?	Fluid resuscitation, antibiotics, nasogastric tube decompression, and surgery
What percentage of patients develop pyloric stenosis?	1%–2% of patients
How do patients with pyloric stenosis typically present?	With nonbilious vomiting, weight loss, a dilated stomach, and electrolyte abnormalities (e.g., a hypochloremic, hypokalemic metabolic acidosis)
What is the treatment for pyloric stenosis?	Admission is usually required. Surgery is sometimes necessary.

INTESTINAL DISORDERS

SMALL BOWEL OBSTRUCTION

What are the signs and symptoms of small bowel obstruction?	Obstipation, nausea, vomiting, abdominal distention, mild abdominal tenderness
What are the most common causes of small bowel obstruction?	Adhesions, cancer, hernias
What are the findings on x-ray?	Scattered air–fluid levels, with rare gas in the colon and rectum
What is the treatment?	Nasogastric tube placement, intravenous hydration, identification of causes, surgical consultation

GASTROINTESTINAL BLEEDING

What is the most common cause of painless rectal bleeding in children?	Meckel's diverticulum
What are the causes of lower gastrointestinal bleeding in adults?	Cancer, arteriovenous malformation, diverticula, colitis, massive upper gastrointestinal bleeding
What are the causes of upper gastrointestinal bleeding in adults?	Peptic ulcer disease, gastritis, Mallory-Weiss tears, varices, esophagitis (rare)

How can you differentiate upper from lower gastro-intestinal bleeding?

Place a nasogastric tube (upper = blood in nasogastric tube, lower = no blood in nasogastric tube)

What is the treatment for gastrointestinal bleeding?

If the bleeding episode is small, especially with an identified cause (e.g., hemor-rhoids), then the patient should be checked for anemia and may be sent home with instructions and precautions. Follow-up should be encouraged to rule out cancer as a cause of bleeding.

If the bleeding episode is significant, large-bore intravenous lines should be placed and consultation with a surgeon and a gastroenterologist should be arranged for diagnosis and treatment. Blood should be available.

ANORECTAL DISORDERS

DIVERTICULITIS

What percentage of patients with diverticula develop diverticulitis?

10%–25%

What are the signs and symptoms of mild diverticulitis?

Left lower quadrant (LLQ) pain and tenderness for several days, low-grade fever, mild leukocytosis, abdominal distension, mild peritoneal irritation, anorexia, nausea, vomiting, history of constipation

What are the complications of diverticulitis?

Obstruction, perforation, abscess

What is the most common complication?

Abscess

What are the signs and symptoms of complicated diverticulitis?

Increased tenderness, leukocytosis [white blood cell (WBC) count > 15,000/mm^3], high-grade fever (> 39°C), bacteriuria, pneumaturia, fecaluria, pyuria, abdominal distension

What is the best diagnostic test?

Abdominal CT with contrast

HEMORRHOIDS

How do you detect the difference between external and internal hemorrhoids?	External hemorrhoids are more likely to be painful and thrombose, originating from the perianal skin. Internal hemorrhoids develop from within the anus, are not painful, and are more likely to bleed and prolapse.
What are the signs and symptoms of thrombosed hemorrhoids?	Extreme pain. On exam, the swelling area is usually dark, tender, and firm.
How are thrombosed hemorrhoids treated?	Anesthesia usually is not needed or effective. Incise directly over the hemorrhoid and squeeze out the clot. There should not be excessive bleeding if other factors are not present.
What other factors may affect treatment?	Portal hypertension, inflammatory bowel disease
What is the medical treatment for symptomatic hemorrhoids?	Pain relief (narcotics, topical agents), Anusol, Tucks pads, stool softeners, sitz baths, reference for surgical evaluation (if necessary)

RECTAL AND PERIRECTAL ABSCESS

What are the signs and symptoms of perirectal abscess?	Severe pain on defecation and sitting, history of previous disease, diabetes, rectal trauma, inflammatory bowel disease
What are the physical findings?	A very tender, firm mass in the perianal region on palpation; can be inside the rectum or on the anal skin
What is the treatment?	Surgery. Perirectal abscess should not be treated in the emergency department (ED) without a surgical evaluation.
Why are suprasphincteric and infrasphincteric abscesses treated differently?	It is often difficult to differentiate suprasphincteric and infrasphincteric abscesses. An abscess below the sphincter can be drained without injuring the sphincter; however, incising and draining a trans- or suprasphincteric abscess can

injure the anal sphincter, leading to
permanent incontinence.

ANAL FISSURE

What is an anal fissure and how is it diagnosed?	A disruption of the anorectal skin, usually in the midline. It usually causes severe pain on defecation and can form an abscess. It is recognized as a linear disruption in the skin at the posterior midline position.
What is the medical treatment?	Stool softeners, pain relief, sitz baths. Usually, pain is relieved by decreasing constipation and softening stool. In some cases, surgical treatment may be necessary.
What is the sentinel pile?	An edematous skin tag at the distal end of the fissure

PERITONITIS AND MESENTERIC ISCHEMIA

What is the best diagnostic test for abdominal sepsis if surgery is not immediately indicated?	Abdominal and pelvic CT with oral and intravenous contrast
What are the signs and symptoms of peritonitis?	Anorexia, obstipation, diffuse abdominal pain, rare or absent bowel sounds, rigidity, rebound tenderness
What are the signs and symptoms of mesenteric ischemia?	History of vascular disease or emboli, atrial fibrillation, weight loss, satiety, pain out of proportion to physical findings, amylasemia, lactic acidemia, acidosis, dehydration, conditions requiring *Digitalis* medication
What is the workup if mesenteric ischemia is suspected?	Mesenteric angiography
What are the signs and symptoms of abdominal abscess?	High WBC count (usually greater than 20,000 WBC/mm^3), fever with spikes, malaise, anorexia, weight loss, abdominal pain

What are the signs and symptoms of a pelvic abscess?	Same as for a regular (i.e., abdominal) abscess: tenesmus, lower abdominal pressure
What are the signs and symptoms of upper abdominal or subphrenic abscess?	Shoulder pain, early satiety (from pressure on the stomach), nausea, vomiting, pleural effusions

BILIARY DISORDERS

What is cholecystitis?	Infection of the gallbladder, usually caused•by stasis and bacterial overgrowth
What is biliary colic?	Right upper quadrant (RUQ) pain caused by the obstruction of the cystic duct; there is usually no evidence of infection
What are the symptoms of cholangitis?	Fever, jaundice, and RUQ pain (Charcot's triad)
What other signs are associated with cholecystitis that differentiate it from biliary colic?	Patients with cholecystitis exhibit leukocytosis, a mild fever, and elevated bilirubin levels. Patients with colic are afebrile, have normal levels of WBCs, and usually have normal levels of bilirubin.
What does jaundice indicate?	Long-standing or severe biliary obstruction; patients require further evaluation and likely hospital admission
What are the other causes of jaundice?	Hepatitis, congenital condition, drug reaction, hepatic failure (cirrhosis)
What is the simplest, most sensitive diagnostic test for RUQ pain?	RUQ ultrasound
What should you look for in the ultrasound that indicates cholecystitis?	Gallbladder wall thickening, pericholecystic fluid, sonographic Murphy's sign, gallstones
What is Murphy's sign?	Place your hand on the RUQ and press down gently while asking the patient to breath. There should be pain and interruption of inspiration when the patient's gallbladder hits your hand in a positive test.

Does a positive Murphy's sign always indicate cholecystitis?	No. Patients with severe biliary colic may have a Murphy's sign and RUQ pain for several days after the stone has passed.
What is seen on ultrasound with choledocholithiasis?	Stone in the common bile duct, dilatation of the common bile duct, possibly signs of cholelithiasis
Does common duct obstruction require surgical consult?	Yes, in every case, unless it is a well-documented preexisting condition.
Why?	The risk of cholangitis is high with common duct obstruction.

APPENDICITIS

What is the lifetime incidence of appendicitis (i.e., the chance of a patient having this condition during his lifetime)?	7%
What are the initial signs and symptoms of appendicitis?	1. Anorexia and vomiting 2. Pain that begins peri-umbilically and then moves to the right lower quadrant (RLQ) and only subsides when the patient does not move 3. Rebound or peritoneal signs
How does the presentation of appendicitis in children differ from that in adults?	The pain is often poorly localized. In addition, of children with appendicitis, 15% have diarrhea, which often delays the diagnosis.
What is the psoas sign and what causes it?	Pain when the right hip is extended; associated with the irritation of the psoas muscle where it contacts the appendix
What is the obturator sign?	Pain on internal and external rotation of the right hip
What is Rovsing's sign?	Pain in the LLQ resulting in pain in the RLQ; associated with appendicitis
What is the "hamburger" sign?	Ask the patient if she wants a hamburger to eat. If she does, seriously question the diagnosis of appendicitis.

What is McBurney's point?

A point one-third from the anterior iliac spine to the umbilicus; often the point of maximal tenderness in appendicitis

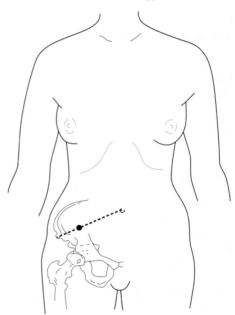

What are some ways to differentiate appendicitis from pelvic inflammatory disease (PID)?

PID is found in young women with a history of sexual activity. These patients often have a history of sexually transmitted diseases. In patients with PID, the pain may be more diffuse in the lower abdomen, associated with cervical motion tenderness and with pus exuding from the cervical os.

What are some other causes of RLQ pain in young women?

1. Ectopic pregnancy (check serum or urine HCG levels)
2. Endometriosis
3. Mittelschmerz (pain during ovulation)
4. Round ligament pain in pregnant women

What infections can mimic appendicitis?

Urinary tract infection (UTI) and pyelonephritis

What lab tests should be obtained in a patient with suspected appendicitis?

CBC, urinalysis, and serum electrolytes levels

Is appendicitis usually associated with leukocytosis?

Yes.

What does a WBC count of more than 20,000 cells/mm³ in a patient with RLQ pain indicate?

Appendiceal abscess

What plain x-rays should be performed?

1. Chest x-ray (to rule out pneumonia)
2. Abdominal x-ray (may reveal a fecalith or kidney stone)

What other diagnostic tests can be performed?

Often, the surgeon must act on the basis of the physical exam findings, medical history, and lab results alone. However, an abdominal CT scan or ultrasonography can be useful. A barium enema may be helpful if the entire appendix can be seen, but in many normal appendices, the entire appendix does not fill with contrast.

What may be seen on a CT scan?

Fecalith, dilated appendiceal lumen, peri-appendiceal fluid, abscess

What may be seen on an ultrasound?

A dilated tender appendix or a normal non-dilated appendix

What is the "two out of three" rule regarding appendicitis?

This rule states that patients who have classic findings in two of three areas (medical history, physical examination, and laboratory test results) most likely have appendicitis.

How many appendices are found to be normal during surgery?

20%

22

Vascular Emergencies

What are the signs and symptoms of acute vascular insufficiency?

The five Ps: pain, pallor, paresthesias, pulselessness, and paralysis

What are the most common causes of acute ischemia?

Embolus (e.g., atheroma, myxoma, thrombus from atrial fibrillation) and thrombosis of chronic occlusion

What is the initial treatment?

Heparin is administered to prevent further emboli and propagation of the present clot. Angiography is usually needed immediately to determine if thrombolytics will be useful.

What is the optimal way of administering thrombolytics?

Through an intraarterial catheter (venous thrombolysis is less effective)

What are the contraindications to thrombolytic therapy?

Recent surgery, history of hemorrhagic stroke, recent history of head trauma (relative), distal vasculature that is not conducive to revascularization

What are the typical signs and symptoms of claudication?

Predictable pain, usually in the calf, that presents after exercise and is abated by rest

What is the ankle:brachial index (ABI)?

The ratio of the systolic pressure in the ankle to the systolic pressure in the brachial artery

What is a concerning ABI?

An ABI less than 0.75 indicates mild to moderate arterial insufficiency usually associated with claudication. An ABI less than 0.5 is often associated with rest pain. An ABI less than 0.25 is usually associated with gangrene and tissue loss.

What is the responsibility of the emergency medicine (EM) physician in these cases?

To determine that an acute event has not occurred. Routine claudication, or even rest pain, is not a true emergency unless it is of sudden onset. These patients should be referred for vascular evaluation. Patients with evidence of acute ischemia or rapidly progressing ischemic symptoms must undergo immediate referral.

What is Paget-Schroetter syndrome?

Effort thrombosis of the subclavian vein that usually occurs in athletic young men and presents as acute swelling and pain of the involved extremity; ultrasound reveals the lesion

How is Paget-Schrötter syndrome treated?

Anticoagulation and possibly thrombolysis are usually effective.

What should be done with a renal patient with an acutely thrombosed arterio-venous fistula?

Surgical consultation should be obtained. Immediate surgery is not always necessary, but the patient should be evaluated so surgery can be scheduled within 12–24 hours.

How do you control bleeding from an arteriovenous fistula?

Direct pressure usually works; however, you must be very careful to avoid thrombosing the shunt. Very rarely, a stitch may need to be placed, but a surgeon should probably do this.

REST PAIN

What is rest pain?

Pain at rest usually occurs in the forefoot and lower leg.

What does rest pain indicate?

Impending ischemia and necrosis. It is usually associated with an ABI of less than 0.5. A work-up is required, but not necessarily as an emergency.

What is gangrene?

Dead tissue. This condition is serious; patients require surgery in most cases.

How is gangrene diagnosed?

No capillary refill or discernable blood flow, blue to black discoloration, tough leathery skin, loss of hair

What is the difference between dry and wet gangrene?	Dry gangrene is not grossly infected. Wet gangrene is.
How is gangrene treated?	Infected, dead tissue must be débrided; patients with wet gangrene require surgical consultation. Patients with dry gangrene and pain can be treated symptomatically and referred as long as no signs of systemic infection are present.
What other studies are needed?	Vascular studies to determine blood flow, plain x-rays to rule out osteomyelitis

VENOUS DISEASE

What is Virchow's triad?	Virchow's triad is stasis, endothelial injury, and hypercoagulability associated with venous thrombosis.
Which patients are at high risk for deep venous thrombosis (DVT)?	Patients with cancer, obese patients, patients who are older than 45 years, and those who have just undergone surgery Patients who have suffered lower extremity trauma, spinal cord injury, or head injury Patients with impaired mobility, known venous disease, congestive heart failure (CHF), myocardial infarction, or hypercoagulable states Patients who take estrogen
Overall, what is the most common condition associated with DVT?	Pregnancy
What is the most significant complication of DVT?	Pulmonary embolism
What is the most common cause of death in pregnant women?	Pulmonary embolism
When should a diagnosis of DVT or pulmonary embolism be considered in a postoperative patient?	When the patient has dyspnea

What are the long-term sequelae of DVT?	Postphlebitic syndrome, recurrence
Where do most DVTs begin?	The deep veins of the calf
What is the source of most pulmonary emboli?	The iliac and femoral veins
What are the signs and symptoms of DVT?	Calf pain and leg swelling, shortness of breath (a common finding in patients with pulmonary embolism), "heaviness" in the legs, bluish discoloration of the toes
What is Homans' sign?	Pain in the calf on forced dorsiflexion
How do you diagnose DVT?	Duplex sonography is useful for evaluating thigh veins but poor for evaluating those in the calf. A negative study in a high-risk patient should be repeated in several days. Venography reliably detects calf and proximal DVT but is expensive. It is best used for confirming the results of an equivocal duplex exam. Physical exam has very poor sensitivity and specificity.
What is the treatment for DVT?	Many centers treat uncomplicated DVT with outpatient therapeutic low-molecular-weight heparin, and switch to outpatient warfarin therapy (for 3–6 months) after anticoagulation is achieved. Other hospitals still admit these patients and treat with intravenous heparin and subsequent warfarin therapy.
What anticoagulant is used to treat DVT or pulmonary embolus in a pregnant woman?	Heparin
What is phlegmasia cerulea dolens?	Massive swelling and bluish discoloration of the lower extremity
What causes phlegmasia cerulea dolens?	Complete or near complete occlusion of the femoral vein, leading to massive venous hypertension in the affected extremity

Is phlegmasia cerulea dolens more dangerous than a typical DVT?	Yes, because it can lead to venous gangrene of the extremity.
What occurs in phlegmasia alba dolens?	Venous hypertension increases enough to prevent arterial inflow, turning the leg white.
What is the treatment for phlegmasia alba dolens?	Immediate elevation, vascular surgery consult, and anticoagulation—this is a true emergency.

AORTIC DISEASE

AORTIC DISSECTION

What is an aortic dissection?	Rupture of the intima of the aorta with bleeding into the subintimal layers of the vessel
What are the risk factors for aortic dissection?	Hypertension, Marfan syndrome, Ehlers-Danlos syndrome, pregnancy, ather-sclerosis, bicuspid aortic valve, and coarctation of the aorta
What are the complications of aortic dissection?	Occlusion of the major aortic branches, rupture and exsanguination
What are the signs and symptoms?	Excruciating, tearing substernal pain that radiates to the back, with associated dyspnea, diaphoresis, and nausea or vomiting
What might be seen on a chest x-ray?	Widening of the aortic knob
What studies are helpful in diagnosing thoracic aortic dissection?	Aortography, chest computed tomography (CT), transthoracic or transesophageal echocardiography
What is the emergent treatment?	Vascular consultation, antihypertensive therapy, and β blockade

AORTIC ANEURYSM

What is an aortic aneurysm?	A dilatation of the aorta, most commonly associated with atherosclerosis. All layers of the aorta are involved (i.e., a true aneurysm).

Where does this most commonly occur?	In the infrarenal aorta, but it can occur anywhere throughout the aorta
What is the presentation?	Patients are often asymptomatic and the aneurysm is found during a routine health exam. Patients may notice a pulsatile mass in their midabdomen. Some patients present with distal embolization (i.e., "trash foot").
What is a leaking aneurysm?	An aneurysm that has lost its integrity and has started to bleed into the surrounding tissues
What are the presenting features of a leaking aneurysm?	Severe back pain in a patient with a known aneurysm; abdominal pain; hypotension; abdominal distention
Should these patients undergo immediate surgery?	If a patient has a known aneurysm and a classic presentation of leak or rupture, some vascular surgeons proceed directly to surgery. Stable patients can undergo abdominal ultrasound or CT scanning.
How is a leaking aneurysm treated in the emergency department (ED)?	Obtain a rapid history (including evaluation of old records), perform a diagnostic evaluation, establish large lines, administer blood, and arrange for a consultation and rapid transfer to an appropriate facility if needed. Do not waste time; these patients can die very quickly.
What are the signs and symptoms of aortocaval fistula from an aortic aneurysm?	Massive lower extremity swelling, CHF

CAROTID DISEASE

What is amaurosis fugax?	Transient loss or change in vision caused by transient loss of blood flow, most often caused by cholesterol emboli
What is a transient ischemic attack (TIA)?	A reversible neurologic event that resolves completely within 24 hours and is associated with carotid or embolic disease

What is the physical sign of carotid stenosis?   Carotid bruit

What is the screening test of choice for carotid disease?   Carotid duplex sonography

What other tests are used to evaluate patients with carotid disease?   Ocular plethysmography, carotid angiography

What is the treatment for TIA?   Work-up of carotid and cardiac disease, possible antiplatelet therapy

23

Unique Injuries

BLAST INJURIES

What determines whether a patient survives an explosion?

1. The patient's distance from the bomb (primary blast effect)
2. Whether the patient was struck by a piece of shrapnel (secondary blast effect)
3. Whether the patient was thrown into a stationary object with great force (tertiary blast effect)

What is "blast lung?"

A condition associated with the change in air pressure that occurs with explosions and characterized by alveolar rupture, intra-alveolar hemorrhage, and pulmonary contusion

What is the treatment for "blast lung?"

Close observation, supplemental oxygen, and sometimes intubation and positive-pressure ventilation

What is the most common cause of neurologic injury following blasts other than direct trauma?

The introduction of air bubbles into the vascular system (i.e., air embolism)

Regarding lung injury, is it safer to be in an enclosed area or outside during an explosion?

To avoid lung injury, it is preferable to be outside. Being outside also keeps you away from a building collapse, which is another major cause of death and disability.

What other injuries are unique to blasts?

Ruptured eardrums and intestinal rupture

Is intestinal rupture more common in blast injuries or after routine blunt trauma?

Intestinal rupture is much more common in patients who have sustained a blast injury.

How is intestinal rupture diagnosed?

Using computed tomography (CT) or diagnostic peritoneal lavage; empiric

laparotomy may be indicated for patients
with severe physical signs

BALLISTICS

**What is the definition of a
high-velocity weapon?**

Muzzle velocity is greater than 2000 feet
per second (fps)

**Do any handguns reach this
velocity?**

Some very special weapons and loads may
come close, but usually only rifles reach
this velocity.

**How is the energy delivered
by the projectile deter-
mined?**

$KE = 1/2 \, M \, V^2$, where KE = kinetic
energy; M = mass of bullet; and V =
velocity of bullet

**How do wounds created by
high- and low-velocity
weapons differ?**

High-velocity weapons create a larger
temporary cavity around the projectile
when the bullet enters the body. Thus, a
greater amount of the weapon's kinetic
energy is released within the victim or on
exit.

**Which is usually larger, the
entrance or the exit wound?**

The exit wound is usually (but not always)
larger.

**What are the problems
associated with wounds
caused by high-power (e.g.,
Magnum) or high-velocity
weapons?**

The amount of damaged tissue may be
extensive. The bullet wound should be
debrided and the underlying tissue
carefully examined to ensure that necrosis
is not present. Formal irrigation and
debridement may be required
(particularly for patients with shotgun
wounds).

**How can a close-range
wound be identified?**

There are often powder burns around the
wound (i.e., black tattooing of the skin
around the entrance wound). In shotgun
wounds, the wadding from the shell may
be in the victim, indicating close
proximity of the weapon.

**What is the treatment for a
simple extremity gunshot
wound with no evidence of
bony, nervous, or vascular
injury?**

After other injuries have been ruled out,
treatment includes débridement of the
wound, thorough irrigation, tetanus
prophylaxis, antibiotics effective against
Gram-positive organisms, and close
follow-up.

HAZARDOUS MATERIALS

List four important consid-erations when dealing with hazardous materials.

1. Identification of the agent
2. Prevention of spread
3. Protection of the patient and health care workers
4. Adequate medical treatment of the patient

How can hazardous mater-ials be identified?

These materials are usually seen in tractor-trailer or train crashes, but can be seen in any crash. The material is usually identified at the scene. If the substance is being transported legally, the substance will be identified by a placard on the vehicle and a manifest. If the substance is being transported illegally, a high index of suspicion is needed. Some jurisdictions have special HazMat personnel or equipment to deal with these problems.

What signs may indicate that hazardous materials are involved?

Strong odors, tearing of the eyes, coughing, burning sensation

What measures must be taken immediately?

1. Immediate protection of health care workers
2. Isolation of involved victims
3. Identification of the offending agent
4. Rapid treatment
5. Consultation with experts
6. Notification and evaluation of those personnel who worked at the scene

24

Burns

INCIDENCE AND PATIENT PROFILE

What two age groups are most often associated with burn injuries?

Children under 6 years are the largest group of burn patients; adults ages between the ages of 25 and 35 years constitute the second largest group of burn patients.

Are most burn patients male or female?

Males are most often burned, except in the elderly population (more than age 65 years).

TYPES OF BURNS

What type of burn typically occurs in children?

More than 80% of burns involving children younger than 5 years are scald burns.

Besides temperature, what consideration affects the severity of a burn?

Heat capacity; moist heat has a much higher capacity and causes a more severe burn than dry heat.

Which chemical burn is worse, an acid or alkali burn?

Generally, alkali burns are worse because the body cannot provide a buffer against alkaline substances, allowing them to burn longer.

What is damaged in patients with first-degree burns?

The epidermis only

What are the signs of a first-degree burn?

The skin is erythematous and very tender; there is no blistering and no permanent damage to the underlying dermal layer. A minor sunburn is an example of a first-degree burn.

What is damaged in patients with second-degree burns?

The epidermis and varying levels of dermis

How are partial-thickness burns (i.e., first- and second-degree burns) further divided?

Superficial partial-thickness burns
Deep partial-thickness burns

What are the signs of a second-degree burn?

Superficial partial-thickness burns:
The hair follicles, sweat glands, and sebaceous glands are intact. The areas affected are extremely painful and hypersensitive to light touch. The wound appears red and mottled with edema and blistering. The surface is typically moist and weepy.

Deep partial-thickness burns:
Necrosis spreads well into the dermis and skin appendages are involved. These wounds may appear similar to superficial burns but are tougher and less sensitive to the touch.

What is damaged in patients with third-degree burns?

Third-degree burns are full-thickness burns that penetrate the entire depth of the dermis. All dermal elements are destroyed, including nerve endings, dermal appendages, and blood vessels.

What are the signs of third-degree burns?

The wound surface appears a waxy white or gray, dark and leathery, or charred. The affected area is usually dry, and thrombosed vessels may be visible. The lesions are painless and insensate to touch because the nerve endings have been destroyed.

BURN SEVERITY

How is the severity of a burn determined?

Burn severity is determined by the depth of the burn and the total body surface area (TBSA) affected by second- and third-degree burns.

How is the TBSA estimated?

The "rule of nines" can be used to estimate the TBSA and determine what percentage of the body is burned:

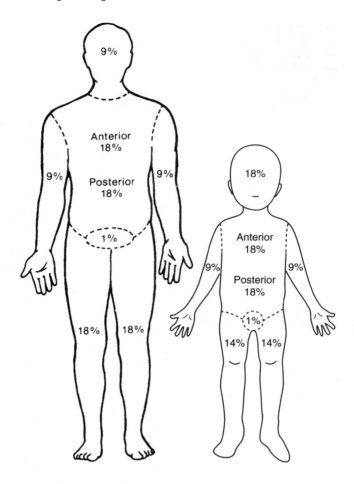

What is the "the rule of the palm?"

The palm is approximately 1% of the TBSA.

What are the criteria for a burn patient's admission to the hospital?

The criteria for hospital admission include:

Full-thickness burns affecting more than 10% of the TBSA

Partial-thickness burns affecting more than 20% of the TBSA

Burns affecting more than 10% of the TBSA in children and elderly patients

Burns of the face, hands, feet, and perineum

Partial- or full-thickness burns of major flexion creases (to minimize

contractures and other related
problems)
Suspected inhalation injury
Burns with associated trauma
Electrical burns
Chemical burns
Burns caused by suspected abuse

SMOKE INHALATION

What factors suggest smoke inhalation?

A history of confinement in a closed
    space, an explosion, or a decreased
    level or loss of consciousness
Charring or carbon deposits around the
    mouth, nose, or in the oropharynx, or
    carbonaceous sputum
Dyspnea
Inflammatory changes to the oropharynx
Facial burns or singed facial or nasal hair
Circumferential burns of the trunk
Alteration in the patient's voice
Low oxygen saturation

What lab values should be ordered to assess smoke inhalation?

Arterial blood gases should be obtained in
patients who are severely burned. Carbon
monoxide levels should be obtained if
there is a history of exposure to noxious
fumes or smoke inhalation is suspected. A
carboxyhemoglobin level greater than
10% is considered significant, and the
treatment is 100% oxygen.

MANAGEMENT OF THE BURN PATIENT

What is the first step in the treatment of burns?

Stop the burning process. Remove
burning clothing, and remove the patient
from the area of the fire.

What principles are followed in the initial management of a burn patient?

As with a trauma patient, it is important
to follow the ABCs (airway, breathing,
circulation).

How should the airway be managed in patients with inhalation injuries?

Intubation should be performed early
because management of the airway
becomes more difficult as swelling
increases.

FLUIDS AND MONITORING

How is the dosage of intravenous fluid initially determined?	The Parkland formula (volume = % TBSA burned × body weight (kg) × 4 ml) is used to estimate the volume of crystalloid necessary in the first 24 hours for the resuscitation of burn patients. TBSA of second- and third-degree burns are used in this calculation.
Over what time period is the intravenous fluid administered?	Half of the estimated volume should be given in the first 8 hours after the burn, with the remainder given over the next 16 hours. Resuscitation fluids should be administered via two large-bore (< 16 gauge) intravenous lines or a central line if necessary.
What type of fluid should be given during the first 24 hours after injury?	Isotonic fluid (e.g., lactated Ringer's solution)
Why are glucose-containing intravenous fluids contraindicated in burn patients in the first 24 hours?	The normal stress response causes an elevation of serum glucose.
What type of fluid should be given to burn patients after the first 24 hours?	5% Dextrose in water (D5W) and colloid, if necessary
How is fluid status monitored?	Urine output must be monitored with a Foley catheter. Adult patients must have a minimum urine output of 0.5 ml/kg/hr, and children must have an output of 1–2 ml/kg/hr. The rate estimated by the Parkland formula is adjusted to achieve these goals. Central venous pressures and pulmonary capillary pressure monitoring may be necessary in severely injured patients.
Which electrolyte must be closely followed after a burn?	Sodium
Why is it important to monitor the temperature of a burn patient?	A burn patient's body temperature tends to be very labile because of the loss of the skin barrier and exposure, fluid loss via

evaporation, the administration of large volumes of hypothermic fluids, and central temperature instability.

WOUND CARE

How are minor burns treated?	First-degree burns require only minor care, such as the application of bacitracin to the injured area. Analgesics may be needed for pain. Healing is complete and without scar formation or skin discoloration.
What is the treatment of superficial partial-thickness burns?	Superficial partial-thickness burns are initially cleaned with an antiseptic soap to remove foreign material and dead skin. Blisters generally are unroofed, and topical antibiotics are applied before dressing the wounds. Dressings need to be changed one to two times daily. Analgesics are administered because these wounds can be very painful. There is little to no scar formation and no major change in skin pigmentation.
What is the treatment of deep partial-thickness burns and full-thickness burns?	Deep partial-thickness burns and full-thickness burns are initially managed similarly to superficial second-degree burns (i.e., cleansing, topical antibiotic agents, dressing changes). These wounds need surgical intervention to minimize complications of the burn injury. The excision of burn wounds and coverage within 72 hours allow for early mobilization and rehabilitation, improved joint function, and shorter hospitalization. The gold standard of burn wound closure is split-thickness skin graft (autograft).
Should IV antibiotics be given to a burn patient upon presentation?	No.
What is an escharotomy and how is it performed?	This procedure entails full-thickness longitudinal incisions, extending through

the eschar to the level of healthy adipose tissue with either a scalpel or an electrocautery knife.

Why is an escharotomy performed?

Escharotomies are performed to prevent circulatory and respiratory compromise, particularly in the presence of circumferential, full-thickness burns.

MANAGEMENT OF COMPLICATIONS

What complications are burn patients susceptible to?

Infection, myoglobinuria, Curling's ulcers (i.e., gastric or duodenal ulcers), ileus

What major infectious complications occur in burn patients?

Post-**B**urn **C**omplications
Pneumonia
Burn-wound infections
Central-line infections

What are the clinical signs of a burn-wound infection?

Fever; increased white blood cell (WBC) count with a left shift; green pigmentation, discoloration, or change of burned areas; and the conversion of second-degree burns to full-thickness burns

Which organisms most commonly cause burn-wound infections?

Staphylococcus aureus, Pseudomonas, Streptococcus, and *Candida albicans*

What are some topical antibiotics?

Silver sulfadiazine, Sulfamylon

Should burn patients receive tetanus prophylaxis?

Yes

In which type of metabolic state are burn patients?

A burn patient is in a hypermetabolic state that is unsurpassed by any other form of trauma or illness.

What is "conservative therapy?"

"Conservative therapy" involves waiting until the burn wound forms an eschar separation. Generally, this type of therapy is not practiced because it is associated with a higher mortality than early excision.

How is myoglobinuria treated?

Hydration and alkalinization of the urine with IV bicarbonate are important to avoid renal injury.

What treatment can minimize the risk of developing Curling's ulcers?

Histamine-2 (H_2) blocker

When should nasogastric tubes be placed in burn patients?

Any patient with more than 20% TBSA will likely develop an ileus and be at risk of vomiting. These patients require nasogastric tubes.

25

Otolaryngologic and Dental Emergencies

EAR DISORDERS

OTITIS

Otitis media (see Chapter 15, "Pediatric Emergencies")

Otitis externa

What is otitis externa?	Infection of the external ear canal and sometimes the tympanic membrane; known as "swimmer's ear"
What is the patient profile for otitis externa?	Swimmers, people with hearing aids
What are the signs and symptoms?	Ear pain, erythema, pain on moving the ear, swelling of the ear and the canal
What is the treatment for otitis externa?	Keep the ear dry, administer acetic acid drops, remove any debris in the canal, and apply topical antibiotics.

BULLOUS MYRINGITIS

What is bullous myringitis?	A vesicular infection of the tympanic membrane and the ear canal
What are the symptoms of bullous myringitis?	Acute, severe ear pain; serous drainage; and fever
What are the signs?	Large, red blebs on the tympanic membrane and the adjacent canal
What is the treatment for bullous myringitis?	Oral antibiotics and analgesics; usually resolves in 24–36 hours

492

TYMPANIC MEMBRANE PERFORATION

What is tympanic membrane perforation?	Disruption of the tympanic membrane caused by blunt force or a sharp instrument.
How is tympanic membrane perforation diagnosed?	This disorder usually occurs after trauma. The patient presents with pain, conductive hearing loss, and tinnitus.
How is this treated?	Keep the ear dry, and use antibiotics only if there is evidence of infection. Refer the patient to an ear, nose, and throat (ENT) specialist for follow-up.
What is the prognosis for tympanic membrane perforation?	Although these perforations occasionally may require surgery, 90% heal spontaneously.
What causes a tympanic membrane rupture?	Increased pressure in the auditory canal resulting from a direct blow, an explosion, scuba diving, or penetrating injuries
What are the signs and symptoms?	Bloody drainage from the ear, hearing loss, otalgia, and possibly vertigo
What does the Rhine-Weber test reveal in patients with a ruptured tympanic membrane?	Conductive hearing loss in the affected ear, bone conduction greater than air conduction
What is the treatment for tympanic membrane rupture?	If there is no evidence of infection, the rupture will heal spontaneously. Patients should be advised to prevent water from entering the ear. Patients with a contaminated perforation require treatment with polymyxin B otic suspension and referral to an otolaryngologist.

FOREIGN BODY IN THE EAR

What is the most common insect caught in the ear?	The cockroach
How can an insect lodged in the ear be killed to facilitate its removal?	Instill mineral oil or lidocaine into the ear canal.

What are the methods for removing foreign bodies from the ear?	The simplest method of removal is irrigation. If necessary, forceps and suction can be used, being careful to avoid perforating the eardrum.
What should be included in follow-up care?	Steroid or antibiotic drops to treat irritation; follow-up or hospital admission if the object cannot be simply removed

FACIAL DISORDERS

FACIAL PARALYSIS

What are causes of facial nerve paralysis?	Trauma, Lyme disease, upper respiratory infection, cholesteatoma, tumor, herpes zoster infection
How is this paralysis diagnosed?	Physical exam findings (e.g., loss of nasolabial fold, frontalis paralysis, drooping corner of the mouth) are diagnostic.
What is the most common cause of bilateral facial nerve paralysis?	Lyme disease
What is Bell's palsy?	Sudden, unilateral facial weakness or paralysis of unidentifiable cause; the most common cause of unilateral facial nerve paralysis
What commonly precedes Bell's palsy?	Upper respiratory infection
What is the treatment for Bell's palsy?	The condition usually resolves spontaneously in 1 month. Protect the eye with drops if it cannot be closed. Evaluation and follow-up by an otolaryngologist are recommended.

FACIAL FRACTURES

What are the most common fractures of the face?	Nasal fractures
What are the signs and symptoms?	Pain, swelling, and deformity

What are the major pitfalls when diagnosing facial fractures?	Missing septal hematoma, missing intracranial extension, missing a cerebrospinal fluid (CSF) leak
How can septal hematoma be ruled out?	Nasal speculum examination
What is the treatment for facial fractures?	**Minimally displaced:** External splint **Severely displaced:** Immediate reduction by a facial surgeon if there is hemorrhaging or if the patient has a major deformity Delayed reduction is usually best. If packing is used, administer antibiotics.
What are indications for hospital admission for patients with facial fractures?	Failure to stop bleeding, CSF leak, other injuries requiring admission

NASAL DISORDERS

EPISTAXIS

What is epistaxis?	Nasal bleeding
What causes epistaxis?	Trauma, sinus infection, tumor
Where does the bleeding occur most commonly?	Anteriorly
Which is more serious, anterior or posterior epistaxis?	Posterior epistaxis is more serious because it is associated with hypertension in elderly patients and may be more difficult to control.
What is the treatment for epistaxis?	Direct pressure, anterior nasal packing Some patients may need posterior nasal packing (consult an ENT physician first). The packs should be removed within 5 days.

NASAL FOREIGN BODY

How is a foreign body in the nose diagnosed?	Foul-smelling nasal discharge, direct visualization during nasal speculum examination
How is a nasal foreign body removed?	Forceful expulsion (close the other naris and have the parent blow into the child's mouth)

Suction catheter

Forceps (when the foreign body is a bead,
remember to rotate the bead until the
hole in the bead is visible, then grab at
the hole)

THROAT DISORDERS

TONSILLITIS

What is tonsillitis?	Acute or chronic infection of lymphoid tissue in the naso-or oropharynx
What are the signs and symptoms of tonsillitis?	Red tonsils, exudate on tonsils, adenopathy Sore throat, fever, adenopathy, chills
Which organism most commonly causes bacterial tonsillitis?	β-Hemolytic *Streptococcus;* can be polymicrobial
What laboratory tests should be performed?	Complete blood cell count (CBC), throat culture, monospot test
What are the major complications of bacterial tonsillitis?	Peritonsillar cellulitis and abscess, rheumatic fever
What is the treatment for tonsillitis?	**Viral:** Acetaminophen, warm saline gargle, Cetacaine **Bacterial:** 10 days of penicillin (erythromycin if the patient is allergic to penicillin)

ABSCESSES

What are the signs and symptoms of a peritonsillar abscess?	Severe throat pain, trismus, enlarged cervical nodes, dysphagia, fever, chills, odynophagia, drooling, dysphonia, referred pain to the ear
What is trismus?	A spasm of the muscles of mastication
How is an abscess identified?	Finding of pus on needle aspiration of the tonsillar pillar
What is seen on oral examination?	Peritonsillar abscesses usually begin at the superior pole and are characterized

by a large, red, bulging tonsil and swelling and lateral displacement of the uvula. In cellulitis, the pillar is softer than in an abscess.

What are the differential diagnoses?

Lymphoma, epiglottitis, diphtheria, viral infections

What is the treatment for peritonsillar abscess?

The abscess must be drained via needle aspiration, gentle opening of the pillar, or emergency tonsillectomy (remember the carotid artery). Oral penicillin G or clindamycin therapy should be initiated. If the patient is dehydrated, intravenous rehydration therapy should be initiated, and antibiotics can be given intravenously instead of orally. Gargling with salt water and taking acetaminophen can provide symptomatic relief. Follow-up is with an otolaryngologist.

What is Ludwig's angina?

Abscesses caused by infection in the submaxillary, sublingual, and submental spaces, accompanied by the elevation of the tongue

What causes this condition?

Oral flora invade the submaxillary, sublingual, and submental spaces, usually at the second or third molars.

Is this a life-threatening infection?

Yes. Airway compromise, extension into the mediastinum, or both can occur and be fatal.

What are the symptoms of Ludwig's angina?

Swelling in the jaw, trismus, stiff tongue, fever, chills, odynophagia

What is found on exam?

Swelling beneath the chin, upwardly displaced tongue, cavities at the second or third molars

What is the treatment?

Maintenance of an adequate airway. Otolaryngologic drainage of the abscesses IV antibiotics (penicillin G, clindamycin, cefoxitin)

What are parapharyngeal abscesses and retropharyngeal abscesses?

Parapharyngeal: Abscess of the lateral pharyngeal space
Retropharyngeal: Abscess of the fascial

plane between the posterior
pharyngeal and paraspinous muscles

**How are these abscesses
diagnosed and treated?**

Diagnosis and treatment are similar to
Ludwig's angina, only the location differs.
A computed tomography (CT) scan of the
neck is often needed to isolate the
location of the abscess.

DENTAL EMERGENCIES

**How can you distinguish a
dental abscess from a cavity?**

A dental abscess is often associated with
caries. The abscess often has a fluctuant
area at the base of the infected tooth.

What is the treatment?

Drainage of the abscess and antibiotics
(usually penicillin VK)

**What are the different
classes of tooth fractures?**

Ellis class I: A chip or sharp edge
    without pain
Ellis class II: Temperature and air
    sensitivity; a yellow spot in the center
    of the fracture is visible
Ellis class III: Exposed nerve, fracture
    has pink center

**What is the treatment for
subluxed or avulsed teeth?**

Subluxed teeth can be reduced into their
    normal position (after administering
    anesthesia) and secured with wax. The
    patient should be referred for dental
    follow-up.
Avulsed teeth should be reimplanted as
    soon as possible. Each minute out of
    the socket reduces the viability of the
    tooth by 1%.

**What do you do with an
avulsed tooth before
reimplantation?**

If it is a permanent tooth, it can be placed
under the tongue, in milk, or in a tooth
preservative until you are ready to place it
in its socket. When ready, place the tooth
in the socket and stabilize it with dental
wax; refer the patient immediately to a
dentist.

26

Ophthalmologic Emergencies

What does the Snellen chart test?	Visual acuity
How is the test performed?	The patient stands 20 feet from the chart with one eye covered and reads the chart. The smallest line that can be read with only a few mistakes is recorded, and then the other eye is tested.
What ocular muscles are responsible for the following movements?	
Adduction?	The medial and inferior rectus muscles
Abduction?	The lateral rectus, inferior and superior oblique, and superior rectus muscles
Elevation?	The superior rectus and inferior oblique muscles
Depression?	The inferior rectus and superior oblique muscles

RETINAL DISORDERS

What are the symptoms of central retinal artery occlusion?	Sudden, painless, monocular loss of vision
What are the signs on physical examination?	Patient is only able to perceive light Relative afferent pupillary defect Pale retina with a red spot Possible appearance of emboli in the retinal arteries
What tests should be performed?	If emboli are seen, carotid and cardiac disease must be excluded by sonogram or

echocardiogram. An erythrocyte sedimentation rate (ESR) should be ordered
in elderly patients to rule out giant cell or
temporal arteritis.

**What is the treatment for
central retinal artery
occlusion?**

Digital pressure to force fluid through
    Schlemm's canal and reduce intra-
    ocular pressure
Carbonic anhydrase inhibition with
    acetazolamide 500 mg orally or β
    Blockade with timolol 0.5%, 1 drop
    every 12 hours

**What are the symptoms of
branch retinal artery
occlusion?**

Partial loss of vision from the embolus
lodged in the branch of the retinal artery

**What tests should be
performed?**

A fundoscopic exam reveals a pale area on
the fundus.

**What is the treatment for
branch retinal artery
occlusion?**

Treatment is similar to that of central
retinal artery occlusion: exclude cardiac
or carotid sources, apply pressure,
administer carbonic anhydrase inhibition
and β-blockers.

**What is the pathophysiol-
ogy of retinal detachment?**

A tear in the retina allows vitreous to seep
behind the retina, separating it from the
underlying choroid.

What are the symptoms?

Flashing lights in peripheral visual fields,
"spider webs" moving across the visual
field, a "curtain" drawn across the vision
field

**What are the findings on
physical exam?**

Blindness in the peripheral fields; central
    vision can be affected if the macula is
    involved
Undulating, pale, detached retina on
    fundoscopic exam
Hemorrhage (as a result of tearing of the
    choroid vessels)

**How is a detached retina
treated?**

Immediate evaluation and
photocoagulation by an ophthalmologist is
indicated. If the detachment is inferior,
the patient should rest with the head
elevated. If the detachment is superior,
the patient's head should not be elevated.

BACTERIAL AND VIRAL DISORDERS

What is blepharitis?	Chronic inflammation of the lid margins
What causes blepharitis?	The infection is caused most commonly by *Staphylococcus aureus* or *Staphylococcus epidermidis.*
What are the symptoms?	Irritation, burning, and itching of the lid margins
What does a physical exam reveal?	Scaling of the lids with debris hanging from the eyelashes
What is the treatment for blepharitis?	**Cleansing:** Use baby shampoo and a cotton swab to remove debris. **Antibiotics:** Administer sulfacetamide ophthalmic drops. **Follow-up:** The patient should see her primary care physician in 1–2 weeks.
What are the causes of orbital cellulitis?	*Haemophilus influenzae* is the most common causative organism. 75% of patients have had recent sinus infection or otitis media.
What are the physical findings?	Lid edema, erythema, proptosis, a tender globe, decreased visual acuity, pupillary paralysis, increased intraocular pressure
What tests should be performed?	Computed tomography (CT) of the orbit to look for orbital involvement of abscesses Blood cultures Lumbar puncture if the patient has an altered mental status or a stiff neck
What is the treatment for orbital cellulitis?	This is a true emergency. Intravenous antibiotic therapy should be started immediately. **Children:** Administer cefuroxime plus a penicillinase-resistant synthetic penicillin. Children allergic to penicillin can be treated with chloramphenicol or trimethoprim–sulfamethoxazole. **Adults:** Administer first-generation cephalosporin or penicillinase-

resistant synthetic penicillin. Vancomycin can be used if the patient is allergic to penicillin.

Which type of conjunctivitis is usually bilateral, viral or bacterial conjunctivitis?

Viral conjunctivitis

What test should be performed in patients with conjunctivitis to rule out corneal ulcers?

Fluorescein staining

Lymphocytes are seen in the Gram stain of which type of conjunctivitis, bacterial or viral?

Viral conjunctivitis

What is the treatment for the following types of conjunctivitis?

Viral?

Warm compresses, antibacterial treatment if the diagnosis is in doubt, frequent handwashing to prevent the spread of infection

Bacterial?

Antibiotic ointment (e.g., bacitracin, gentamicin)
Neisseria gonorrhoeae conjunctivitis needs to be treated with IV ceftriaxone

How are corneal ulcers differentiated from conjunctivitis?

Fluorescein staining shows uptake in the denuded area of the cornea if the ulcer is present.

What is the treatment for corneal ulcers?

Gram staining and cultures should be done to help identify the organism; however, topical antimicrobial treatment should be instituted immediately with gentamicin or tobramycin ointment (0.3%).

ACUTE ANGLE CLOSURE GLAUCOMA

What are the symptoms of acute angle closure glaucoma?

Severe eye pain, blurred vision, seeing halos around lights, lacrimation, nausea, vomiting, and headache

What are the findings of a physical examination?	Lid edema, conjunctival hyperemia, and circumcorneal infection
What causes acute angle closure glaucoma?	Increased pressure within the eye caused by obstruction of the outflow of aqueous humor
How is this disorder treated?	**Hyperosmotic agents:** 50% Glycerin or isosorbide orally, mannitol intravenously **Carbonic anhydrase inhibitors:** Acetazolamide (500 mg initially, then 250 mg every 6 hours) **β Blockers:** Timolol 0.5% drops (1 drop every 12 hours) **Miotics:** Pilocarpine 2%–4% drops (1 drop every 12 hours) **Corticosteroids** **Antiemetics**

ANTERIOR UVEITIS

What is anterior uveitis?	Inflammation of the anterior segment of the eye
What are the symptoms of anterior uveitis?	Deep eye pain, decreased visual acuity, and photophobia
What are the physical findings?	Ciliary flush (circumcorneal injection of the episcleral and scleral vessels) and conjunctival injection
What causes anterior uveitis?	Systemic disease (e.g., autoimmune disorders, sarcoidosis, Lyme disease), infection (e.g., tuberculosis, syphilis), or trauma
What is the treatment?	Treatment of the underlying disease Cyclopegics (e.g., homatropine hydrobromide, scopolamine, cyclopentolate) Steroids (prednisolone acetate 1% drops)

OPTIC NEURITIS

What is optic neuritis?	Inflammation of the optic nerve
What are the causes of optic neuritis?	Multiple sclerosis, sarcoidosis, leukemia, viral illness, tuberculosis, heavy metal intoxication

What are the symptoms?	Loss of visual acuity over time (approximately 1 week); color vision is more affected Pain in the region of the globe
What are the findings on physical exam?	There may be no findings ("patient sees nothing, doctor sees nothing"). The patient may have an afferent pupillary defect.
What is the treatment for optic neuritis?	Treatment is focused on the underlying cause. Steroids are the treatment of choice for retrobulbar neuritis.

OCULAR TRAUMA

What are the symptoms of a corneal abrasion?	Foreign body sensation in the eye; a sharp, stabbing pain aggravated by eyelid movement
How is a corneal disorder quickly diagnosed?	Place one drop of tetracaine in the eye; if the pain is immediately relieved, a corneal problem is likely.
What is a diagnostic test for corneal trauma?	Fluorescein reveals corneal trauma under cobalt blue light.
What is the treatment for a corneal abrasion?	Foreign body removal (if necessary) Cycloplegia with cyclopentolate 1% or homatropine 5% Bacitracin ointment Patching Pain relief (over-the-counter medicines usually suffice) Follow-up with an ophthalmologist in 24 hours
How does a corneal laceration differ from an abrasion?	A foreign body laceration of the cornea can allow a foreign body to penetrate the inner chamber of the eye, a much more serious condition than corneal abrasion. In patients with corneal lacerations, avoid pressure on the eye, and refer the patient to an ophthalmologist immediately.
What is a "teardrop" pupil?	An irregularity in the outline of the iris, often from a laceration, and protrusion of the iris near the limbus

Should you obtain a magnetic resonance imaging (MRI) scan if an iron intraocular foreign body is suspected?	No. MRI may cause the object to move, resulting in further damage.
What is a hyphema?	Blunt injury to the eye can tear the small blood vessels supplying the iris, causing blood to accumulate in the anterior chamber. This injury can lead to staining (i.e., red discoloration) of the corneal epithelium and possibly glaucoma (by blocking the trabecular meshwork).
How is hyphema diagnosed?	On physical exam, a bloody fluid level is seen in the anterior chamber.
What is the treatment?	Patients should be admitted to the hospital for cycloplegia, bedrest, and daily monitoring of the eye to look for evidence of further bleeding. Intraocular pressure should also be monitored.
What is the weakest part of the orbit?	The floor
What muscle can be entrapped in an orbital fracture?	The inferior rectus muscle
What are the physical findings of an orbital fracture?	Swelling, enophthalmos, upward and lateral gaze problems, anesthesia in the distribution of the infraorbital nerve
Which radiographic view is best for demonstrating orbital fractures?	Waters' view
What is the treatment for an orbital fracture?	If hyphema is present, admit the patient to the hospital. If not, discharge the patient with an ophthalmology follow-up appointment.

Index

Abdomen
    acute, 384–386
    surgical evaluations of, 406–408
    trauma, 419–420
Abdominal pain
    differential diagnosis, 8
    diffuse, 8
    evaluation of
        imaging studies, 9
        laboratory tests, 9
        physical examination, 7–8
        surgical, 9–10
    referred, 6–7
    somatic, 7
    types of, 6–7
    visceral, 7
Abortion, spontaneous, 139
Abruptio placentae, 140–141
Abscess
    abdominal, 469
    bartholinian, 165, 168
    Bartholin's gland, 157
    brain, 275
    definition of, 165
    dental, 498
    diagnosis of, 166
    incision and drainage of, 166–168
    parapharyngeal, 497–498
    pathogens that cause, 166
    pelvic, 470
    perirectal, 165–166, 168, 468–469
    peritonsillar, 496–498
    pilonidal, 165, 168
    rectal, 468–469
    retroparapharyneal, 497–498
    scrotal, 127–128
    subphrenic, 470
    treatment of, 166–167
    types of, 165–166
Absolute neutrophil count, 232, 242

Acetaminophen, 325
Achilles reflex, 424
Achilles tendon injury, 438
Acquired immunodeficiency syndrome,
    186–187
Activated charcoal, for poisoning, 310
Acute abdomen, 384–386
Acute angle closure glaucoma, 502–503
Acute chest syndrome, 223
Acute compartment syndrome, 433–434
Acute coronary syndromes
    angina pectoris (see Angina pectoris)
    description of, 48–50
    diagnosis of, 50–54
    myocardial infarction (see Myocardial
        infarction)
    symptoms of, 50
    treatment of,
        goals, 54
        myocardial oxygen demand reduc-
            tions, 55
        oxygen delivery supplementation,
            54
        platelet glycoprotein IIb/IIIa recep-
            tor inhibitors, 57–58
        thrombus formation prevention,
            55–58
Acute dystonic reaction, 302
Acute hemolytic transfusion reaction,
    212–213
Acute hemorrhage, 465
Acute mountain sickness, 361
Acute otitis media, 373–374
Acute pancreatitis, 110–113
Acute periodic paralysis, 284–285
Acute renal failure, 121–122
Acute splenic sequestration, 223
Acute tubular necrosis, 312
Acute vascular insufficiency, 474
Adenovirus infection, 383

Adrenal crisis, 251
Adrenal gland
  congenital hyperplasia of, 15
  congenital hypoplasia of, 366
  insufficiency, 249–251
Aeromedical transport, 441–443
Affective disorders
  bipolar disorder, 296–297
  complications of, 295
  major depression, 295–296
  prevalence of, 295
Airway
  cricothyrotomy, 38–39
  examination of, 34
  intubation of (*see* Intubation, of airway)
  nasopharyngeal, 34
  obstruction of, 40
  oropharyngeal, 34
  trauma evaluations, 410–411
Akathisia, 302
Albumin, 211–212
Alcohol
  ethanol, 330–331
  ethylene glycol, 333–334
  isopropanol, 330–331
  methanol, 331–332
  types of, 330
Alcohol abuse, 293
Alcoholic myopathy, 284
Aldosterone, 250
Alkali ingestion, 342
Allergic reactions, 200–201
Allergic transfusion reaction, 213
Altered mental status, 29–32
Alveolar-arterial gradient, 65
Amaurosis fugax, 479
Amebiasis, 102
Amniotic sac, premature rupture of, 147
Amphetamines, 328–329
Anal fissure, 469
Analgesics
  acetaminophen, 325
  description of, 324
  nonsteroidal anti-inflammatory drugs, 326
  opioids, 326–327
  salicylates, 326
Anal reflex, 424
Anaphylactoid reaction, 201, 358–359
Anaphylaxis, 200–201
Ancylostoma infection, 175
Anemia

aplastic, 218–219
  diagnostic criteria, 214
  hemolytic (*see* Hemolytic anemia)
  iron deficiency, 215–216
  megaloblastic, 216–218
  sickle cell, 221–224
  sideroblastic, 216
  signs and symptoms of, 214
Aneurysm, aortic, 478–479
Angina pectoris
  classification of, 49
  Prinzmetal's, 49
  stable, 49
  unstable, 49
  variant, 49
Angulated fracture, 431
Anhidrosis, 356
Anion gap, 15, 252, 313
Ankle:brachial index, 474
Anorexia nervosa, 299–300
Ant bites, 358–359
Anterior cerebral artery stroke, 261
Anterior cord syndrome, 423
Anterior uveitis, 503
Antibiotics
  for burn patient, 490
  for *Clostridium difficile* colitis, 101
  for invasive diarrhea, 101
  for pneumonia, 82
Anticholinergic agent poisoning, 313–314
Anticholinergic syndrome, 313
Anticonvulsants, for seizures, 276–277
Antidepressants
  atypical second generation, 306–308
  tricyclic
    therapeutic uses, 305
    toxicity, 322–323
Antimony poisoning, 337
Antipsychotics
  atypical, 303–304
  contraindications, 301
  indications, 301
  side effects, 301–303
Antiretroviral therapy, 188
Antisocial personality disorder, 298
Antithrombin III, 212
Anxiolytics, 304
Aorta
  aneurysm, 478–479
  coarctation of the, 370–371
  dissection, 478
  traumatic rupture of, 418–419

Aortic valve
   disorders of, 67–68
   insufficiency, 67
   stenosis, 67, 371
Apgar score, 146
Aphasia, 261
Aplastic anemia, 218–219
Aplastic crisis, 223–224
Appendicitis, 471–473
Arachnid bites, 358–360
Arrhythmias
   description of, 345
   in hypothermic patients, 351–352
Arsenic poisoning, 282, 336
Arteriovenous fistula, 475
Arthritis
   crystal-induced synovitis, 201–203
   diagnosis of, 201
   osteoarthritis, 204–205
   in pediatric patients, 386
   rheumatoid, 203–204
   septic, 171, 386
Ascariasis, 174–175
Ascaris lumbricoides infestation,
      174–175
Aspergillosis, in bone marrow transplant
      patient, 243
Aspirin
   for acute coronary syndromes, 55
   toxicity, 326
Asthma
   definition of, 74
   early-onset, 74
   evaluation of, 75
   pathophysiology of, 74
   risk factors, 74
   severity assessments, 76
   signs and symptoms of, 75
   treatment of, 76
Asystole, 41
Atherosclerosis, 260
Atrial fibrillation, 43
Atrial flutter, 43
Atrioventricular block, 44
Aura, 265
Autoimmune hemolytic anemia, 226
Avulsed tooth, 498
Avulsion fracture, 431
Azathioprine, 234

β Blockers, 316–317
Babinski sign, 425
Bacillus cereus poisoning, 95

Bacteremia, 15, 381
Bacterial vaginosis, 154–155
Balanoposthitis, 130
Ballistics, 482
Barbiturates
   side effects, 37
   toxicity, 324
Bartholinian abscess, 165, 168
Bartholin's gland abscess, 157
Beck's triad, 73, 413
Bee stings, 358–359
"Bell clapper" deformity, 125
Bell's palsy, 283, 494
Benign paroxysmal positional vertigo,
      278–279
Bennett's fracture, 431
Benzodiazepines
   for airway intubation, 36
   mechanism of action, 324
   psychiatric uses, 304
   side effects, 37
   toxicity, 324
Biceps reflex, 424
Biliary colic, 470
Biliary pancreatitis, 113–114
Bipolar disorder, 296–297
Black widow spider bite, 359
Bladder, rupture of, 421
Blast injuries, 481–482
Blepharitis, 501
Blood (*see also* Circulation)
   elevated pressure (*see*
         Hypertension)
   loss, in trauma patient, 413
   volume
      in adults, 40
      in children, 45
      normal, 40
      resuscitation of, 40–41
Blood transfusion
   blood products
      albumin, 211–212
      antithrombin III, 212
      cryoprecipitate, 211
      fresh frozen plasma, 210–211
      immunoglobulins, 212
      packed red blood cells, 208–209
      platelets, 209–210
      whole blood, 207–208
   complications of
      acute hemolytic transfusion reac-
            tion, 212–213
      allergic transfusion reaction, 213

Blood transfusion—*Continued*
  febrile nonhemolytic transfusion
    reaction, 213
  infection, 213–214
  description of, 207
"Blue dot" sign, 126
Body temperature
  of burn patient, 488–489
  factors that determine, 354
  monitoring of, 352–353
Boerhaave's syndrome, 462
Bone, anatomy of, 427
Botulism, 285–286
Boutonnière deformity, 438
Boxer's fracture, 431
Boyle's law, 443
Bradyarrhythmia, 44
Bradycardia, in newborn, 46
Brain abscess, 275
Braxton-Hicks contractions, 136
Breath-holding spells, 21
Breathing
  resuscitation assessments, 39–40
  trauma assessments of, 411–412
Breech presentation, of fetus, 148–149
Bronchiolitis, 376
Brown-Séquard syndrome, 424
Brudzinski's sign, 271
Buckle fracture, 429
Bulbocavernosal reflex, 414
Bulbocavernosus reflex, 424
Bulimia, 299–300
Bullous myringitis, 492
Bullous pyoderma gangrenosum, 400
Bupropion, 306–307
Burns
  complications of, 490–491
  first-degree
    definition of, 484
    management of, 489
  hospital admittance criteria, 486–487
  incidence of, 484
  management approach
    airway, 487
    fluids, 488–489
    principles, 487
    wound care, 489–490
  patient profile, 484
  second-degree
    definition of, 484–485
    management of, 489
  severity determinations, 485–487
  smoke inhalation associated with, 487

  third-degree
    definition of, 485
    management of, 489
  total body surface area determina-
    tions, 485–486
Burst fracture, 426
Buspirone, 304

Cadmium poisoning, 337–338
Calcium channel blockers, 317
Cancer
  metastatic, 126
  penile, 133
Candida albicans, 153
Candidiasis
  in bone marrow transplant patient,
    243
  esophageal, 194
  oropharyngeal, 193–194
  vulvovaginitis secondary to, 153–154
Carbamate poisoning, 340–341
Carbon monoxide poisoning, 341–342
Carbuncle, 165
Cardiac arrhythmias, 345
Cardiac syncope, 19–20
Cardiac tamponade, 73, 413
Cardiogenic shock, 12–14, 59
Cardiomyopathy
  dilated, 70–71
  hypertrophic, 71
  restrictive, 71
Cardiopulmonary arrest, 45
Carotid arteries
  disease of, 479–480
  stenosis of, 480
Cathartics, 310
Catheter
  femoral access, 451–452
  Foley, 451
  Hickman, 451
  jugular access, 452
  subclavian access, 452
  Tenckhoff, 451
Cauda equina syndrome, 424
Cellulitis, 162–164
Central cord syndrome, 423
Central lines, 451–452
Central nervous system
  infections of
    brain abscess, 275
    encephalitis, 272–275
    meningitis, 270–272
  toxins that affect, 311–312

tumors of, 269–270
Central venous access, 40
Cerebellar hemorrhage, 262
Cerebral blood flow, 259
Cerebral crisis, 256
Cerebral edema
   characteristics of, 256
   high-altitude, 361–362
Cerebral perfusion pressure, 258
Cerebrovascular disease, 260–264
Cerebrovascular stroke, 260–261
Cervicitis, 150
Cesarean delivery, 145
Chadwick's sign, 135
Chance fracture, 425
Chandelier sign, 151
Charles' law, 443
Chest pain
   causes of, 4
   evaluation of, 4–5
   physical examination findings, 4–5
   somatic, 3
   types of, 3
   visceral, 3
Chest trauma, 417–419
Chest tubes
   insertion of, 445–446
   Pleurovac connection, 446–448
   for pneumothorax, 449
Chickenpox, 379
Chigger bites, 360
Child abuse
   neglect and, differences between, 388
   physical, 388–390
   sexual, 390–391
Childbirth (*see* Labor)
Children (*see also* Infant; Neonate)
   congenital heart defects
      characteristics of, 369–370
      diagnosis of, 369–370
      hypoplastic left heart syndrome,
         371–372
      left-sided, 370–372
      right-sided, 372
      tetralogy of Fallot, 372
      total anomalous pulmonary venous
         return, 371
      transposition of the great arteries,
         372
   exanthems
      chickenpox, 379
      Duke's disease, 378
      erythema infectiosum, 378

German measles, 378
      hand-foot-and-mouth disease, 379
      measles, 377
      pityriasis rosea, 379
      roseola infantum, 378–379
      scarlet fever, 377–378
   fever in, 366, 381–382
   fluid and electrolyte replacement,
      367–369
   gastrointestinal disorders in
      acute abdomen, 384–386
      gastroenteritis, 382–383
      intussusception, 385–386
      malrotation, 384–385
      Meckel diverticulum, 385
      pyloric stenosis, 383–384
   orthopedic disorders in
      arthritis, 386
      congenital hip dislocation, 387
      Legg-Calvé-Perthes disease, 387
      slipped capital femoral epiphysis,
         388
      synovitis, 387
   respiratory tract infections in
      acute otitis media, 373–374
      bronchiolitis, 376
      epiglottitis, 375–376
      laryngotracheobronchitis, 375
      pharyngitis, 375
      pneumonia, 377
      sinusitis, 372–373
   shock in, 14–15, 365–366
   syncope in, 19–21
Chlamydia trachomatis, 150
Chloral hydrate, 37
Cholangitis, 470
Cholecystitis, 470
Choledocholithiasis, 471
Cholelithiasis, 113
Cholinergic crisis, 286–287
Chorioamnionitis, 147
Chronic obstructive pulmonary disease,
   77–78
Chronic pancreatitis, 114–115
Chronic renal failure, 122–123
Circulation (*see also* Blood)
   resuscitation goals
      blood volume, 40–41
      cardiac rhythm, 41–42
   trauma evaluations, 412–414
Claude's syndrome, 261
Claudication, 474
Clay shoveler's fracture, 431

Closed fracture, 427
Clostridium spp.
    C. difficile colitis, 101
    C. perfringens poisoning, 96
    C. tetani, 285
Clozapine, 303–304
Cluster headache, 266
Coagulation disorders
    hemophilia, 229–230
    laboratory evaluation, 228
    von Willebrand disease, 230
Coarctation of the aorta, 370–371
Cocaine, 328
Cold-related illness
    frostbite, 353–354
    hypothermia
        definition of, 350
        mild, 351
        moderate, 351
        rewarming treatment of, 352–353
        severe, 351
        toxins that induce, 312
Colic
    biliary, 470
    esophagus, 94–95
    renal, 118
Colles' fracture, 431
Coma, 29
Comminuted fracture, 427
Community-acquired pneumonia,
        79–80, 197
Compartment syndrome, 433–434
Compression fracture, 426
Computed tomography
    for abdominal pain evaluations, 9
    for appendicitis evaluations, 473
Condyloma acuminatum (*see* Genital
        warts)
Congenital adrenal hyperplasia, 15
Congenital adrenal hypoplasia, 366
Congenital heart defects
    characteristics of, 369–370
    diagnosis of, 369–370
    hypoplastic left heart syndrome,
        371–372
    left-sided, 370–372
    right-sided, 372
    tetralogy of Fallot, 372
    total anomalous pulmonary venous re-
        turn, 371
    transposition of the great arteries, 372
Congenital heart disease
    cyanosis and, 17

    shock and, 15
    types of, 67
Congenital hip dislocation, 387
Congestive heart failure
    causes of, 59
    classification of, 59
    diagnosis of, 60–61
    diastolic, 60
    high-output, 60
    signs of, 51
    systolic, 60
    treatment of, 61
Conjunctivitis
    bacterial, 502
    in neonate, 367
    viral, 502
Conscious sedation, 35–36
Conversion disorder, 298
Coombs' test, 226
Cornea
    abrasion of, 504
    laceration of, 504
    ulcers of, 502
Coronary artery disease
    myocardial infarction and, 50
    risk factors, 48
Corpus luteum cyst, 156
Corticosteroids
    for asthma, 76
    in transplantation patient, 234
Cortisol, 249
Cremaster reflex, 424
Cricoid pressure, 40
Cricothyrotomy, 38–39
Crohn's disease, 28, 105
Croup, 375
Cryoprecipitate, 211
Cryptococcal meningitis, 193
Cryptosporidium spp., 190
Crystal-induced synovitis, 201–203
Curling's ulcers, 491
Cushing's triad, 422
Cyanosis, 16–17
Cyclosporine, 233–234, 239
Cysticercosis, 177
Cystocele, 158
Cytomegalovirus
    retinitis, 193
    in transplantation patient, 237–238,
        242

Dalton's law, 443
Decerebrate posturing, 414

Decorporation, 350
Decorticate posturing, 414
Deep venous thrombosis, 476–477
Deferoxamine, 339–340
Dehydration, 367
Delirium
  causes of, 292
  definition of, 292
  dementia and, differentiation be-
    tween, 30
  high-risk populations, 292
  signs and symptoms of, 30, 292–293
  treatment of, 293
Delivery (*see* Labor)
Delusions, 294
Dementia
  AIDS-related, 192–193
  characteristics of, 291–292
  delirium and, differentiation between,
    30
  signs and symptoms of, 30
Dental abscess, 498
Dental emergencies, 498
Depression, 295–296
Dermoid cysts, 156
Diabetic ketoacidosis, 254–256
Dialysis
  for acute renal failure, 122
  emergencies related to, 123–124
  hemodialysis (*see* Hemodialysis)
  peritoneal, 123
Dialysis disequilibrium syndrome, 123
Diarrhea
  acute, 97–98
  causes of, 97
  Clostridium difficile colitis, 101
  definition of, 97
  in HIV-infected patient, 190
  invasive, 97, 99–101
  noninvasive, 98–99
  parasitic, 101–103
  traveler's, 99
Digitalis toxicity, 314–316
Dilated cardiomyopathy, 70–71
Dislocation
  elbow, 435
  hip
    congenital, 387
    trauma-induced, 435
  knee, 435
  patellar, 435
  shoulder, 434
Displaced fracture, 429

Disseminated intravascular coagulation,
    352
Diverticulitis, 467
Diverticulosis
  lower gastrointestinal bleeding associ-
    ated with, 24
  in transplantation patient, 236
Dizziness, 277
Dobutamine, for congestive heart fail-
    ure, 61
Dopamine, for congestive heart failure, 61
Drawer test, 436
Drowning, 363–364
Duke's disease, 378
Duodenal ulcer, 465
Duroziez's murmur, 68
Dysfunctional uterine bleeding, 160
Dyspnea, 5–6
Dystocia, 149

Ears
  bullous myringitis, 492
  foreign body in, 493–494
  otitis externa, 492
  otitis media, 373–374
  tympanic membrane perforation, 493
Eating disorders, 299–300
Eaton-Lambert syndrome, 287
Ebstein-Barr virus, 238
Eclampsia, 141–142
Ecthyma gangrenosum, 399
Ectopic pregnancy, 138
Edema (*see* Cerebral edema; Pulmonary
    edema)
Ehrlichiosis, 184–185
Elbow injuries, 435
Electrical injuries, 344–348
Electric shock, 345
Electrocardiography
  diagnostic uses
    acute coronary syndromes, 51–53
    chronic renal failure, 123
    congestive heart failure, 61
    hypothermia, 351
    myocarditis, 70
    pericarditis, 72
    pulmonary embolism, 64
    Q waves, 53
    ST segment, 53
Electrocution, 347
Electrolytes
  for burn patient, 488
  for pediatric patient, 367–369

Embolism
  cerebrovascular stroke secondary to, 260
  paradoxical, 260
  pulmonary
    diagnosis of, 64–66, 476–477
    risk factors, 63–64
    treatment of, 66
Emergency medical systems
  aeromedical transport, 441–443
  multi-tiered, 440–441
  personnel, interactions with physicians, 441
  single-tiered, 440
  training, 439–441
  triage, 444
Encephalitis
  causes of, 272
  definition of, 272
  diagnosis of, 272
  rabies and, 273–275
  signs and symptoms of, 272
Endocarditis
  causes of, 68–69
  infective, 68–69
  risk factors, 68
Endometriosis, 160
Endometritis, 149
Endotracheal tube
  for adult, 37
  for children, 45
Enterobius vermicularis infection, 173–174
Epididymitis, 129–130
Epidural hematoma, 423
Epiglottitis, 375–376
Epistaxis, 495
Ergotamine, for migraine headaches, 265
Erysipelas, 164–165
Erythema infectiosum, 378
Erythema multiforme
  major (*see* Stevens-Johnson syndrome)
  minor, 393–394
Escharotomy, 489–490
Escherichia coli infection, 100
Esophagogastroduodenoscopy, 22
Esophagus
  candidiasis of, 194
  colic, 94–95
  disorders of, 88–90, 462
  foreign body ingestion, 91–93

hemorrhage, 88–89
  Mallory-Weiss syndrome, 89
  perforation of, 89–90
  trauma, 89
  varices, 27, 90
Ethambutol, for tuberculosis, 85
Ethanol, 330–331
Ethylene glycol, 333–334
Exanthems, in pediatric patients
  chickenpox, 379
  Duke's disease, 378
  erythema infectiosum, 378
  German measles, 378
  hand-foot-and-mouth disease, 379
  measles, 377
  pityriasis rosea, 379
  roseola infantum, 378–379
  scarlet fever, 377–378
Exertional syncope, 67
Eyes
  acute angle closure glaucoma, 502–503
  anterior uveitis, 503
  bacterial infection of, 501–502
  blepharitis, 501
  foreign body in, 505
  muscles, 499
  optic neuritis, 503–504
  orbital cellulitis, 501–502
  retinal disorders, 499–500
  Snellen chart test evaluations, 499
  trauma, 504–505
  viral infection of, 501–502

Facial area
  fractures, 494–495
  lacerations of, 460–461
  paralysis of, 494
  trauma, 414–417, 461, 494–495
Failure to thrive, 388
Fecal occult blood testing, 24
Felon, 437
Female genital tract
  lower, infections of
    genital ulcer disease, 155
    genital warts, 155
    vulvovaginitis, 153–155
  upper, infections of
    cervicitis, 150
    Fitz-Hugh-Curtis syndrome, 152
    pelvic inflammatory disease, 150–152
Femoral fractures, 437

Femoral vein, for central venous access, 40–41, 451–452
Fetomaternal hemorrhage, 144
Fetus
  breech presentation of, 148–149
  heart rate
    baseline, 146
    detection of, 135
Fever
  in children, 366, 381–382
  description of, 32–33
  in neonate, 366, 381–382
  postpartum, 149
  seizures, 277, 382
  in transplantation patient, 236
Fifth disease (*see* Erythema infectiosum)
First-degree burns
  definition of, 484
  management of, 489
Fitz-Hugh-Curtis syndrome, 152
Flail chest, 411
Fluids maintenance
  in burn patient, 488–489
  in pediatric patient, 367–369
Flumazenil, 324
Fluoroquinolones, for invasive diarrhea, 100
Folate deficiency, 217
Foley catheter, 120, 451
Follicular cysts, 156
Food-borne botulism, 285–286
Food poisoning
  Bacillus cereus, 95
  characteristics of, 95
  Clostridium perfringens, 96
  definition of, 95
  mechanism of action, 95
  scombroid, 96–97
  Staphylococcus aureus, 96
Foreign body
  in ear, 493–494
  in esophagus, 91–93
  in eye, 505
  ingestion of, 91–93
  in nose, 495–496
Fournier's gangrene, 128–129
Fourth disease (*see* Duke's disease)
Fractures
  angulated, 431
  avulsion, 431
  Bennett's, 431
  boxer's, 431
  buckle, 429

  burst, 426
  Chance, 425
  clay shoveler's, 431
  closed, 427
  Colles', 431
  comminuted, 427
  compression, 426
  descriptive terminology for, 426
  displaced, 429
  facial, 494–495
  femoral, 437
  Galeazzi's, 432
  greenstick, 429
  hangman's, 425, 431
  intra-articular, 431
  Jefferson's, 425
  Jones, 431
  Le Fort classification system, 415–416
  mandibular, 414–415
  Monteggia's, 432
  oblique, 428
  odontoid, 426
  open, 427, 433
  orbital, 505
  pathologic, 428
  pelvic, 420
  penile, 133
  Pott's, 432
  rib, 418
  simple, 427
  skull, 422
  Smith's, 431
  spiral, 428
  tooth, 498
  torus, 429
  transcervical, 431
  transverse, 428
  treatment of, 432–433
  vertebral, 425–426
Fresh frozen plasma, 210–211
Frostbite, 353–354
Frostnip, 354
Furuncle, 165

Galeazzi's fracture, 432
Gangrene, 475–476
Gastric lavage, for poisoning, 309–310, 342
Gastroenteritis, 382–383
Gastroesophageal reflux disease, 93–94
Gastrointestinal bleeding
  characteristics of, 466–467

Gastrointestinal bleeding—*Continued*
  lower
    in adults, 24–26
    in children, 27–28
  upper
    in adults, 21–24
    in children, 26–27
Gastrointestinal disorders, in children
  acute abdomen, 384–386
  gastroenteritis, 382–383
  intussusception, 27, 385–386
  malrotation, 27–28, 384–385
  Meckel diverticulum, 385
  pyloric stenosis, 383–384
Genital ulcer disease, 155
Genital warts, 155
Genitourinary system
  bladder rupture, 421
  female (*see* Female genital tract)
  kidneys (*see* Kidneys)
  penis (*see* Penis)
  trauma, 420–421
  vagina (*see* Vagina)
German measles, 378
Giardiasis, 102–103
Glasgow Coma Scale, 422
Glaucoma, 502–503
Glucose metabolism disorders
  description of, 253
  diabetic ketoacidosis, 254–256
  hypoglycemia, 253–254, 312
  nonketotic hyperosmolar coma,
    256–257
Gold poisoning, 336
Goodpasture's syndrome, 122
Graft-versus-host disease, 243–245
Greenstick fracture, 429
Group A β-hemolytic streptococcal in-
    fection, 375, 378
Guillain-Barré syndrome, 282
Gunshot wounds, 482

Hallpike maneuver, 278
Hallucinations, 294
Hallucinogens
  description of, 329
  lysergic acid diethylamide, 330
  phencyclidine, 329–330
Hamman's sign, 5
Hampton's hump, 65
Hand-foot-and-mouth disease, 379
Handgun wounds, 482
Hangman's fracture, 425, 431

Hazardous materials, 483
Headache
  cluster, 266
  conditions that cause
    central nervous system tumors,
      269–270
    subarachnoid hemorrhage, 268–269
    temporal arteritis, 268
    trigeminal neuralgia, 267
  description of, 264
  migraine, 264–266
  tension, 266
  toxic metabolic, 267
Head trauma, 421–423
Heart (*see* Congenital heart defects;
    Congenital heart disease; Con-
    gestive heart failure)
Heartburn, 94
Heart disease (*see* Congenital heart dis-
    ease)
Heat exhaustion, 355
Heat rash, 355
Heat-related illness, 354–356
Heat stroke, 355
Heavy metal poisonings, 282, 335–340
Hectic fever, 32
Heel-strike test, 405
Hegar's sign, 135
Helminthic infections
  Ancylostoma, 175
  Ascaris lumbricoides, 174–175
  diagnostic sign of, 173
  Enterobius vermicularis, 173–174
  pinworms, 173–174
  Strongyloides stercoralis, 175–176
  strongyloidiasis, 175–176
  tapeworms, 176–177
  Trichinella spiralis, 176
  trichinosis, 176
Hematochezia, 24
Hemodialysis
  description of, 123
  for ethylene glycol poisoning, 334
  for poisonings, 310
Hemolytic anemia
  autoimmune, 226
  causes of, 219
  extravascular, 220
  intravascular, 220
  microangiopathic, 226–227
  sickle cell anemia, 221–224
  signs and symptoms of, 219
  thalassemia, 224–226

treatment of, 220
Hemoperfusion, for poisonings, 311
Hemophilia, 229–230
Hemoptysis, 28–29
Hemorrhage
    acute, 465
    cerebellar, 262
    esophageal, 88–89
    fetomaternal, 144
    intracerebral, 262–263
    pontine, 263
    putamen, 263
    retinal, 390
    subarachnoid, 268–269
    thalamic, 263
Hemorrhagic pancreatitis, 114
Hemorrhoids, 468
Hemothoraces, 417–418
Hemothorax, 412
Henoch-Schönlein purpura, 401
Henry's law, 443
Hepatitis
    A, 107–108
    B, 107–108, 214
    C, 107–108, 214
    causes of, 106
    cholestatic, 109
    D, 107–108
    definition of, 106
    diagnostic workup for, 106
    differential diagnosis, 106
    E, 107–108
    hospital admittance criteria, 106–107
    symptoms of, 106
    toxic, 109
    viral, 107–109
Herpes simplex virus
    in HIV-infected patients, 195
    in transplantation patients, 238–239
Herpes zoster, 393
Heterocyclic antidepressants, 305
Hickman catheter, 451
Hidradenitis suppurative, 165, 168
High-altitude illness
    acute mountain sickness, 361
    description of, 360–361
    high-altitude cerebral edema,
        361–362
    high-altitude pulmonary edema, 362
    Monge's disease, 362–363
    pathophysiology of, 360
    pregnancy effects, 360
Highway Safety Act of 1966, 439

Hip dislocation
    congenital, 387
    trauma-induced, 435
Histamine-2 antagonists, for upper gas-
        trointestinal bleeding, 23
Hollow viscus injury, 420
Homans' sign, 477
Honeymoon cystitis, 116
Horizontal mattress stitch, for suturing,
        455
Human chorionic gonadotropin, 136
Human immunodeficiency virus
        infection
    acquired immunodeficiency syndrome
        and, differences between,
        186–187
    antiretroviral therapy, 188
    from blood transfusion, 213–214
    CD4 count, 187–188
    cutaneous disorders associated with
        description of, 194
        herpes simplex virus, 195
        Kaposi's sarcoma, 194–195
        varicella-zoster virus, 195
    diarrhea, 189–190
    febrile findings, 189
    gastrointestinal disorders associated
        with, 193–194
    hematologic disorders associated with,
        199
    from needle-stick injury, 188–189
    neurologic disorders associated with
        CNS lymphoma, 192
        CNS toxoplasmosis, 191–192
        cryptococcal meningitis, 193
        dementia, 192–193
        diagnostic workup, 190–191
    occupational exposure, 189
    ophthalmologic disorders associated
        with, 193
    prevalence of, 186
    respiratory disorders associated with
        community-acquired pneumonia,
            79–80, 197
        *Mycobacterium avium-intracellu-
            lare* complex, 198–199
        Pneumocystis carinii pneumonia,
            81, 195–197
        tuberculosis, 197–198
    sexually transmitted diseases associ-
        ated with, 199
    viral load assessments, 188
Humeral shaft fractures, 436

Hydatidiform mole, 139
Hydrocarbon poisoning, 334–335
Hydrocele, 126–127
Hydrocephalus, 259
Hydrofluoric acid, 342–343
Hyperbilirubinemia, 366–367
Hypercalcemia, 233
Hyperemesis gravidarum, 139
Hyperinfection syndrome, 237
Hyperkalemia, 123
Hypersensitivity reaction, 200
Hypertension
    in aortic dissection patients, 63
    causes of, 61
    definition of, 61
    secondary, 61–62
Hypertensive emergency
    catecholamines sensitivity and, 62
    definition of, 62
    signs and symptoms of, 62–63
    treatment of, 63
Hypertensive encephalopathy, 62–63
Hyperthermia, 312
Hyperthyroidism, 246
Hypertonic saline, 413
Hypertrophic cardiomyopathy, 71
Hyphema, 505
Hypoglycemia, 253–254, 312
Hypoplastic left heart syndrome,
    371–372
Hypothermia
    definition of, 350
    mild, 351
    moderate, 351
    rewarming treatment of, 352–353
    severe, 351
    toxins that induce, 312
Hypothyroidism, 248
Hypovolemic shock, 11, 14
Hysterical syncope, 20

Idiopathic hypertrophic subaortic steno-
    sis, 19–20
Immunity
    cell-mediated, 233
    humoral, 233
Immunoglobulins, 212
Immunosuppression, 233
Inborn error of metabolism, 15
Increased intracranial pressure, 31,
    258–259, 414, 422
Infant (see also Children)
    blood volume of, 14

botulism, 285–286
    shock in, 14–15
Infection (see also specific infection)
    in burn patient, 490
    in oncologic patients, 232
    opportunistic, 235
    in transplantation patient, 234–236
Infective endocarditis, 68–69
Inflammatory bowel disease
    Crohn's disease, 28, 105
    definition of, 103
    differential diagnosis, 103
    epidemiology of, 103
    pathogens that cause, 103
    ulcerative colitis, 104–105
Insect bites, 358–360
Intermittent fever, 32
Internuclear ophthalmoplegia, 281
Interstitial lung disease, 78–79
Interstitial pneumonitis, 244
Intestinal perforation, 465–466
Intra-articular fracture, 431
Intracerebral hemorrhage, 262–263
Intracerebral mass lesion, 270
Intracranial pressure, increased, 31,
    258–259, 414, 422
Intravenous pyelogram, 119
Intubation, of airway
    medications for, 35, 410
    nasotracheal, 38
    orotracheal, 37–38
    rapid sequence, 35–37
Intussusception, 27, 385–386
Iron deficiency anemia, 215–216
Iron poisoning, 338–340
Ischemic stroke, 260–261
Isoimmunization, 144
Isoniazid, for tuberculosis, 85
Isopropanol alcohol, 330–331

Jaundice
    in adult, 470
    in neonate, 366–367
Jefferson's fracture, 425
Jellyfish sting, 360
Jones fracture, 431
Jugular access, for central lines, 452

Kaposi's sarcoma, 194–195
Kawasaki disease, 20, 379–381
Kehr's sign, 420
Keraunographic skin marking, 347
Kernig's sign, 271

Ketamine, for airway intubation, 36
Kidney
    failure of (*see* Renal failure)
    transplantation of, 239–240
Kidney stones, 119
Killip-Kimball classification system, 50
Kleihauer-Betke assay, 143–144
Knee injuries, 435–436
Knot tying, 457–460

Labetalol, for hypertensive emergency,
        63
Labor
    complications of
        abnormal fetal presentation,
            148–149
        meconium aspiration syndrome,
            147–148
        premature labor, 147
        umbilical cord prolapse, 148
    fetal assessments during, 146
    postpartum complications, 149
    premature, 147
    stages of, 146
Lacerations
    corneal, 504
    facial, 460–461
Lachman's test, 436
Lactic acidosis, 252
Lacunar infarcts, 262
Laryngotracheobronchitis, 375
Lavage
    gastric, 309–310, 342
    peritoneal, 144
Lead poisoning, 336
Le Fort system, for fracture classifica-
        tion, 415–416
Legg-Calvé-Perthes disease, 387
Lhermitte's sign, 204, 280
Lice
    bites, 359–360
    diseases caused by (*see* Pediculosis)
Lidocaine, for acute myocardial infarc-
        tion, 58
Lightening, 136
Lightning injuries, 347–348
Lithium
    therapeutic uses of, 307–308, 319
    toxicity, 319–320
Lochia, 146
Loperamide, for traveler's diarrhea, 99
LSD (*see* Lysergic acid diethylamide)
Ludwig's angina, 497

Lumbar puncture, indications, 32
Lung
    abscesses, 82
    "blast," 481
Lyme disease, 181–182
Lysergic acid diethylamide, 330

Major depression, 295–296
Maladaptive behavior, 299
Malaria
    causes of, 178
    cyclical fever associated with, 179
    definition of, 177
    diagnostic workup, 179
    prevention of, 180
    symptoms of, 178–179
    transmission of, 178
    treatment of, 179–180
Malignancies
    complications of
        infections, 232
        superior vena cava syndrome, 232
        tumor lysis syndrome, 231
    types of, 230–231
Mallet finger, 437–438
Mallory-Weiss syndrome, 89
Malrotation, 27–28, 384–385
Mandibular fracture, 414–415
Marine animal stings, 360
Marjolin's ulcer, 170
Mass casualty incident, 444
Mastitis, 149
McBurney's point, 472
Mean corpuscular hemoglobin, 214
Mean corpuscular hemoglobin concen-
        tration, 214
Mean corpuscular volume, 214
Measles, 377
Meckel diverticulum, 28, 385
Meconium aspiration syndrome, 47,
        147–148
Medical direction, 441
Megaloblastic anemia, 216–218
Melena, 24
Ménière's disease, 279
Meningitis
    aseptic, 270
    cryptococcal, 193
    definition of, 270
    diagnostic workup, 271–272
    lumbar puncture evaluations, 271
    meningococcal, 271
    neonatal, 271

Meningitis—*Continued*
  risk factors, 270
  signs and symptoms of, 271
  treatment of, 272
  tuberculous, 84
Meningococcal meningitis, 271
Meperidine, for airway intubation, 36
Mercury poisoning, 336–337
Mesenteric ischemia, 469–470
Metabolic acidosis, 251–253
Metabolic syncope, 18
Methanol, 331–332
Methemoglobinemia, 17
Methysergide maleate, for migraine
      headaches, 266
Metronidazole
  for Crohn's disease-related complica-
      tions, 105
  for giardiasis, 102–103
Microangiopathic hemolytic anemia,
      226–227
Middle cerebral artery stroke, 261
Midgut volvulus, 27
Migraine headache, 264–266
Miscarriage (*see* Spontaneous abortion)
Mitral valve
  disorders of, 66
  insufficiency, 66
  stenosis, 66
Mittelschmerz, 159
Molar pregnancy, 139
Monge's disease, 362–363
Monoamine oxidase inhibitors
  mechanism of action, 320
  psychiatric uses, 305–306
  toxicity, 321–322
Mononeuritis multiplex, 282–283
Monteggia's fracture, 432
Mucocutaneous lymph node syndrome
      (*see* Kawasaki disease)
Multiple sclerosis
  chronic progressive, 282
  definition of, 279
  diagnosis of, 281–282
  epidemiology of, 279–280
  inactive, 282
  relapsing, 282
  signs and symptoms of, 280
Munchausen syndrome by proxy,
      388–389
Murphy's sign, 7, 470–471
Myasthenia gravis, 286–287
Myasthenic crisis, 286

Mycobacterium avium-intracellulare
      complex, 198–199
Myocardial infarction
  acute, 50, 54
  complications of
    description of, 50
    treatment of, 58–59
  coronary artery disease and, 50
  diagnosis of, 51
  incidence of, 49
  Killip-Kimball classification system, 50
  non-Q wave, 53
  pacing for, 58
  shock in, 12–13
  treatment of, 54
  vasopressin and, 23
Myocardial oxygen demand
  decreases in, 55
  description of, 48
Myocarditis, 70
Myoglobinuria, 490
Myonecrosis, 169–170
Myopathies
  acquired, 283–284
  acute periodic paralysis, 284–285
Myxedema coma, 248–249

Nägele's rule, 135
Naloxone, 327
Nasal disorders
  epistaxis, 495
  foreign body, 495–496
Nasogastric tubes
  in burn patient, 491
  description of, 450
Nasotracheal intubation, of airway, 38
Near drowning, 363–364
Neck trauma, 417
Necrotizing fasciitis, 168–170
Neisseria gonorrhoeae, 150
Neonate (*see also* Children; Infant)
  congenital heart defects
    characteristics of, 369–370
    diagnosis of, 369–370
    hypoplastic left heart syndrome,
        371–372
    left-sided, 370–372
    right-sided, 372
    tetralogy of Fallot, 372
    total anomalous pulmonary venous
        return, 371
    transposition of the great arteries,
        372

conjunctivitis in, 367
fever in, 366
"fussing" in, 365
gastrointestinal bleeding in
    lower, 27
    upper, 26
jaundice in, 366–367
resuscitation in, 46
shock in, 365–366
Nephrolithiasis, 118
Neurogenic shock, 12
Neuroleptic malignant syndrome, 303
Neuroleptics
    therapeutic uses, 301
    toxicity, 323
Neuromuscular transmission disorders
    botulism, 285–286
    Eaton-Lambert syndrome, 287
    myasthenia gravis, 286–287
    tetanus, 285
Neuropathies
    Bell's palsy, 283, 494
    Guillain-Barré syndrome, 282
    heavy metal intoxications, 282
    mononeuritis multiplex, 282–283
    Volkmann's ischemic paralysis, 283
Newborn (*see* Neonate)
Nickel poisoning, 337
Nikolsky's sign, 396
Nonanion gap acidosis, 252–253
Nonketotic hyperosmolar coma,
    256–257
Nonsteroidal anti-inflammatory drugs,
    326
Nystagmus, 278

Oblique fracture, 428
Obturator sign, 471
Odontoid fracture, 426
Ohm's law, 344
Oncologic emergencies, 230–231
Open fracture, 427, 433
Opioids, 326–327
Optic neuritis, 281, 503–504
Orbit
    cellulitis of, 501–502
    fractures of, 505
Orchitis, 130
Organophosphate poisoning, 340–341
Oropharyngeal candidiasis, 193–194
Orotracheal intubation, of airway, 37–38
Orthopedic disorders, in children
    arthritis, 386

congenital hip dislocation, 387
    Legg-Calvé-Perthes disease, 387
    slipped capital femoral epiphysis, 388
    synovitis, 387
Orthopedic trauma
    ankle, 438
    description of, 426–427
    dislocations (*see* Dislocation)
    elbow, 435
    emergencies, 433–434
    fractures (*see* Fractures)
    knee, 435–436
    long bones, 436–437
    shoulder, 434–435
    wrist, 437–438
Orthostatic hypertension, 301–302
Osborne waves, 351
Osmolar gap, 252
Osteoarthritis, 204–205
Osteomyelitis, 170, 224
Otitis media, 373–374
Ovaries, disorders of
    cysts, 155–156
    masses, 155–156
    torsion, 156–157
Oxygen delivery
    for acute coronary syndromes, 54
    supplemental systems, 40
Oxyhemoglobin dissociation curve, 352

Packed red blood cells, 208–209
Paget-Schroetter syndrome, 475
Pain
    abdominal (*see* Abdominal pain)
    chest (*see* Chest pain)
    pelvic, 159–160
    peritoneal, 7
    rest, 475–476
    scrotal, 124
Pancreatic trauma, 420
Pancreatitis
    acute, 110–113
    biliary, 113–114
    chronic, 114–115
    definition of, 109
    hemorrhagic, 114
    types of, 109–110
Panic disorder, 297–298
Pannus, 204
Papilledema, 281
Paralysis
    acute periodic, 284–285
    facial, 494

Paralysis—*Continued*
Todd's, 277
Volkmann's ischemic, 283
Parapharyngeal abscess, 497–498
Paraphimosis, 132
Parasite bites, 359–360
Parasitic infections
helminthic infections
Ancylostoma, 175
Ascaris lumbricoides, 174–175
diagnostic sign of, 173
Enterobius vermicularis, 173–174
pinworms, 173–174
Strongyloides stercoralis, 175–176
strongyloidiasis, 175–176
tapeworms, 176–177
Trichinella spiralis, 176
trichinosis, 176
high-risk populations, 171–172
malaria
causes of, 178
cyclical fever associated with, 179
definition of, 177
diagnostic workup, 179
prevention of, 180
symptoms of, 178–179
transmission of, 178
treatment of, 179–180
pediculosis, 172–173
scabies, 172
tick-borne diseases
description of, 180
ehrlichiosis, 184–185
Lyme disease, 181–182
Rocky Mountain spotted fever,
182–184
tick paralysis, 186
tularemia, 185–186
in transplantation patient, 237
Parkinsonian syndrome, 303
Paronychia, 437
Parotid duct injury, 461
Partial thromboplastin time, 228
Patellar dislocation, 435
Pathologic fracture, 428
Pediculosis, 172–173
Pelvic inflammatory disease, 150–152,
472
Pelvis
abscess of, 470
fracture of, 420
pain of, 159–160
Pemphigus vulgaris, 399–400

Penetrating trauma
to abdomen, 419
to chest, 418
Penis, disorders of
balanoposthitis, 130
cancer, 133
fracture, 133
lesions, 132–133
paraphimosis, 132
phimosis, 130–131
priapism, 133–134
urethritis, 130
Peptic ulcer disease
causes of, 463
complicated, 464–466
definition of, 462–463
differential diagnosis, 464
pain associated with, 463
symptoms of, 463
uncomplicated, 464
Percutaneous transluminal coronary
angioplasty
for acute coronary syndromes, 57
indications, 57
Pericardial effusion, 73
Pericardial friction rub, 5
Pericardiocentesis
for cardiac tamponade, 73
complications associated with, 73
Pericarditis, 71–72, 124
Perirectal abscess, 165–166, 168,
468–469
Peritoneal dialysis, 123
Peritoneal lavage, during pregnancy, 144
Peritoneal pain, 7
Peritonitis, 123–124, 469–470
Peritonsillar abscess, 496–497
Personality disorders
antisocial, 298
complications of, 299
definition of, 298
treatment of, 299
Pharyngitis, 375
Phencyclidine, 329–330
Phimosis, 130–131
Phlegmasia cerulea dolens, 477–478
Phobic avoidance, 297
Physostigmine, for anticholinergic syn-
drome, 313
Pilonidal abscess, 165, 168
Pinworms, 173–174
Pityriasis rosea, 379
Placenta previa, 139–140

Plasmodium spp., 178
Platelet glycoprotein IIb/IIIa receptor
    inhibitors, 57–58
Platelets
    blood transfusion of, 209–210
    disorders (*see* Thrombocytopenia)
Pleurovac system, 446–448
Pneumocystis carinii pneumonia
    in HIV-infected patient, 81, 195–197
    in transplantation patient, 237
Pneumonia
    atypical, 80
    in children, 377
    community-acquired, 79–80, 197
    complications associated with, 81
    high-risk populations, 79
    nosocomial, 80
    organisms that cause, 79
    in pediatric patients, 377
    Pneumocystis carinii (*see Pneumocys-
        tis carinii* pneumonia)
    treatment of, 81–82
Pneumonitis, interstitial, 244
Pneumothorax
    characteristics of, 85–87, 412
    chest tubes for, 449
Poisoning
    analgesics
        acetaminophen, 325
        description of, 324
        nonsteroidal anti-inflammatory
            drugs, 326
        opioids, 326–327
        salicylates, 326
    anticholinergic agents, 313–314
    antimony, 337
    arsenic, 336
    cadmium, 337–338
    carbamates, 340–341
    carbon monoxide, 341–342
    cardioactive agents
        β blockers, 316–317
        calcium channel blockers, 317
        digitalis, 314–316
    caustic ingestions, 342–343
    ethanol, 330–331
    ethylene glycol, 333–334
    food (*see* Food poisoning)
    general management guidelines,
        309–311
    gold, 336
    hallucinogens
        description of, 329

    lysergic acid diethylamide, 330
    phencyclidine, 329–330
    heavy metal, 335–340
    hydrocarbon, 334–335
    iron, 338–340
    isopropanol, 330–331
    lead, 336
    mercury, 336–337
    methanol, 331–332
    nickel, 337
    organophosphates, 340–341
    psychopharmacologic agents
        lithium, 307–308, 319–320
        monoamine oxidase inhibitors,
            320–322
        neuroleptics, 323
        selective serotonin reuptake in-
            hibitors, 320
        tricyclic antidepressants, 305,
            322–323
    sedative-hypnotic agents, 324
    silver, 338
    systemic effects of
        cardiovascular, 311
        endocrine, 312–313
        gastrointestinal, 312
        neurologic, 311–312
        renal, 312
        respiratory, 312
    types of, 330
    xanthines, 317–318
Polymyositis, 284
Polyps, in children, 27
Pontine hemorrhage, 263
Portacath, 451
Posterior fossa tumor, 270
Postpartum complications, 149
Postural syncope, 18
Pott's fracture, 432
Pre-eclampsia, 141–142
Pregnancy
    early, complications during
        ectopic pregnancy, 138
        hyperemesis gravidarum, 139
        molar pregnancy, 139
        spontaneous abortion, 139
        vaginal bleeding, 137
    ectopic, 138
    late, complications during
        abruptio placentae, 140–141
        eclampsia, 141–142
        placenta previa, 139–140
        preeclampsia, 141–142

Pregnancy—*Continued*
  milestones during, 135–136
  molar, 139
  normal, 135–137
  physiologic changes during, 136–137
  radiographic evaluations during,
      144–145
  trauma during
    blunt, 142–143
    causes of, 142
    evaluations, 143–145
    incidence of, 142
    resuscitation and care, 145
Prehn's sign, 129
Premature labor, 147
Premature rupture of membranes, 147
Priapism, 133–134, 224
Prinzmetal's angina, 49
Propofol, 37
Prothrombin time, 228
Pruritus ani, 174
Pseudodementia, 30, 292
Pseudomonas infection, 162
Psoas sign, 471
Psychiatric disorders
  bipolar disorder, 296–297
  cognitive
    delirium, 292–293
    dementia, 291–292
  conversion disorder, 298
  depression, 295–296
  evaluations, 289–290
  panic disorder, 297–298
  phobic avoidance, 297
  prevalent types of, 289
  substance abuse, 293
  suicide, 291
  violent behavior, 290
Psychotic disorders, 294–295
Pulmonary arrest, 346
Pulmonary edema
  characteristics of, 59
  high-altitude, 362
Pulmonary embolism
  diagnosis of, 64–66, 476–477
  risk factors, 63–64
  treatment of, 66
Pulse
  in children, 45
  in newborn, 46
Pulseless electrical activity, 41–42
Pulse oximetry, for breathing assess-
    ments, 39

Pulsus paradoxus, 73
Purified protein derivative skin test, for
    tuberculosis evaluations, 83–84,
    198
Purpura fulminans, 400–401
Putamen hemorrhage, 263
Pyelonephritis, 117, 240
Pyloric stenosis, 383–384, 466
Pyrazinamide, for tuberculosis, 85

QRS complex tachyarrhythmia, 42–43
Quadriceps reflex, 424
Quickening, 136
Quincke's sign, 68

Rabies, 273–275
Radiation injuries, 348–350
Radiograph, diagnostic and evaluative
    uses of
  abdominal pain, 9
  acute pancreatitis, 112
  aortic dissection, 478
  appendicitis, 473
  asthma, 76
  cellulitis, 163
  chronic obstructive pulmonary dis-
      ease, 77
  congestive heart failure, 60
  infection endocarditis, 69
  interstitial lung disease, 79
  Legg-Calvé-Perthes disease, 387
  osteoarthritis, 205
  Pneumocystis carinii pneumonia, 196
  rheumatoid arthritis, 203
  spinal trauma, 426
  trauma, 144–145, 410
  tuberculosis, 83, 198
Ramsay Hunt syndrome, 393
Ranson's criteria, for acute pancreatitis,
    113
Rape, 160–161
Rapidly progressive glomerulonephritis,
    121–122
Rapid sequence induction, of airway,
    35–37
Rectal abscess, 468–469
Rectocele, 158–159
Red blood cell distribution width, 214
Renal calculi, 118
Renal colic, 118
Renal failure
  acute, 121–122
  chronic, 122–123

description of, 120–121
    intrinsic, 121
    oliguric, 120
    postrenal, 121
    prerenal, 121
Renal transplantation, 239–240
Respiratory failure, 39
Respiratory syncytial virus, 376
Respiratory tract infections, in children
    acute otitis media, 373–374
    bronchiolitis, 376
    epiglottitis, 375–376
    laryngotracheobronchitis, 375
    pharyngitis, 375
    pneumonia (*see* Pneumonia)
    sinusitis, 372–373
Rest pain, 475–476
Restrictive cardiomyopathy, 71
Resuscitation
    in adults, 34–44
    airway
        cricothyrotomy, 38–39
        examination of, 34
        intubation of (*see* Intubation, of airway)
        nasopharyngeal, 34
        oropharyngeal, 34
    breathing, 39–40
    in children, 45–46
    circulation, 40–44
    in neonates, 46
    of pregnant trauma patient, 145
Reticulocyte count, 214–215
Retina
    detachment of, 500
    disorders of, 499–500
    hemorrhage, in shaken-baby syndrome, 390
Retinal artery occlusion, 499–500
Retroparapharyneal abscess, 497–498
Retroperitoneum, 142
Rewarming, for hypothermic patients, 352–353
Rheumatoid arthritis, 203–204
Rh immune globulin, for isoimmunization, 144
Rhinosinusitis, 373
Rib fractures, 418
Rifampin, for tuberculosis, 85
Risperidone, 304
Risus sardonicus, 285
Rocky Mountain spotted fever, 182–184
Roseola infantum, 378–379

Rotator cuff injury, 434–435
Rotavirus infection, 383
Rovsing's sign, 7, 471
Rubella (*see* German measles)
Rubeola (*see* Measles)

Salicylates, 326
Salter classification, of orthopedic fractures, 436–437
Scabies, 172, 360
Scarlet fever, 377–378
Schizophrenia, 294–295
Sclerotherapy, for esophageal varices, 90
Scombroid, 96–97
Scorpion bites, 358
Scrofula, 85
Scrotum, disorders of
    abscess, 127–128
    epididymitis, 129–130
    Fournier's gangrene, 128–129
    infections, 127–129
    pain, 124
    testes
        hydrocele, 126–127
        metastatic cancer of, 126
        torsion of, 124–126
        tumors, 126
Second-degree burns
    definition of, 484–485
    management of, 489
Sedative-hypnotic agents, 324
Seizures
    diagnostic workup, 277
    differential diagnosis, 275
    febrile, 277, 382
    generalized, 276
    management of, 276–277
    partial, 276
    syncope and, differential diagnosis between, 19
    toxins that induce, 312
Selective serotonin reuptake inhibitors
    psychiatric uses of, 306
    toxicity, 320
Septic arthritis, 171, 386
Septic shock
    characteristics of, 13–14
    in neonate, 365
Serotonin syndrome, 320
Sexual abuse, 390–391
Sexual assault, 160–161
Sexually transmitted diseases (*see specific disease*)

Shaken-baby syndrome, 390
Shock
    cardiogenic, 12–14, 59
    in children, 14–15
    compensated, 10
    definition of, 10
    distributive, 14
    hypovolemic, 11, 14
    maternal, 143
    in neonate, 365–366
    neurogenic, 12
    septic (*see* Septic shock)
    signs of, 10
    types of, 10–11
    uncompensated, 10
Shoulder dystocia, 149
Shoulder injuries
    dislocation, 434
    rotator cuff, 434–435
Sicca syndrome, 244
Sickle cell anemia, 221–224
Sickle cell disease, 15
Sick sinus syndrome, 43–44
Sideroblastic anemia, 216
Silver poisoning, 338
Simple fracture, 427
Simple interrupted stitch, for suturing,
    455
Simple running stitch, for suturing, 456
Sinusitis, 372–373
Skull fracture, 422
Slipped capital femoral epiphysis, 388
Small bowel obstruction, 466
Smith's fracture, 431
Smoke inhalation, 487
Snake bites, 356–358
Snellen chart test, 499
Spider bites, 359
Spinal cord injury, 425
Spinal trauma, 423–426
Spiral fracture, 428
Spontaneous abortion, 139
Spontaneous pneumothorax, 86–87
Spontaneous ventilation, in newborn, 46
St. Anthony's Fire (*see* Erysipelas)
Staphylococcal scalded skins syndrome,
    398–399
Staphylococcus aureus poisoning, 96
Status epilepticus
    definition of, 276
    management of, 276
    nonconvulsive, 32
Stevens-Johnson syndrome, 394–395

Stings, 358–359
Stridor, 375
Stroke
    description of, 260–261
    hospital admittance criteria, 264
    ischemic, 260–261
    vertebrobasilar, 262
Strongyloides stercoralis, 175–176
Strongyloidiasis, 175–176
Subarachnoid hemorrhage, 268–269
Subclavian access, for central lines, 452
Subclavian steal, 18
Subcuticular stitch, for suturing, 456
Subdural hematoma, 423
Subphrenic abscess, 470
Substance abuse, 293
Succinylcholine, 35
Sucking chest wound, 411–412
Suicide, 291
Sulfhemoglobinemia, 17
Sulfonylureas, 254
Superior vena cava syndrome, 232
Supratentorial herniation syndromes,
    259
Supraventricular tachycardia, 42
Surgical patient, evaluation of, 405–407
Sutures
    absorbable, 453–454
    "catgut," 453
    definition of, 453
    nonabsorbable, 454
    polydioxanone, 454
    techniques, 454–457
    vicryl, 454
Syncope
    in adults, 17–19
    in children, 19–21
    hysterical, 20
    types of, 18
Synovitis, 387
Syphilis, in HIV-infected patients, 199
Systemic lupus erythematosus, 205–206

Tachyarrhythmia
    QRS complex, 42–43
    unstable, 43
Tachycardia
    supraventricular, 42
    ventricular, 42
Tacrolimus, 234
Tactile fremitus, 81
Taper point needle, 454
Tapeworms, 176–177

Tardive dyskinesia, 303
Teeth
    avulsed, 498
    fractures, 498
Temperature (*see* Body temperature)
Temporal arteritis, 268
Tenckhoff catheter, 451
Tensilon test, 286
Tension headache, 266
Tension hemothorax, 412
Tension pneumothorax, 86–87, 412
Terminal ileitis, 103
Testes
    epididymitis, 129–130
    hydrocele, 126–127
    metastatic cancer of, 126
    orchitis, 130
    torsion of, 124–126
    tumors, 126
Tetanus, 285
Tetralogy of Fallot, 372
Tet spell, 372
Thalamic hemorrhage, 263
Thalassemia, 224–226
Theophylline, 318
Third-degree burns
    definition of, 485
    management of, 489
Thoracotomy, 412, 414
Three-bottle system, 446–447
Thrombocytopenia, 227–228
Thrombolytic therapy
    for acute coronary syndromes, 56
    contraindications, 56
    indications, 474
    for thrombus prevention, 55–56
Thrombus formation, 55–58
Thyroid storm, 247
Thyrotoxicosis (*see* Hyperthyroidism)
Tick-borne diseases
    description of, 180
    ehrlichiosis, 184–185
    Lyme disease, 181–182
    Rocky Mountain spotted fever,
        182–184
    tick paralysis, 186
    tularemia, 185–186
Todd's paralysis, 277
Tonsillitis, 496
Tophi, 202
Torus fracture, 429
Total anomalous pulmonary venous re-
    turn, 371

Toxic epidermal necrolysis, 395–396
Toxic megacolon, 104–105
Toxic metabolic headache, 267
Toxic shock syndrome, 396–398
Toxoplasmosis, 191–192
Tracheostomy, 39
Transcervical fracture, 431
Transfusion reaction
    acute hemolytic, 212–213
    allergic, 213
    febrile nonhemolytic, 213
Transient ischemic attack, 479–480
Transplantation
    bone marrow
        allograft, 241
        autologous, 241
        complications associated with
            graft-versus-host disease,
                243–245
            infectious, 242–243
        description of, 240–241
        indications, 240
        rejection, 241
    kidney, complications associated with,
        239–240
    post-transplant emergencies
        description of, 233–234
        infection
            bacterial, 236–237
            description of, 234–236
            parasitic, 237
            viral, 237–239
        rejection, 239–240
Transposition of the great arteries, 372
Transverse fracture, 428
Trauma
    abdominal, 419–420
    blast injury, 481–482
    chest, 417–419
    cosmetic repairs after, 460–461
    facial, 414–417, 461
    genitourinary, 420–421
    head, 421–423
    high-risk mechanisms of injury,
        409
    initial evaluation
        airway, 410–411
        breathing, 411–412
        circulation, 412–414
        description of, 409–410
        disability, 414
    neck, 417
    neurotrauma, 421–426

Trauma—*Continued*
  ocular, 504–505
  orthopedic (*see* Orthopedic trauma)
  pancreatic, 420
  penetrating
    to abdomen, 419
    to chest, 418
  spinal, 423–426
  wound closure after (*see* Wound closure)
Trauma center, 408–409
Triage, 444
Triceps reflex, 424
Trichinella spiralis infection, 176
Trichinosis, 176
Trichomoniasis, 154
Tricuspid valve
  disorders of, 68
  insufficiency, 68
  stenosis, 68
Tricyclic antidepressants
  therapeutic uses, 305
  toxicity, 322–323
Trigeminal neuralgia, 267
Tripod fracture, 416–417
Trismus, 496
Tuberculosis
  classification of, 82
  definition of, 197
  diagnostic workup for, 83, 198
  disseminated, 84
  high-risk populations, 82, 197
  in HIV-infected patients, 197–198
  miliary, 85
  primary, 82–83
  purified protein derivative skin test, 83–84, 198
  reactivation, 84
  renal, 85
  signs and symptoms of, 197–198
  treatment of, 85, 198
Tuberculous meningitis, 84
Tubes (*see* Chest tubes; Endotracheal tube; Nasogastric tubes)
Tularemia, 185–186
Tumor lysis syndrome, 231
Tumors
  central nervous system, 269–270
  description of, 230
  posterior fossa, 270
  scrotal, 126
Tympanic membrane perforation, 493
Tyramine, 320

Ulcerative colitis, 104–105
Ultrasound, for abdominal pain evaluations, 9
Umbilical cord, prolapse of, 148
Uremic pericarditis, 124
Urethral injury, 421
Urethritis, penile, 130
Urinary alkalinization, for poisonings, 311
Urinary bladder (*see* Bladder)
Urinary calculi, 118–120
Urinary stones, 120
Urinary tract infection, 116–117
Urine
  output, in children, 46
  retention of, 120
Urticaria, 392–393
Uterus
  contractions of, trauma-induced, 143
  dysfunctional bleeding of, 160
  prolapse of, 158
  rupture of, 143
Uveitis, anterior, 503

Vagina
  bleeding of, 137
  masses
    Bartholin's gland abscess, 157
    cystocele, 158
    differential diagnosis, 157
    rectocele, 158–159
    uterine prolapse, 158
Valgus deformity, 433
Varicella-zoster virus
  in HIV-infected patients, 195
  in transplantation patient, 238, 242
Varus deformity, 432
Vasopressin, for upper gastrointestinal bleeding, 23
Vasovagal syncope, 18
Venlafaxine, 307
Venous disease, 476–478
Ventricular fibrillation, 41
Ventricular tachycardia, 42
Ventriculoperitoneal shunt malfunction, 259
Vertebral fractures, 425–426
Vertebrobasilar migraine, 279
Vertebrobasilar stroke, 262
Vertical mattress stitch, for suturing, 455
Vertigo
  central, 279
  definition of, 277
  peripheral, 277–279

Violent behavior, 290
Virchow's triad, 476
Visceral nerves, 3
Vitamin B_{12} deficiency, 217–218
Vitamin K, 26
Volkmann's ischemic paralysis, 283
von Willebrand disease, 230
Vulvovaginitis
  bacterial vaginosis, 154–155
  candidiasis, 153–154
  causes of, 153
  definition of, 153
  signs and symptoms of, 153
  trichomoniasis, 154

Wasp stings, 358–359
Weber's syndrome, 262
Westermark's sign, 64
Wheezing, 75

Whispered pectoriloquy, 81
Wound closure
  knot tying, 457–460
  sutures
    absorbable, 453–454
    "catgut," 453
    definition of, 453
    nonabsorbable, 454
    polydioxanone, 454
    techniques, 454–457
    vicryl, 454
  types of, 452–453
Wrist injuries, 437–438

Xanthines, 317–318

Zone of coagulation, 353
Zone of hyperemia, 353
Z-plasty, 457